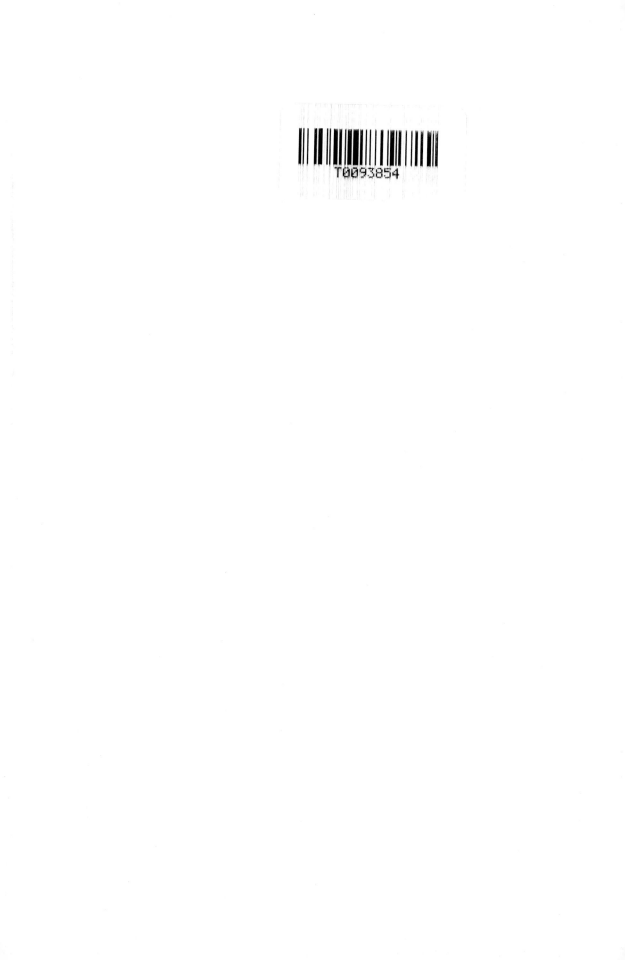

T0093854

Neonatal Nursing: A Global Perspective

Julia Petty • Tracey Jones
Agnes van den Hoogen • Karen Walker
Carole Kenner
Editors

Neonatal Nursing: A Global Perspective

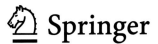

Editors
Julia Petty
Department of Nursing
Health and Wellbeing
School of Health and Social Work
University of Hertfordshire
Hatfield, Hertfordshire, UK

Agnes van den Hoogen
University Medical Centre
of Utrecht (UMCU)
Wilhelmina Children's Hospital
Utrecht, The Netherlands

Carole Kenner
School of Nursing, Health, and Exercise
Science, The College of New Jersey
Ewing, NJ
USA

Tracey Jones
Division of Nursing, Midwifery and
Social Work
School of Health Sciences
University of Manchester
Manchester, UK

Karen Walker
University of Sydney
Sydney, Australia

ISBN 978-3-030-91338-0   ISBN 978-3-030-91339-7   (eBook)
https://doi.org/10.1007/978-3-030-91339-7

This Springer imprint is published by the registered company Springer Nature Switzerland AG
The registered company address is: Gewerbestrasse 11, 6330 Cham, Switzerland

Neonatal Nursing: A Global Perspective - Introduction

Neonatal morbidity and mortality rates globally continue to be high. In 1990 the World Health Organization (WHO) reported that five million newborns died during the neonatal period—the first 28 days of life. By 2019 this number was 2.4 million. While progress has been made, more needs to be done. There is an array of factors that contribute to the current state of newborn health globally; these include poor quality care at or immediately after birth, premature births, and complications during the labor and birth. Prominently and importantly, there is also a significant issue with a lack of standardized training and education for the workforce who provide care for small and sick newborns. The ten countries with the highest neonatal death rates in 2019 were: India, Nigeria, Pakistan, Ethiopia, Democratic Republic of the Congo, China, Indonesia, Bangladesh, Afghanistan, and United Republic of Tanzania (WHO 2020).

The Council of International Neonatal Nurses, Inc. (COINN) have worked for some time with countries around the globe to improve newborn care, and part of this work included developing competencies for neonatal nurses providing care in middle- and low-resource countries. These were designed after reviewing many documents and standards in high-resource countries for both midwifery and neonatal nursing education. This was an important scheme of work and placed high on COINN's strategic agenda to address one of the key factors impacting neonatal outcomes specifically in countries where there is, and continues to be, no specific neonatal education or training. Following this work, the COINN board recognized that more needed to be done to assist those working around the globe to understand the differences in practice and education. As a result, this book was produced. Utilizing teams from across the globe who are actively working in neonatal practice and education, the book offers the reader an opportunity to examine how neonatal education is structured in addition to gaining knowledge around the demographics and challenges of specific parts of the world. The book focuses on the WHO regions approach, to present stories from the six regions of the world: Africa, the Americas, South-East Asia, Europe, Eastern Mediterranean, and Western Pacific. While these vast regions have many variations within them, examples of countries from specific areas are offered to highlight key aspects of neonatal nursing care, neonatal nurse education and training.

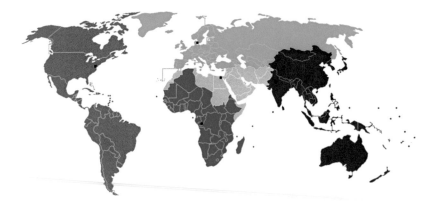

World Health Organization regions represented in this book. https://commons.wikimedia.org/wiki/File:World_Health_Organisation_regional_offices.PNG

Importantly, this textbook is written in line with the Council of International Neonatal Nurses, Inc. (COINN) vision for global unity for neonatal nursing. The core values and goals of COINN are based on excellence and advocacy for high-quality newborn care, as well as respecting diversity by integrating cultural norms and values within the care of newborns and their families. The book promotes neonatal nursing as a global speciality through evidence, research, and education of neonatal nurses and offers key examples of the millennium goals and global outcomes, as well as variations in outcomes for babies.

The authorship of this textbook is the COINN Board, and it is aimed at neonatal nurses across the world as well as current and aspiring students in this field. Overall, the intended audience for this book is anyone interested in global neonatal/maternal health, health professionals, public health officials, policymakers, regulators, students and faculty in any of these areas, and families that receive neonatal/maternal care. The chapters offer a comprehensive introduction to the topic of neonatal care, offering an understanding of the local and national drivers and touching on political and financial influences. To offer the reader a grasp of how both charitable and government stakeholders impact on care provision, this has been considered throughout the chapters. Case studies have been integrated to offer a personal approach to the discussion and enable the reader to hear stories from both those working in the field of neonatal care and parents who have experienced a neonatal journey.

The first part sets the context for the book as a whole. Secondly (Part I: Global Regions), the book focuses on global perspectives of neonatal nursing from different continents aligning with the World Health Organizations' global regions: The Americas (USA, Canada, and South America), Western Pacific region (Australia and New Zealand), European region (UK and Europe), African region, South-East Asia, and Eastern Mediterranean region. For each region, education and competencies, challenges and opportunities, research and evidence-based practice (EBP) as well as practice regulations are described. The next part (Part II: Key Topics for Neonatal Nursing Across the Globe) elaborates on key topics for neonatal nursing across the globe, such as the continuity of neonatal care in the community, patient- and family-centered care in neonatal settings, sleep and brain development, the fundamental care needs of the neonate and family, and global perspectives on hypothermia, hypoglycemia, and hypoxia. Compared to Part I that is written in a more formal academic but readable style using key literature and evidence, the writing style of Part II varies and is written according to the individual style of each chapter author, taking on a more reflective stance. Overall, the varied styles taken within this textbook enable an understanding from a diverse audience with varying academic levels and experience, both staff and students, bedside nurses, advanced practice nurses, midwives, allied professionals, and even parents. In addition, first person story-based reflective narratives are interspersed throughout the book to capture the perspectives of nurses, staff, and parents in the form of vignettes.

Book Features

- This is the very first global neonatal nursing textbook.
- The book offers reflective real-life stories and vignettes written by parents and nurses to support the main content.
- The book presents knowledge sharing across boundaries from all continents.
- Each chapter includes "think points" to guide reflective reading and learning.
- This textbook is written in line with the Council of International Neonatal Nurses, Inc. (COINN) vision for global unity for neonatal nursing as well as core values and goals based on excellence and advocacy for high-quality newborn care.

Reference

World Health Organization (WHO) (2020) Newborns: Improving survival and well-being. https://www.who.int/news-room/fact-sheets/detail/newborns-reducing-mortality

Manchester, UK   Tracey Jones
Yardley, PA, USA

Yardley, PA, USA   Julia Petty
Hatfield, UK

Yardley, PA, USA   Carole Kenner
Ewing, NJ, USA
Honolulu, HI, USA

About the Book

Collectively we are a global network of neonatal nurses with careers dedicated to the field of neonatal care. We have a passion for improving and optimizing the care of babies and families globally and supporting/educating the international neonatal nursing workforce. Our Vision is global unity for neonatal nursing. We aim to facilitate the growth of neonatal nursing and to advocate for our babies and families across the globe. The COINN Board members work as experts in the field in one, some, or all the following areas: clinical practice, education, management/leadership, research, and advanced practice. We represent the Board on key, high-profile international platforms and meetings of other international organizations to ensure neonatal nursing has a voice. Between us we have contributed and/or authored a significant number of international journal articles, chapters, and textbooks.

The contributors of this book comprise both the COINN Board and key experts that we network closely with. They are listed alphabetically by surname in the list of contributors.

Contents

Part I Global Regions

1 USA... 3
Carole Kenner, Mary Pointer, Deb Discenza,
and Carol B. Jaeger
1.1 Introduction....................................... 3
1.2 Organization of Neonatal Care....................... 4
1.3 Education and Training.............................. 4
1.4 Evidence-Based Practice............................ 5
1.5 Neonatal Care in the 1960s and 1970s................. 7
1.6 Neonatal Care in the 1980s and 1990s................. 7
1.7 Neonatal Care in the 2000s.......................... 8
1.8 Summary.. 9
1.9 Conclusion.. 10
References.. 10

2 Canada... 11
Marsha Campbell-Yeo, Tanya Bishop, Danica Hamilton,
Fabiana Bacchini, and Leah Whitehead
2.1 Introduction....................................... 11
2.2 Organization of Neonatal Care....................... 12
2.3 Education and Training.............................. 13
2.4 Five Decades of Neonatal Care in Canada.............. 14
2.5 Evidenced-Based Care: Priority Areas................. 15
2.6 Conclusion.. 20
References.. 20

3 South America.. 23
Andréia Cascaes Cruz, Flavia Simphronio Balbino,
and Ana Paula Dias França Guareschi
3.1 Introduction....................................... 23
3.2 Organization of Neonatal Care....................... 24
3.3 Hospital Organization for Neonatal Care.............. 25
3.4 Role of Professional Associations.................... 27
3.5 Education and Training.............................. 27
3.6 Evidence-Based Practice............................ 28
3.7 Conclusion.. 30
References.. 30

4   Australia... 31
Karen Walker, Jennifer Dawson, Kylie Pussell,
and Karen New
  4.1   Introduction 31
  4.2   Australian Population Data 31
  4.3   Australian Neonatal Healthcare System 32
  4.4   Evolution of Neonatology and Neonatal Nursing 33
  4.5   Education and Training 33
  4.6   Professional Organizations 34
  4.7   Parent Support Organizations 35
  4.8   Australian Nurses' Contribution 35
  4.9   2020 in Australia 35
  4.10 Conclusion... 38
  References... 38

5   New Zealand 39
Debbie O'Donoghue, Petra Harnett, and Joanne Clements
  5.1   Introduction 39
  5.2   Cultural Awareness and Cultural Safety Within Nursing and
        Neonatal Nursing in New Zealand: Debbie O'Donoghue.... 39
  5.3   Nursing Education and Training: Petra Harnett........... 42
  5.4   Organization of Neonatal Care 44
  5.5   Evidence-Based Practice: Joanne Clements 49
  5.6   Conclusion... 51
  References... 51

6   UK... 53
Tracey Jones, Jennifer Lowe, and Kirstin Webster
  6.1   Introduction 53
  6.2   Organization of Neonatal Care 55
  6.3   Neonatal Structure in the Devolved Nations 55
  6.4   The Multidisciplinary Team......................... 56
  6.5   Education and Training 57
  6.6   Professional Registration 58
  6.7   Neonatal Nursing Career Progression 58
  6.8   Continuing Professional Development 59
  6.9   Evidence-Based Practice 59
  6.10 Data Collection and National Audit................... 60
  6.11 Dissemination of Evidence-Based Practice............... 60
  6.12 Emerging Evidence into Practice...................... 60
  6.13 Conclusion... 64
  References... 64

7   Western Europe.. 67
Agnes van den Hoogen, Ingrid Hankes Drielsma, Ellis Eshuis,
and Joke Wielenga
  7.1   Introduction 67
  7.2   Education and Training 68
  7.3   Evidence-Based Practice 70

7.4 Conclusion 71
References... 72

8 Eastern Europe 73
Marina Boykova
8.1 Introduction 73
8.2 Organization of Neonatal Care 73
8.3 Nursing Education and Competencies................... 74
8.4 Challenges and Opportunities 75
8.5 Research and Evidence-Based Practice................. 75
8.6 Professional Associations............................ 75
8.7 Conclusion 80
References... 80

9 South Africa.. 81
Carin Maree
9.1 Introduction 81
9.2 Education and Training 82
9.3 The Organization of Neonatal Care 83
9.4 Evidence-Based Practice 84
9.5 Conclusion 85
References... 85

10 Eastern Africa 87
Andre Ndayambaje, Fauste Uwingabire, Pacifique Umubyeyi,
Ruth Davidge, Bartholomew Kamiewe, Geralyn Sue Prullage,
Carole Kenner, and Noreen Sugrue
10.1 Introduction 87
10.2 Neonatal Nursing.................................. 87
10.3 Structure of Neonatal Care Provision 88
10.4 Conclusion 92
References... 92

11 Asia (Japan).. 93
Wakako Eklund, Miki Konishi, Aya Nakai, Aya Shimizu,
Kazuyo Uehara, and Noriko Nakamura
11.1 Introduction 93
11.2 Organization of Neonatal Care 94
11.3 Multidisciplinary Team in NICU (Shimizu and Uehara).... 95
11.4 Role of Professional Associations (Shimizu and Uehara)... 96
11.5 Practice Regulation (Konishi) 97
11.6 Education and Training (Nakai and Konishi) 97
11.7 Evidence-Based Practice (Nakai and Konishi) 101
11.8 Future Challenges 104
11.9 Conclusion 107
References... 107

12 Middle East (Lebanon)................................ 111
Lina Kordahl Badr, Lama Charafeddine, and Saadieh Sidani
12.1 Introduction 111
12.2 Background 111

12.3   Care and Design.................................. 112
12.4   Transport 113
12.5   Neonatal Staff 113
12.6   Policies... 114
12.7   Parents 114
12.8   Monitoring of Outcomes and Physical Parameters 114
12.9   Infection Control, Sepsis 114
12.10   Feeding... 115
12.11   Intravenous Lines................................. 115
12.12   Thermoregulation................................. 115
12.13   Developmental Care............................... 115
12.14   Pain Management................................. 116
12.15   Discharge Planning 116
12.16   Long-Term Follow-Up.............................. 116
12.17   Conclusion...................................... 116
References.. 117

Part II   Key Topics for Neonatal Nursing Across the Globe

13   Continuity of Neonatal Care in the Community: Post-discharge Care for Preterm, Small, and Sick Babies 121
Andre Ndayambaje
13.1   Continuity of Neonatal Care at Community
        and Home Level................................. 122
13.2   Role of Community Health Workers in
        Promotion of Continuum Newborn Care................ 123
13.3   Conclusion...................................... 124
References.. 124

14   Patient and Family Centered Care in Neonatal Settings....... 127
Andréia Cascaes Cruz, Luciano Marques dos Santos, and
Flavia Simphronio Balbino
14.1   Introduction 127
14.2   Newborn Hospitalization in the NICU
        and Impact on the Family 128
14.3   Definition of Patient and Family Centered Care (PFCC) ... 128
14.4   Principles of the PFCC approach and its
        Interface with the NICU............................ 129
14.5   Implementation of PFCC in the Clinical Practice
        of Nurses in the NICU............................. 129
14.6   Benefits from the Implementation of the PFCC
        as a Care Model in the NICU........................ 131
14.7   Conclusion...................................... 132
References.. 132

15   Brain Development, Promoting Sleep and Well-Being in the Context of Neonatal Developmental Care.................. 135
Julia Petty and Agnes van den Hoogen
15.1   Introduction 135

15.2   Model and Definitions 136
15.3   Brain Development 136
15.4   Causes of Neonatal Stress and Sleep Disruption 137
15.5   Promoting and Protecting Sleep 137
15.6   Other Components of the Integrated Developmental
        Care Model 140
15.7   Conclusion 147
        References 148

16   **Hypoxia, Hypoglycemia, Hypothermia; The Three
      Hs - A Global Perspective on Early Care of the Newborn** 151
      Judy Hitchcock
      16.1   Introduction 151
      16.2   The Pink, Sweet and Warm Infant 153
      16.3   The Blue, Hungry and Cold Infant 154
      16.4   What Are the Signs of Hypothermia? 155
      16.5   What Is this Negative Cascade? 156
      16.6   How to Keep the Infant Warm 156
      16.7   Hypoxia 156
      16.8   What Is Hypoxia? 157
      16.9   What Is Hypoglycaemia? 158
      16.10   Managing Hypoglycaemia 158
      Glossary 159
      Further Reading 160

17   **Nursing Mana: Intuitive Effects on Nurse and Patient Care** . . . 161
      Leilani Kupahu-Marino Kahoano,
      Myrahann K. Kanahele-Gerardo, Susan Kau,
      and Alakai Georgiana N. Kahale
      17.1   Introduction 161
      17.2   Intuition 162
      17.3   Mana 162
      17.4   Inherited Mana 162
      17.5   Acquired Mana 163
      17.6   Native Mind, Heart and Spiritual Scientists 166
      17.7   Mo'oku'auhau: Genealogy 167
      17.8   Nursing School Curriculum 167
      17.9   Infant Mental Health 167
      17.10   Pu'ukohola Heiau 168
      17.11   Uniki Training 168
      17.12   White Coat Ceremony 168
      17.13   Conclusion 169
      References 169

18   **Global Research to Advance Neonatal Nursing
      and Neonatal Outcomes** 171
      Wakako Eklund
      18.1   Introduction 171
      18.2   Strength of Global Collaboration 172

18.3   Hot Research Topics in 2021/2022 175
18.4   Conclusion 178
References 178

Part III   Final Words

19   Key Messages and the Way Forward 183
Julia Petty
References 187

Index 189

Contributors

Fabiana Bacchini Canadian Premature Babies Foundation, Toronto, ON, Canada

Lina Kordahl Badr Azusa Pacific University, Azusa, CA, USA

The American University of Beirut, Beirut, Lebanon

Flavia Simphronio Balbino School of Nursing, Federal University of Sao Paulo, Sao Paulo, Brazil

Tanya Bishop Council of International Neonatal Nurses, Inc. (COINN), Yardley, PA, USA

IWK Health, Halifax, NS, Canada

Marina Boykova School of Nursing and Health Sciences, Holy Family University, Philadelphia, PA, USA

Council of International Neonatal Nurses, Inc. (COINN), Yardley, PA, USA

Marsha Campbell-Yeo School of Nursing Dalhousie University, Halifax, NS, Canada

IWK Health, Halifax, NS, Canada

Council of International Neonatal Nurses, Inc. (COINN), Yardley, PA, USA

Lama Charafeddine The American University of Beirut, Beirut, Lebanon

Joanne Clements Kidz First Children's Hospital, Middlemore Hospital, Counties Manukau District Health Board, Auckland, New Zealand

Andréia Cascaes Cruz School of Nursing, Federal University of Sao Paulo, Sao Paulo, Brazil

Council of International Neonatal Nurses, Inc. (COINN), Yardley, PA, USA

Ruth Davidge Kwa-Zulu Natal Department of Health, Neonatal Nurses Association of Southern Africa (NNASA), Johannesburg, South Africa

Jennifer Dawson The Royal Women's Hospital, Melbourne, VIC, Australia

Deb Discenza Preemieworld, LLC, Springfield, VA, USA

Luciano Marques dos Santos Estadual University of Feira de Santana, Feira de Santana, Bahia, Brazil

Ingrid Hankes Drielsma Workplace Bureau TOPZ and Path Project, Amsterdam, The Netherlands

Wakako Eklund Pediatrix Medical Group of Tennessee, Nashville, TN, USA

School of Nursing, Bouvé College of Health Sciences, Northeastern University, Boston, MA, USA

Council of International Neonatal Nurses, Inc. (COINN), Yardley, PA, USA

Ellis Eshuis Leids Universitair Medisch Centrum, Leiden, The Netherlands

Ana Paula Dias França Guareschi School of Nursing, Federal University of Sao Paulo, Sao Paulo, Brazil

Danica Hamilton Families in Recovery (FIR) Program, BC Women's Hospital + Health Centre, Vancouver, BC, Canada

Petra Harnett Christchurch NICU, Canterbury District Health Board, Christchurch, New Zealand

Judy Hitchcock Capital and Coast District Health Board, Wellington, New Zealand

Council of International Neonatal Nurses, Inc. (COINN), Yardley, PA, USA

Carol B. Jaeger Advanced Practice Nursing Programs, The Ohio State University College of Nursing, Columbus, OH, USA

Tracey Jones Division of Nursing, Midwifery and Social Work, School of Health Sciences, University of Manchester, Manchester, UK

Council of International Neonatal Nurses, Inc. (COINN), Yardley, PA, USA

Susan Kau Kapiolani Medical Center for Women & Children Caring for Hawaii Neonates, Honolulu, HI, USA

Queen Julia Kapiolani Hawaiian Civic Club (QJKHCC), Honolulu, HI, USA

Leilani Kupahu-Marino Kahoano Hawaii Healthcare I Cradles and Crayons Pediatric Nursing Agency, Ewa, HI, USA

Mālama o Nā Keiki I Caring for Hawai'i Neonates (C4HN), Honolulu, HI, USA

Alliance of Global Neonatal Nursing (ALIGNN), Honolulu, HI, USA

Queen Julia Kapiolani Hawaiian Civic Club (QJKHCC), Honolulu, HI, USA

Council of International Neonatal Nurses, Inc. (COINN), Yardley, PA, USA

Bartholomew Kamiewe YML, Lusaka, Zambia

Myrahann K. Kanahele-Gerardo Mālama o Nā Keiki I Caring for Hawai'i Neonates Kekaha, Kauai, HI, USA

Queen Julia Kapiolani Hawaiian Civic Club (QJKHCC), Honolulu, HI, USA

Carole Kenner School of Nursing, Health, and Exercise Science, The College of New Jersey, Ewing, NJ, USA

Council of International Neonatal Nurses, Inc. (COINN), Yardley, PA, USA

Alliance of Global Neonatal Nursing (ALIGNN), Honolulu, HI, USA

M. Konishi School of Nursing, Dokkyo Medical University, Tochigi, Japan

Jennifer Lowe North West Neonatal Operational Delivery Network, Manchester, UK

Carin Maree Department of Nursing Science, University of Pretoria, Pretoria, South Africa

Council of International Neonatal Nurses, Inc. (COINN), Yardley, PA, USA

A. Nakai Graduate School of Nursing, Chiba University, Chiba-City, Chiba, Japan

N. Nakamura Seirei Hamamatsu General Hospital, Naka-ku, Hamamatsu, Shizuoka, Japan

Andre Ndayambaje University of Global Health Equity (UGHE), Kigali, Rwanda

Council of International Neonatal Nurses, Inc. (COINN), Yardley, PA, USA

Karen New School of Health and Behavioural Science, University of the Sunshine Coast, Sippy Downs, QLD, Australia

Debbie O'Donoghue Christchurch NICU, Canterbury District Health Board, Canterbury & West Coast, Christchurch, New Zealand

Council of International Neonatal Nurses, Inc. (COINN), Christchurch, New Zealand

Julia Petty Department of Nursing, Health and Wellbeing, School of Health and Social Work, University of Hertfordshire, Hatfield, Hertfordshire, UK

Council of International Neonatal Nurses, Inc. (COINN), Yardley, PA, USA

Alakai Georgiana N. Kahale Lei Poina ole - Poe Niihau (people of Niihau), A Program of Mālama o Nā Keiki | Caring for Hawai'i Neonates Kekaha, Kauai, HI, USA

Queen Julia Kapiolani Hawaiian Civic Club, Honolulu, HI, USA

Mary Pointer Council of International Neonatal Nurses, Inc. (COINN), Yardley, PA, USA

Frontier State Bank, Oklahoma City, OK, USA

Geralyn Sue Prullage Council of International Neonatal Nurses, Inc. (COINN), NNP SIU School of Medicine, Alton, IL, USA

Kylie Pussell CEO Miracle Babies Foundation, Sydney, NSW, Australia

A. Shimizu Graduate School of Nursing, Kyoto Tachibana University, Kyoto-City, Kyoto, Japan

Saadieh Sidani The American University of Beirut, Beirut, Lebanon

Noreen Sugrue Latino Policy Forum, Chicago, IL, USA

K. Uehara Child Health Nursing, Okinawa Prefectural College of Nursing, Naha, Okinawa, Japan

Pacifique Umubyeyi Rwanda Military Hospital, Kigali, Rwanda

Fauste Uwingabire College of Medicine and Health Sciences, School of Nursing and Midwifery, University of Rwanda, Kigali, Rwanda

Agnes van den Hoogen University Medical Centre of Utrecht (UMCU), Wilhelmina Children's Hospital, Utrecht, The Netherlands

Council of International Neonatal Nurses, Inc. (COINN), Yardley, PA, USA

Karen Walker University of Sydney, Sydney, Australia

Royal Prince Alfred Hospital, Sydney, Australia

President, Council of International Neonatal Nurses, Inc. (COINN), Yardley, PA, USA

Kirstin Webster ANNP Lead for the Scottish Neonatal Nurses Group (SNNG), Fife, Scotland, UK

National Maternity and Perinatal Audit (NMPA), Royal College of Obstetricians, London, UK

Leah Whitehead IWK Health, Halifax, NS, Canada

Joke Wielenga IC Neonatology, Emma Children's Hospital/Amsterdam University Medical Center, Amsterdam, The Netherlands

Part I

Global Regions

USA

1

Carole Kenner, Mary Pointer, Deb Discenza, and Carol B. Jaeger

1.1 Introduction

Neonatal care from the United States perspective represents a small specialization under the American Academy of Pediatrics (AAP). *Guidelines for Perinatal Care* originally published in 1983, now in its eight edition, provides guidelines for high-risk obstetrical care and all levels of neonatal care. One nurse serves on the Committee of Fetus and Newborn AAP to give input into nursing care. Neonatal nursing care

C. Kenner (✉)
School of Nursing, Health, and Exercise Science, The College of New Jersey, Ewing, NJ, USA

Council of International Neonatal Nurses, Inc. (COINN), Yardley, PA, USA

Alliance of Global Neonatal Nursing (ALIGNN), Honolulu, HI, USA
e-mail: kennerc@tcnj.edu

M. Pointer
Council of International Neonatal Nurses, Inc. (COINN), Yardley, PA, USA

Frontier State Bank, Oklahoma City, OK, USA

D. Discenza
Preemieworld, LLC, Springfield, VA, USA

C. B. Jaeger
Advanced Practice Nursing Programs, The Ohio State University College of Nursing, Columbus, OH, USA

and standards for neonatal nursing education are set by the National Association of Neonatal Nurses (NANNs) and certification for staff nurses and neonatal nurse practitioners available by NCC. NANNs also have a group for Nurse Practitioners (master's or doctorally prepared advanced practice nurses) (NANNPs) who set the competencies and requirements for education and practice. Cultural differences do exist throughout the United States. There is a large group of Native Americans—many Indian tribes including Alaskan natives. The United States is a mix of Central and South American natives, large Asian populations—especially Japan, China, Thailand, Viet Nam, the Caribbean; European—especially United Kingdom, Ireland, Scotland, Russia, and most Eastern and Western Europe; Middle East—Israel, Pakistan, United Arab Emirates; and African—Nigeria, Egypt, Kenya, South Africa in particular. Depending on where care is given, these cultural differences along with religious differences—Jewish, Protestant, Catholic, Orthodox, Muslim, and many others must be incorporated into the nursing care. This chapter will describe neonatal nursing practice/care and education and give exemplars to illustrate the US perspective.

1.2 Organization of Neonatal Care

In the 1970s, a movement in perinatal/neonatal care called for a regionalization model. This meant that levels of care would be created. Level I was a newborn nursery for well, term infants; Level II was an intermediate or special care nursery that would offer lower technological care-intravenous lines, oxygen by nasal cannula, head hoods, incubators or radiant warmers, and tube feedings. There might or might not be an in-house neonatologist 24 h per day, but there would be laboratory and radiologic services. The most intensive care was Level III usually housed in a Children's specialty or university teaching hospital. These units might care for surgical neonates too. Over the next decades, as survival of neonates as small as 400 g and 23-week gestation grew and technology advances increased, there came a need for Level IV units and Maternal Fetal Units. The Level IV regional unit is the most advanced care and offers surgical care, transports between hospitals, and outreach education to other levels of care personnel in the region. The Maternal Fetal Units—most often found in specialty hospitals—offer fetal surgery for such conditions as congenital diaphragmatic hernia, congenital cystic adenomatoid malformation, and other life-threatening conditions. Levels III, IV, and Maternal Fetal Units all require a team approach to care coordination including the families as partners in the care team. The team consists of neonatologists, pediatricians, neonatal nurse practitioners, staff nurses, respiratory therapists, child life specialists, lactation consultants, lab technologists, pediatric physical therapists, occupational therapists, geneticists, surgeons, social workers, and clergy, to name a few. These specialists create a plan of care, and updates are given during handoffs, report between shifts by nurses and in interdisciplinary rounds where in many units, parents can participate.

1.3 Education and Training

In undergraduate or basic nursing education, students only receive basic maternal newborn content. Some opt to do a rotation in the neonatal intensive care unit. Many hospitals will not hire new nurses directly into the NICU because of the lack of experience during their nursing school clinicals. They must spend 1–2 years in medical surgical nursing and then go into the NICU. Some hospitals have extensive nurse residency programs where new nurses spend 6 months to a year with a mentor. These healthcare organizations generally start nurses out on general medical surgical units and not in areas such as the NICU. Other healthcare organizations have extensive unit orientations. The exact orientation for neonatal nurses varies from hospital to hospital. However, the suggested content for orientation for neonatal nurses is outlined by NANN. The *Essentials of Neonatal Nurses—Orientation Lecture Series Modules 1–10: Streaming Video* (NANN 2012) is available for purchase. The content covers cardiac, gastroenterology, genitourinary, hematologic, immunology and infection, maternal fetal issues, newborn assessment, nutritional and metabolic, and pulmonary issues.

Advanced practice neonatal nurses are called either nurse practitioners or clinical nurse specialists—both minimally prepared at the master's level. That education means 1.5–2 years beyond basic education. The master's focuses on content specific to neonatal care, role development, advanced health assessment and pharmacology, as well as leadership development. Many regions of the country have opted to eliminate the clinical nurse specialists as they cannot get reimbursed for services the way nurse practitioners can. Nurse practitioners can be either master's or doctorally prepared. There are some nurses who already are advanced practice NPs and want to change specializations so they can take a course of study—about 1 year to gain a post—master's certificate in this specialization. The doctoral preparation is either as a Doctor of Nursing practice (DNP) or Doctor of Philosophy (PhD). The DNP focuses on neonatal content if the nurse is not already a neonatal nurse practitioner (NNP) with emphasis on quality improvement, evidence-based practice, research methods as related to evidence-based practice, leadership development, health policy, population health, use of technology, clinical scholarship, organizational systems leadership, and scientific underpinnings for practice outlined by the American Association of Colleges of Nursing (AACN) in *The Essentials of Doctoral Education for Advanced Nursing Practice* (2006). NNPs prescribe medications and must meet board of nursing requirements for maintaining prescriptive authority, which at the very least includes recent continuing education units in pharmacology for license renewal. The DNP is a practice doctorate that culminates in a capstone evidence-based project. The PhD prepared nurse is expected to advance the science of nursing. The course of study focuses on nursing theory, advanced research-qualitative, quantitative, mixed methods, statistics, grant writing, various elective courses, and conduct of a high-level research study for the dissertation. The PhD is a research degree.

Formal educational programs are accredited by national accreditation organizations such as Commission on Collegiate Nursing Education (CCNE) or Accreditation Commission for Education in Nursing (ACEN). In addition, each state board of nursing reviews all nursing programs, and there are regional accrediting bodies for the colleges and universities. Neonatal nursing programs must also adhere to the National Association of Neonatal Nurse Practitioners (NANNP) guidelines for education and NCC

requirements as this organization offers the certification examination nationally for both neonatal staff nurses who hold degrees or preparation (bachelor's degree, or associate degree—2-year community college or diploma—hospital based) less than a master's or doctorate. There are many levels of scrutiny for formal educational programs. To be classified as a neonatal nurse practitioner, you must meet both the educational preparation and, in most states, national certification. NANN also created *Competencies and Orientation Toolkit for Neonatal Nurse Practitioners* that covers advanced, master's or doctorally prepared neonatal nurses for a new role and for the evaluation of their continued competence (NANN 2014). This document provides examples and forms to document skill/competency achievement as well as content on how to put together a professional nursing portfolio to demonstrate experiences and knowledge. There are guidelines for the nurse's mentor or preceptor during orientation and evaluation tools that can be adapted to meet the variations in units and patient complexity. These types of support for the staff nurse, advanced practice nurse, and preceptors or evaluators provide consistent training content and evaluation methods.

1.4 Evidence-Based Practice

Evidence-based practice is ever changing as the research findings to support neonatal nursing care grows. Areas of interest include: skin care guidelines, neonatal abstinence syndrome, breastfeeding practices, infant mental health supports, maternal mental health and its relationship to infant bonding, trauma informed care, transition from hospital to home and to primary care, ethical issues in neonatal care, integrative, family centered developmental care, impact of the NICU environment on neonatal and family outcomes, support for fathers experiencing a NICU stay, perinatal, neonatal hospice and palliative care interventions, and use of probiotics as a necrotizing enterocolitis prevention. This list is not exhaustive but gives some examples of topics that impact nursing care.

Reflective Practice

When I began working in the NICU, we completed tasks that we now know are unnecessary or may be harmful. Unfortunately, we did not have the evidence to support changes. What were these practices? Suctioning an endotracheal tube hourly with saline instillation, placing the baby prone, using all types of tape on even the most fragile skin, always resuscitating using 100% oxygen. Now we know that suctioning an endotracheal tube should be as needed without saline, and ideally with two people performing the procedure-oxygen should be only 10–20% greater than the level the infant is receiving (Goncalves et al. 2015). The American Academy of Pediatrics (AAP) supports the "Back to Sleep" program for neonates unless there is a specific contraindication to reduce the incidence of Sudden Infant Death syndrome. And NANN and AWHONN have reaffirmed the guidelines for neonatal skin care now in its fourth edition (Kuller 2018). These guidelines are very specific about skin care, use of tape, and preventive measures to protect fragile skin in premature infants.

Case Study

An infant born at 35 weeks' gestation was admitted to the NICU with a maternal history of opioid use treated with methadone. The infant appeared irritable, with a high-pitched cry, muscle twitching and upon initiation of feedings experienced vomiting and difficulty sucking. An interprofessional team approach was instituted-that included the family to ensure consistency in the treatment plan. This plan is based on clinical observation of each individual baby's symptoms not on a standardized scoring scale as used in the past. The focused assessment included consolability, sleep-wake patterns, and feeding ability. Both non-pharmacologic and pharmacologic interventions were implemented. Non-pharmacologic interventions included use of a quiet, low light environment with minimal stimulation; encouragement of the family to assist in care including breast-feeding if there was no contraindication, swaddling, and feeding-on demand rather than scheduled. At first the infant was experiencing difficulty breastfeeding and was extremely irritable, so morphine was used only as needed. Over the course of the next few days the parents gained confidence in their caretaking, breastfeeding was successful, and the infant would quiet with reduced stimulation-such as swaddling in the bed with low lights and sounds. The infant was discharged home in 28 days.

Reflective Practice: Carol B. Jaeger

My experience in neonatal care has spanned many decades as an officer in the military and as an employee in not-for-profit, and public civilian systems. My professional nursing roles have included bedside caregiver, neonatal nurse practitioner, educator, manager, policy administrator, neonatal network administrator, and advanced practice nurse faculty. Across my career, my perspective has focused on continuous learning to improve practice delivery to babies and families, with the goal to optimize the physical and psychosocial outcome of babies and families.

The rising global problem of opioid use has heightened the awareness among health professionals of the complex neonatal consequences. The incidence of neonatal abstinence syndrome (NAS) that includes Neonatal Opioid Withdrawal (NOW) is rising too. While we have cared for such infants for decades, we are finally gathering more evidence to support sound evidence-based assessments and interventions.

1.5 Neonatal Care in the 1960s and 1970s

The science of neonatology, and the care of sick and premature babies, was new in the 1960s and 1970s. Pediatricians and nurses specializing in neonatal care were pioneers in the field. I was one of those pioneers. Our neonatal team translated physiologic knowledge and care to the baby from pediatric medicine and nursing practice. We accommodated the evolving care in a limited number of neonatal intensive care units (NICUs) in tertiary teaching hospitals—spaces proximal to newborn nurseries. Some of the early neonatal units and the professional pioneers were military medical facilities staffed with military personnel caring for dependent family members. Initial neonatal air transport within regional care networks were military helicopter and fixed-wing pilots staffed with military and/or civilian neonatal staff.

The new science and care required instrumentation to successfully manage the unique needs of sick and premature babies. Neonatal staff and medical engineers began researching, designing, and trialing the design of equipment, technical devices, and supplies to meet the physiologic needs of babies. Examples of instrumentation devices developed to provide care included transport incubators, incubators, warming beds, ventilators, cardiorespiratory monitors, and intravenous (IV) pumps.

Most continuing education was hands-on learning by the interprofessional healthcare team at the bedside. Gradually, professional nursing programs and hospital orientations began to offer specialized education and training in the pathophysiologic/physiologic support of the sick and premature newborn, and the psychosocial effect of maternal–infant separation.

Neonatologists and nurse caregivers were ill prepared to support parents in the NICU; so, most units were open to "parents as visitors" during prescribed times in the afternoon and eve-

ning. Space and comfortable seating at the bedside were limited, and parental touching was often discouraged. The blinds of viewing windows between the NICU and the corridor were opened only periodically to "allow" parents/families to observe their baby amid the rows of incubators, monitors, and IV poles/pumps. NICU babies were discharged to home, with parents having little experience or knowledge of the behavior of their baby. Neonatal clinics specializing in follow-up of the baby were limited, and parents traveled distances to connect with neonatal teams of interdisciplinary healthcare professionals to receive continuing care.

1.6 Neonatal Care in the 1980s and 1990s

The population of premature babies increased, survivability improved, science expanded, and Level II and III neonatal special care units (NSCU)/NICUs grew in number across the United States. Neonatal interprofessional specialists began to multiply, such as nutritionists, physical and occupational therapists, and social workers. Medical and surgical physicians began to focus on neonatal anomalies, genetic conditions, and premature physiologic management. Over time, building the specialty knowledge and skill among the interprofessional disciplines created silos among and between the specialties and specialists. In the latter years of the 1990s, the value of collaboration among the neonatal team members to coordinate care was recognized to better serve babies and parents.

We began to collect metrics to measure the mortality, morbidity, and diagnostic indices of babies in the NSCU/NICU; as well as descriptors and ratios of the NSCU/NICU workforce. We disseminated and compared data locally, regionally, state-wide, nationally, and internationally. The goal was to change the way we had learned to perform care when the data and the evidence indicated a better way to manage and support the baby. In addition, the shortage of neonatologists and medical residents inspired the development of experienced neonatal nurses as neonatal nurse specialists/practitioners to function with expanded skills, thus extending the "reach" of the neonatologist.

The science proliferated and neonatal professionals reached-out to learn from/with other NSCU/NICU teams. Neonatologists and cardiothoracic surgeons collaborated to implement extracorporeal membrane oxygenation (ECMO) in Level III NICUs as a therapy to manage babies with acute respiratory distress, pulmonary hypertension as the result of elevated pulmonary vascular resistance, and life support before or after cardiac surgery. The development and therapeutic use of natural and, later, synthetic surfactant with babies born with immature lung development positively influenced the short-term and long-term effects of respiratory distress. The use of nasal continuous positive airway pressure (CPAP) compared to extended ventilation via intubation demonstrated a reduction in bronchopulmonary dysplasia (BPD).

The implementation of improvement science methods in the NSCU/NICU was initiated to better utilize the benefits of new knowledge, developing technology, significance of newborn developmental needs, the influence of a supportive physical environment, and parent/family involvement. Evidence-based strategies to control and manage infections in the neonate were employed, and closely monitored, to affect a reduction in central line-associated bloodstream infections and antibiotic resistant infections. The healthcare team began to partner with parents to engage them in the care of their baby and to "open" the NSCU/NICU to parents/families for continuous access, with the exception of the change-of-shift report by professionals. The healing environment of the baby in the NICU, and the space accommodation for parents engaging with their babies in the NICU were recognized as significant to the optimum outcome of the baby. Single family rooms became a viable option to support family centered care in the NICU.

1.7   Neonatal Care in the 2000s

Despite the goal to decrease the incidence of premature birth, the number has continued to increase in the United States. NSCU/NICUs of multiple hospitals have engaged in business agreements to create networks led by specialty medical centers, usually Children's Hospitals affiliated with teaching facilities that include maternal fetal specialty programs. Specialized services for women and babies prompted the designation of Level IV NICUs commensurate with maternal fetal programs.

Collaborations among the neonatal medical and surgical specialties and the maternal fetal specialists have been developed to manage the deliveries of high or at-risk women with a high-risk fetus who needed immediate intervention to manage a life-threatening condition. The nurse practitioner (NP) workforce has grown, and further specialized among the neonatal and pediatric medical/surgical specialties. The NPs have evolved as primary providers of care in all levels of neonatal care and expanded their role in neonatal outpatient clinics. The demand is far greater than the supply in the workforce. Depending on the statutory authority of the state, NPs can be licensed in one of three modes—an independent practitioner, a collaboration arrangement with a physician(s), or a supervisory arrangement with a physician(s).

The evaluation and strength of evidence have become critical to standardize the practice of care, and to structure the competent performance of practice by interprofessionals. Improvement science has proliferated. Studies focus on decreasing the mortality and morbidity of mothers and babies, and the increase of population health within the community. Collaboratives among NSCU/NICUs have organized across regions, states, and the nation, to evaluate evidence, compare metrics, define clinical pathways, monitor clinical implementation, and disseminate results. One example is the collaboration of maternal and newborn professionals to reduce the incidence of late preterm birth at 34–37 weeks gestation caused largely by consumer preference for a planned birth and/or the birth of a smaller baby. Obstetricians convincingly discouraged an early birth option by educating their clients that a term birth will optimize the health of their baby. This limited NICU admissions. Other examples of neonatal collaboration to improve practice through evidence include: (a) pain management of the neonate, (b) management of the extreme low birth weight baby, (c) early feeding with breastmilk, (d) management of babies with neonatal abstinence syndrome (NAS), (e) prevention of bronchopulmonary dysplasia (BPD), (f) NICU single family room design, (g) satisfaction/confidence survey of parents using family-centered care, (h) infant and family-centered developmental care, and (i) transition to home and discharge planning.

The science and the instrumentation of practice have continued to expand. The number of extreme low birthweight (ELBW) babies born at 22–26 weeks gestations increases, and survivability is improving. Babies born with genetic anomalies and/or surgical conditions, such as hypoplastic left heart syndrome (HPLH) and abdominal wall defects, are receiving staged treatment/repair and surviving. Babies diagnosed with hypoxic-ischemic encephalopathy are surviving with the use of cerebral hypothermia, using total body cooling or head cooling.

Continued and continuing education with simulation opportunities is building momentum in formal education programs and medical facilities. Computer-assisted technology augments the simulation learning for skills, procedures, instrumentation use, practice management, decision-making, collaborative team interaction.

Physical environments in NSCU/NICUs are more sensitive to the comfort and support of babies, parents, families, and professionals. Infant and family-centered developmental care has become integral to the physical, environmental, and psychosocial care of the baby, consequently using systems thinking to holistically integrate operations, nutrition, pain and stress management, positioning and touch, sleep and arousal, and skin-to-skin contact.

In many NICUs, parent advisors, who have lived the NICU parent experience, have become members of the collaborative healthcare team to negotiate the relationship between parents/family and health care interprofessionals. Parent advisors, and parent advisory councils, assist with the interpretation and prioritization of parent/family needs, the role/message of the parents as advocates for their baby, cultural orientation

to the unit and health environment, and health education relative to the condition of their baby.

Facility operations are more sophisticated as multiple hospital neonatal networks evolve, and neonatal specialty units develop, such as small baby units, cardiac units, neuro care units, chronic care units. Transport teams are independent, function by ground and air, and service populations within large geographic regions.

1.8 Summary

I have been fortunate to be a part of the innovation that has occurred in many decades of neonatal science and neonatal nursing. The evolution of science, practice, outcome, and education has been demonstrated through outcomes of babies and families. Making a difference through knowledge and experience has made my journey fulfilling. Further, I extend my appreciation to the babies, families, and professionals who have made this journey with me.

The next reflective practice from a parent's perspective illustrates how far we have come from the story Dr. Jaeger shared. Yet as Deb Discenza shares, we still have a long way to go.

Reflective Practice: Parent Perspective: Deb Discenza

Family-Centered Care Has Come a Long Way

My daughter Becky was born at 30 weeks' gestation in 2003. The NICU was noisy, chaotic and bay-structured with a total of four bays. Phones ringing, alarms going off, and we parents clamoured for the precious few rocking chairs to get some bedside time at the already crowded incubator. The focus was on the healthcare of the baby and it looked like the parents were more of an afterthought than a necessary component of the team. Kangaroo Care was something I learned about from my former Registered Nurse (RN) mother-in-

law, not the team of nurses'. Pumping breast milk was something I did myself (without any clue what I was doing) upon spotting the breast pump in my room. Chaos ruled our 38-day stay in the NICU.

Today family-centered care takes on a whole new meaning with private room NICUs, NICU parent classes on special needs care and preparing for discharge day. Kangaroo Care is far more common now than it used to be and with the Baby-Friendly movement, breast milk is center-stage in care.

But we still have a long way to go especially in the face of parent-professional discussions. Empathy is not something a professional learns from a textbook. Parent respect is not an item on a test. Connecting with families on a meaningful level is a key component of success for the NICU professional and more importantly, for the long-term outcome of the NICU infant.

Another Observation About My Daughter's NICU Stay

In our noisy, crowded NICU, I saw amongst my 30-weeker daughter's "neighbours" the tiniest of babies I had ever witnessed: Infants that were micro-preemies at 25 and 26 weeks' gestation. Thinking my 30 weeker girl was lucky by comparison, I had no idea at the time that they would be saving babies even earlier than that shortly thereafter. Saving an infant at 22 weeks was unheard of in 2003 but now is becoming more commonplace.

As we delve into the latest frontier of neonatal medicine, we need to remember that while we are doing the best we can to save every baby earlier and earlier we also need to keep a strong view on long-term outcomes. Yesteryear's premature babies are now adults and the ramifications of neonatal medicine are front and center with these former patients every day. Care

has gotten better over time, but there are side effects to premature birth that continue to plague the community. Everything from complicated lung challenges to mental health challenges to developmental challenges, we need to always view all of these early babies with a keen eye on how to best help their outcomes in the NICU and especially out of the NICU. Otherwise we are increasingly burdening families and the state, regional, and federal programs for the beginning and often the entire life of that child.

1.9 Conclusion

This chapter highlights how neonatal nursing care and education have evolved over the last 60 years. Great strides have been made in our education and the evidence to support our care. We embrace parents as partners in care yet, we still need to truly adopt an infant and family-centered developmental care approach to our work.

References

American Association of Colleges of Nursing (AACN) (2006) The essentials of doctoral education for advanced nursing practice. https://www.aacnnursing.org/Portals/42/Publications/DNPEssentials.pdf

Goncalves RL, Tsuzuki LM, Carvalho GS (2015) Endotracheal suctioning in intubated newborns: an integrative literature review. Rev Bras Ter Intensiva 27(3):284–292

Kuller J (2018) Neonatal evidence-based skin care guidelines, 4th edn. http://apps.nann.org/store/product-details?productId=61672348

National Association of Neonatal Nurses (NANN) (2012) Essentials of neonatal nurses-orientation lecture series modules 1-10-streaming Video. http://apps.nann.org/store/product-details?productId=363

National Association of Neonatal Nurses (NANN) (2014) Competencies and orientation toolkit for neonatal nurse practitioners, 2nd edn. http://apps.nann.org/store/product-details?productId=9876350

Canada

2

Marsha Campbell-Yeo, Tanya Bishop,
Danica Hamilton, Fabiana Bacchini,
and Leah Whitehead

2.1 Introduction

Canada, a geographically large country with just over 37.5 million people, has considerable number of rural areas with pockets of more densely populated regions in each of the ten provinces and three territories. Neonatal care falls within a small specialized field under the Canadian Pediatric Society (CPS). The country has approximately 178 neonatal intensive care units (NICUs). Within the overall healthcare system, neonatal intensive care is structured in different ways across the country. Some structures have the NICU/Special Care Nursery located within a Children's hospital, others within a Women's and Newborn hospital, and some would have a unit within a general health center serving the care needs of all populations. At times the care may be fragmented from ongoing care needs of these infants and families depending on the structure of a particular NICU.

Neonatal nursing care and practice is guided by the Canadian Nurses Association (CNA) and neonatal national competencies (Canadian Nurses Association 2010). Nurses can undertake specialization in neonatal nursing through programs such as the Canadian Nurses Association (CNA) Certification Program. The Canadian Nurses Association (CNA) represents Canadian nurses nationally and globally. CNA offers, as one of the 22 certifications available, a certification in neonatal nursing. In preparation for this certification, neonatal competencies were developed by national representation of 24 subject matter experts in neonatal nursing care (Canadian Nurses Association 2010). To become certified, a nurse must have at least 1950 hours of work experience in the specialty area within the past 5 years or 1000 h of work experience in the specialty area plus 300 hours of formal specialized education in the past 10 years. The candidate will need to pass an online exam to become certified and maintain their certification every 5 years by re-writing the

M. Campbell-Yeo (✉)
School of Nursing Dalhousie University,
Halifax, NS, Canada

IWK Health, Halifax, NS, Canada

Council of International Neonatal Nurses, Inc.
(COINN), Yardley, PA, USA
e-mail: marsha.campbell-yeo@dal.ca

T. Bishop
Council of International Neonatal Nurses, Inc.
(COINN), Yardley, PA, USA

IWK Health, Halifax, NS, Canada

D. Hamilton
Families in Recovery (FIR) Program, BC Women's
Hospital + Health Centre, Vancouver, BC, Canada

F. Bacchini
Canadian Premature Babies Foundation,
Toronto, ON, Canada

L. Whitehead
IWK Health, Halifax, NS, Canada

J. Petty et al. (eds.), *Neonatal Nursing: A Global Perspective*,
https://doi.org/10.1007/978-3-030-91339-7_2

exam or through 100 hours of continuous education credits. Certification in one's specialty area instills a great deal of pride and is shown to improve both patient outcomes and overall satisfaction of care (CNA Certification Program 2021). There are hopes to align specialty certification with national accreditation standards. The Canadian Association of Neonatal Nurses (CANN) established in 2006 is the professional body for neonatal nurses in Canada (Canadian Association of Neonatal Nurses n.d.). CANN is a national association member of the Council of International Neonatal Nurses, Inc. (COINN).

This chapter will provide an overview of Canadian neonatal nursing education and practice, an historical overview of neonatal care, and priority areas for evidence-based practice. Personal reflections from nurses and parents further highlight changes in neonatal care philosophy.

Key "Think Points" for Learning

- Neonatal care encompasses multiple levels of care complexity, training and care environments, and diverse nursing roles and education.
- Neonatal care priorities include:
- Partnering with families to fully integrate them in care provision.
- Optimization of the assessment and management of neonatal pain-related stress.
- Focus on measuring outcomes, quality improvement, and a multidisciplinary approach to care.
- Innovation in partnership with marginalized populations within our country.

2.2 Organization of Neonatal Care

Canadian neonatal units are organized by levels of care, providing a range of care with some caring for Level I/II infants and the larger tertiary units caring up to Level III/IV infants. Subsequent care levels can provide all care for the previous level and then add additional services. The most referenced definitions for levels of care in Canadian NICUs is provided by the Provincial Council on Maternal and Child Health (PCMCH) (Provincial Council for Maternal and Child Health 2013; Shum 2020). Level I care would include phototherapy, antibiotics, and support for feeding difficulties. Much of this care has safely transitioned to postpartum units in the tertiary care centers where NICU staff are able to assist if needed. Level II care can include all that is required to care for infants 30 weeks gestation and greater. This can include oxygen, continuous positive airway pressure (CPAP), short durations of mechanical ventilation, gavage feedings, and peripheral/umbilical/central lines. Level III units provide care to all gestations, weights, and routinely offer mechanical ventilation, high-frequency oscillation, nitric oxide, and surgical care. Level IV care is not referenced in the PCMCH document but is known throughout the country as the ability to offer Extra Corporeal Membrane Oxygenation (ECMO). Several tertiary center NICUs will collaborate with Pediatric Intensive Care Units in their health facilities to offer this level of care. Many regions or provinces of the country will have one identified tertiary referral care center to serve the complex care needs of infants from multiple provinces and territories.

The vast majority of Canadian NICUs continue to offer care within an open bay environment or design, where multiple infants and their families are cared for in one room. Given the associated benefit and in an effort to have families more engaged in the care of their child, more NICUs are being redeveloped each year to either a smaller pod room style (1–4 bed), single-patient room, single family room, or combination of these models (van Veenendaal et al. 2020).

Interprofessional teams within the NICU consist of many skilled healthcare providers. Care is typically overseen by a neonatologist or pediatrician as the most responsible provider. Neonatal nurses provide the majority of direct care in partnership with families. Many other disciplines make up the neonatal care team, such as neonatal nurse practitioners (NNPs), clinical nurse specialists (CNS), clinical associates (CA), residents, allied health team members (respiratory therapy, occupational therapy, physiotherapy, pharmacy, dieticians, lactation consultants, social work), and many more. There is an emergence of newer roles to neonatal care within units such as psychologists, music therapists, and indigenous patient navigators. Teams are proud of the relationships that are built with families in the NICU. An important team member in many units includes a family advisor or parent partner. The latter role was born out of a Family Integrated Care (FiCare) research study that helped shape the philosophy of many NICUs across the country (O'Brien et al. 2018). The parent partner is a parent with lived/living experience of a NICU admitted infant. Parent partners provide invaluable psychosocial "peer" support to families and are often employed as a member of the unit. Parent partners also oversee the ongoing recruitment of parent volunteers and alumni families, as well as participate in unit discussions regarding strategic planning and care philosophy and facilitate family engagement opportunities with current families in the unit. Roles like these serve to innovate, respect the patient/family voice, and challenge the historic hierarchy of the healthcare system.

In most units, clinical goals are planned, implemented, and evaluated on daily rounds for the upcoming 24 h. Families are included in this care planning, recognized as the experts in care who know their infant best. Goal setting with families is a priority, with the main focus on preparing infants and their families for discharge or transition to a center closer to home.

2.3 Education and Training

In Canada, all provinces and territories require nurses to have a bachelor's degree except Quebec, where diploma programs are still offered. As of 2015, the 11 provincial/territorial bodies require the successful completion of a standardized Canadian RN entry-to-practice exam. Registered nurse entry to practice in Canada is based on completion of an accredited university baccalaureate nursing program. Most programs range from 2 to 4 years, based on prior education. For example, students entering immediately following completion of post-secondary education will be expected to complete a 4-year program of study. Students with prior university education or a previous university degree may be accepted into a 2- or 3-year accelerated nursing program. Nursing education programs focus primarily on the care of well newborns with little to no content related to critically ill and/or preterm newborns. Access to clinical placements further exacerbate this knowledge gap with postpartum and pediatric placements prioritized. A compounding variable would be the significantly limited availability of clinical placements in the NICU due to restricted access for nursing students with only a handful being afforded the opportunity for placements. The introduction of a critical care certificate at some universities has piqued greater interest and knowledge in the area; however, global exposure for early learning at NICU settings is uncommon.

There is no national license in Canada, and each province or territory has regulatory bodies (https://www.cna-aiic.ca/en). Each province and territory have a nursing college that oversees and maintains nursing registration. A minimum number of hours must be worked in the profession and the member must remain in good standing. Foundation to the profession would be standards of practice and code of ethics documents (Canadian Nurses Association 2017).

While the hiring of experienced nurses is preferred, there is an increasing trend, due to nursing shortages, of newly graduated nurses being hired to work in NICUs across the country. This trend has led to greater need for employer-based training and mentorship for new staff. The introduction of single-family room NICUs has created concern for new graduate nurses due to the loss of organic mentorship opportunities and learning by osmosis from the experienced practitioners around them.

There are no existing national standards regarding orientation of newly hired nursing staff to NICU settings in Canada. Once a nurse is hired for the NICU, the orientation programs vary in terms of length, content, and delivery, with many using a combination of classroom, simulation and precepted shifts to prepare nurses for neonatal specialty practice based on their previous experience. One province, British Columbia, requires courses in neonatal intensive care before hiring into their NICUs on track for certification. Many NICUs would also have a phased in approach to orientation with care of Level I/II neonates introduced first and then more advanced levels of care introduced after in-unit experience has been gained. Therefore, employers take on the bulk of responsibility for neonatal nurse preparation for clinical care.

NICU settings offer several opportunities for nurses to learn and grow throughout their career, particularly within the tertiary care units. A few of these opportunities include: the emergency or resuscitation nurse which responds to infants requiring assistance at birth; transportation nurse for the acutely ill infant transport or the repatriation of an infant to home health centers; charge nurse or care facilitator role; nurse educator, discharge coordinator, lactation consultant, or part of specialty team such as the intravenous team or Peripherally Inserted Central Catheter (PICC) team who would insert and manage intravenous access or central lines in the unit.

Canada has two advanced practice nursing roles (APN), the clinical nurse specialist (CNS), and the nurse practitioner (NP), both of which require a minimum of a Master of Nursing degree. A PhD in nursing is the most common requirement for a university academic/research position. A Doctor of Nursing Practice (DNP) is less common with only one university in Canada, as of 2021, offering this program.

Advanced practice nurses fulfil leadership roles within the NICU (neonatal/pediatric nurse practitioners (NNPs), clinical nurse specialists (CNSs), etc.). The minimum education is a master's in nursing. Many NICUs rely heavily on NNPs to oversee clinical care of infants and their families; however, the education systems are often unreliable in maintaining the workforce levels that are desired. For instance, some provinces must collaborate with local universities when the need for NNPs arises; taking a very active role in recruitment, education, and clinical requirements. The requirements to practice for the NNP role vary across the country where some provinces do not recognize the neonatal nurse practitioner subspecialty and require a pediatric nurse practitioner who then furthers their training in neonatal care to fulfil licensing requirements.

2.4 Five Decades of Neonatal Care in Canada

Neonatology and the care of infants who are sick or preterm is a relatively young field, primarily taking hold as a recognized area of practice in Canada in the 1960s and 1970s. As with many facets of healthcare, new ways to provide care are often the result of the combination of emerging science and societal/political advocacy with accompanying funding opportunities. Such was the case with neonatology; with increasing knowledge of infant development and physiological needs, extrapolation of knowledge of adult equipment to be used in infants, and the death of Patrick Bouvier Kennedy, the son of President Kennedy and his wife, 39 h after being born 5.5 weeks early. While the latter occurred in the United States, our neighbor to the South, this triad of events led to a surge in interest and funding and was a significant impetus to modern North American neonatal care.

Neonatal care in Canada followed a similar timeline, although there is some controversy as to the exact opening of the first official neonatal care unit. Dr. Bob Usher (1929–2006) became Director of Nurseries at the Royal Victoria Hospital in Montreal in 1959, but it is uncertain when the unit offered "special care" services. A special care nursery at the Hospital for Sick Children in Toronto was opened in 1961 and was credited to the leadership of Paul Swyer (1921–2019). To aid in the provision of regionalized neonatal care delivery, neonatal transports first carried out by pediatric residents occurred in a non-standardized way in the late 1960s. It was not until the mid-1970s that official transport programs (primarily paramedics sometimes with physicians) were created. The first programs were out of Vancouver BC Children's and Women's Hospitals and Toronto Hospital for Sick Children, which began in 1976. More modern-day ground, as well as air medical transport programs, primarily nurse, and/or nurse and respiratory therapist-led, emerged in the 1980s. It was not until 1990 that the Canadian Pediatric Society Section of Neonatal Perinatal Medicine was established. The Canadian Association of Neonatal Nurses (CANN), a non-for-profit organization that represents nurses from across Canada who specialize in the care of newborn infants and their families, was established in 2006.

The focus on neonatal care also led to the simultaneous creation of provincial reproductive outreach programs. One of the first was established in the province of Nova Scotia, in 1973, with the aim of working directly with hospital and community-based hospitals and care providers to promote excellence in perinatal care. Neonatal nurses from tertiary centers provided considerable teaching and training to smaller centers through provision of courses such as S.T.A.B.L.E.® (Park City, Utah) since first introduced in 1996.

2.5 Evidenced-Based Care: Priority Areas

2.5.1 Family-Integrated Care

The concept of family-centered care in neonatal care was raised in the literature in the late 1990s, with the first Canadian commentary written by three neonatal nurses from Winnipeg, Manitoba (Beveridge, Bodnaryk, and Ramachandran) in the Canadian Nurse in 2001 (Beveridge et al. 2001). While there was considerable emphasis, with some success, placed on improving family-centered care in NICUs across the country in the early 2000s, the introduction of the concept of family integrated care in 2013 by Canadian researchers (O'Brien et al. 2018), has led to greatest practice uptake. Family-integrated care is an extension of family-centered care and con-

sists of four primary pillars: training of care providers on effective parent teaching; parent presence in the NICU, generally no less than 6 h/day as well as attendance at parent targeted education sessions; parental inclusion and involvement in team rounds; and incorporation of trained alumni parents of former NICU infants as peer support (Franck and O'Brien 2019). Parent partners are one of the cornerstones of family-integrated care and their inclusion on NICU committees and boards as a voice for families is readily becoming an expected element of care and decision-making across Canadian NICUs. The creation of the Canadian Premature Babies Foundation (CPBF) in 2012, a parent-led, charitable organization, provides education, support, and advocacy for premature babies and their families (Canadian Premature Babies Foundation n.d.). The primary goal of this organization is to help ensure national access to peer support programs, helpful materials, and resources for families and healthcare professionals, and investigate ways to improve the lives and experiences of premature babies and their families.

Parent Reflection: Leah Whitehead

I laid my head back in the light blue leather chair. I imagined I was somewhere else, anywhere else. My baby was nestled into my chest; little Tessa, born at 28 weeks. My mind tried to shut out the sounds of her CPAP machine, the sounds of the monitor and the sounds of life around me in a crowded, open-bay unit. "This is not your home," I whispered to Tessa. "There is a place better than this for you. This is not it." Somewhere beyond me, a neighbouring parent was playing beach sounds. I imagined Tessa and me, being alone for the first time, on a beautiful Nova Scotian beach, safe and secure in the sun.

NICU was a disorienting place for me...a place I was visiting and yet a piece of my heart was living there. It knocked the wind out of me and depleted my usual con-

fidence. This was our first baby. From the very beginning, we wanted to set the tone of our family culture but with a NICU baby, that was not possible. Nearly all the things we valued as a family were beyond our control.

In NICU, the moments which changed my day, my outlook, my ability to participate and cope, were simply that: moments; moments of compassion and kindness. It was the nurse patiently giving us a tour so that we could feel more 'at home;' it was the discharge planner who was comfortable with my emotion and allowed me to cry; it was the neo who did not dismiss my theories but let me talk them through with him; it was the bedside nurse singing Meatloaf's "I Would do Anything for Love" as we arrived in the morning.

It was in these moments, these moments when nothing was required of me, where I could cautiously explore a new environment and a new role, where I felt like I could be a parent and make decisions and look out for Tessa, because someone was looking out for me. As we begin to recognize that health care providers are temporarily occupying a space in a families' life and that it is not families temporarily occupying a space in a health centre, the care shifts to one that is filled with interactions that are kind, compassionate and honouring of people and relationships.

Our NICU was ready to make this kind of radical shift. In 2013, I, alongside another NICU mom and two social workers, began to build the Parent Partner Volunteer Program. The intention of this program was peer support and, while it has created that network, it also has served as a driver for change in our NICU. Over the course of our eight-year journey, thousands of families and a core group of nearly 40 volunteers have bravely and generously shared their voices and their stories to shape the care of our NICU. And our healthcare staff have willingly and graciously listened and continue to listen even when it is not easy. In both cases, this kind of care comes at enormous cost. For the families, it takes an emotional, physical and mental toll to revisit what can be traumatic experiences. For healthcare staff, it can also take an emotional, a relational and a professional toll as they boldly stand up in a system that requires cultural transformation.

To honour a family's preferences and to truly believe they are a leader on their baby's care team takes a considerable amount of commitment. However, with a pioneering spirit and the vulnerability to make mistakes, our families physicians and staff are continuing to pursue excellence in medical, physical and emotional care of families admitted to NICU by moving in pace with each other, always together.

Parent Reflection: Fabiana Bacchini

I was lying on the hospital bed, still wearing the blue gown many hours or days after my C-section, when a doctor walked in. The room was bright and cold. I kept staring at the white board where I had written my goal to carry my pregnancy to 28 weeks.

Next to me, my twin A, Michael was wrapped in a hospital blanket forever sleeping peacefully. My mind was racing, and I questioned how could a baby die before even having a chance to live? He had passed away in utero at 25 weeks due to a heart malformation. At 26 weeks, I went into preterm labour and a few hours later I was rushed to the OR to have an emergency C-section. It was a deafening silence. My surviving twin, Gabriel, was rushed to the NICU before I could even lay my eyes on him.

When the doctor walked in, I was alone. My husband had gone home to care for our

3-year-old son. He came to give me an update on Gabriel's condition. "Your son has a patent ductus arteriosus (PDA), which is a heart condition…". His words faded away. I couldn't control my tears. He asked me why I was crying. He certainly did not know that I had just lost a baby to a heart condition.

I shut down for almost 3 weeks after that day. I did not allow any nurse or doctor to talk to me about Gabriel. My husband would get all the updates and share with me. The nurses were my pillars. They taught me how to touch my 2-pound baby, change his tiny diaper, and clean his eyes. As I became more comfortable with the alarms, they started to 'translate' the NICU to me and invited me to be more involved in his care. I joined a research study called Family Integrated Care (FICare), a model of care that integrates families as partners in the NICU care team. It certainly changed my coping strategy and gave me a new perspective as I became part of the team, presented my son at rounds, and received education to be able to advocate for him. It really prepared me for the long road ahead.

After 146 days, Gabriel was discharged, and I started to volunteer at the hospital providing peer support and as an advisor in different committees. It was my way to express my gratitude for the team who had saved my son's life and helped me to find my voice. Six years as a volunteer led me to the Canadian Premature Babies Foundation (CPBF). The organization provides support and education for families, raises awareness about prematurity, trains parents and hospitals to create peer support programs, and collaborates with health care professionals in research and quality improvement projects.

There are enough parents and health care professionals working together, in true collaboration, pursuing a model of care that not only creates a more compassionate

health care system, but also improves outcomes for babies, their families, and empowers parents to be their babies' advocates in hospital and in the community.

We still have a long way to go until all hospitals consider parents as essential caregivers and partners in care, and until all research projects have a parent at the table, but we have made huge strides in the last decade. Change takes time, but there is no looking back. We have reached a point of no return.

2.5.2 Assessment and Management of Neonatal Pain

Another area of evidence-based neonatal care in which many Canadians were pioneers relates to the assessment and management of neonatal pain, determination of the short- and long-lasting serious consequences associated with untreated pain in early life, and the establishment of an international training consortium for trainees and researchers interested in pediatric pain. With respect to pain assessment, examples include the development and validation of the Premature Infant Pain Profile (PIPP) (Stevens et al. 1996), one of the most commonly used and well-validated composite pain assessment tool used in neonatal care as well as the Premature Infant Pain Profile-Revised (PIPP-R) (Gibbins et al. 2014). With respect to pain management, the first study, examining the effectiveness of the use of skin-to-skin contact for preterm infants, was conducted in Canada (Johnston et al. 2003), as well as numerous Cochrane reviews guiding clinical practice regarding effectiveness of interventions to reduce pain have been led by Canadian researchers (e.g., skin-skin (Johnston et al. 2017), sucrose (Stevens et al. 2016), breastfeeding (Shah et al. 2012)). Studies providing evidence supporting infants' ability to feel and remember pain (Taddio et al. 2006) and serious long-lasting adverse outcomes (e.g., altered brain growth, cognition, emotional regulation and epigenetic expression) have also been led by Canadians (Grunau 2013). Canada is also well known for research training and advocacy regarding neonatal/pediatric pain. The Pain in Child Health (PICH) international training consortium for Canadian and International trainees established in 2002 has trained and continues to train more than 500 trainees and has contributed considerable research productivity (von Baeyer et al. 2014). This global contribution to the field was highlighted in the 2012 State of Science and Technology in Canada Report (The State of Science and Technology in Canada 2012). Neonatal/pediatric pain ranked the highest of Canada's top 10 ranked specialized research clusters in which Canada publishes more than expected based on world publication, accounting for 15.5% of world papers in the field. Lastly, programs such as KidsinPain, Be Sweet to Babies, Power of a Parents Touch, and Solutions for Kids in Pain (SKIP) have had considerable success in increasing advocacy and awareness of the need for improved pain care for sick and preterm infants.

Practice Reflection: Marsha Campbell-Yeo

When I look back at my over three decades of neonatal practice it is difficult to pinpoint any one aspect that stands out. It is interesting as I reflect how I have come full circle on so many things.

I went to work as a neonatal nurse more than 34 years ago because I loved the fast pace, the adrenalin rush and the idea of saving lives using high tech care. To me at that time, providing the best care for babies was all about the best technology had to offer. While it is certainly true that the babies who survive today did not survive when I first started, the bad news is that it comes with many necessary painful medical procedures.

Later, as a clinician scientist, I wanted to find ways to decrease the pain and stress often associated with the life-saving tech-

nology. So why pain? Well, when one considers a typical very preterm baby cared for in an NICU, most endure between 7–17 painful or stressful procedures a day, meaning that the youngest and sickest babies can experience over a thousand procedures, like heel pokes, intravenous insertion and blood collections, during their NICU stay.

Looking back, I am amazed that when I started as a neonatal nurse, it was widely believed that babies did not feel or remember pain. In fact, babies even underwent surgery without pain medication simply receiving medications to keep them from moving. I know that's hard to believe. Thankfully, today we know babies do feel and remember pain, and we know that untreated pain can also impact how babies react to pain later in life, how their brains develop, and even how they will learn and regulate their emotions.

Sadly, recent studies tell us that less than half of babies in the world receive any pain relief for these procedures. We also know that finding solutions to reduce this exposure to pain in early life is not always easy. Simply providing medications is not the answer, as many drugs that work for adults don't work for babies, or in some cases finding the right balance is difficult. We and others knew we had to find other ways. We realized our world had become so reliant on specialized drugs and technology; we were underutilizing our most important resource-parents! We wanted to determine how keeping babies and mothers together could help. Together, with my research team and the support of a world-leader in neonatal pain, Dr. Celeste Johnston, we conducted several studies to test simple parent strategies like the upright holding of a diaper clad baby on the bare chest of a mother, called skin-to-skin contact (SSC) or kangaroo mother care (KMC). Seems natural, right... but it wasn't happening across many NICU's to reduce procedural pain.

Through our research we found incredible things. Human touch for babies provided during routine procedures like heel pokes and needles decreased how a baby felt and responded to pain. Touch stabilized their heart rates and the amount of oxygen in their bodies and helped them recover faster after the procedure was over. We conducted studies with fathers, other adults like grandmothers or aunts, and even tested whether a baby's preterm twin could help reduce the stress associated with these procedures. We determined that it wasn't just a mother's contact that could help. Human touch was the answer and we demonstrated that it was effective throughout a baby's entire NICU stay. And the best part was, it helped parents too. Parents told us that it made them feel closer to their baby. It made them feel better. They felt less stressed, more in control and confident.

We wanted to find ways to tell other scientists and clinicians about what we and others had found. So, we created a synthesis of all the science that had been done around the world about skin-to-skin contact and pain relief—all re-affirming the benefits of human touch. But we needed to tell parents too, as most don't realize how powerful their touch could be. We created a video available globally, translated into 17 languages   https://www.youtube.com/watch?v=3nqN9c3FWn8.

And this is where I have come full circle, because I believe balancing human touch with technology is the answer. Partnering with parents, families, clinicians, policy makers and researchers to use diverse technologies in novel ways to help ensure that we are able to more fully engage parents as active participants not only in pain care but in all aspects of their baby's care. My vision for neonatal care is that parental presence and involvement is no longer considered a nice thing to do but is considered an essential aspect of the care so that all babies' in NICUs have the best of both worlds- parent touch and technology.

2.5.3 Canadian Neonatal Network

A key area of focus in Canada that has led to significant improvement in neonatal outcomes was the creation of the Canadian Neonatal Network™ (CNN), founded in 1995 and currently includes over 30 hospitals and 17 universities (The Canadian Neonatal Network™ n.d.). The Network maintains a national database of participating sites which allows national tracking of neonatal outcomes as well as opportunity for collaboration between researchers and clinicians nationally and internationally to determine areas for improvement of neonatal care. The establishment of the CNN also provided the opportunity for benchmarking across sites and led to the establishment of two additional national programs, the Canadian Neonatal Follow-up Network (CNFUN) (The Canadian Neonatal Follow-Up Network n.d.) and the Evidence-based Practice for Improving Quality (EPIQ) program (EPIQ n.d.). The CNFUN consists of multidisciplinary teams of participating Neonatal and Perinatal Follow-Up Programs, and the program creates opportunities to share data to help guide practice to improve long-term neurodevelopmental outcomes of preterm or at-risk neonates. The EPIQ program includes 27 Canadian centers with a broad/diverse membership (e.g., neonatal nurses, neonatal nurse practitioners, clinical nurse specialists, neonatologists, physio and occupational therapists and pharmacists, respiratory therapists, social workers). Since 2018, family parent partners have been consistently added and participate as full members of the QI teams. It is this philosophy of working together which offers the best chance of success for optimal outcomes of neonates, their families, and care providers.

2.5.4 Striving for More Holistic Care for Infants with Neonatal Abstinence Syndrome and Their Families

As the opioid epidemic continues, our care approach to infants exposed to substances in utero and at risk for Neonatal Abstinence Syndrome (NAS) or Neonatal Opioid Withdrawal Syndrome (NOWS) varies across the country. We recognize that substance use is multifactorial and, depending on the region, perceived as a health care or legal issue with various levels of child protective agency involvement. Many units are reliant on a modified Finnegan score, first introduced in the 1970s by American Dr. Roberta Finnegan, as a subjective scoring tool to quantify the withdrawal symptoms an infant experiences. The Families In Recovery (FIR) unit at BC Women's Hospital in Vancouver, British Columbia was the first of its kind to keep mothers who use substances and their infants together (B.C. Women's Hospital + Health Centre and Provincial Health Services Authority 2020). The approach looks to care for these infants and their withdrawal symptoms through a functional assessment, the infant's qualitative experience and not the healthcare provider's quantitative determination. The research validated Eat Sleep Console model is the belief that the family is the primary non-pharmacological treatment for their infant (Grossman et al. 2018). There is a need for ongoing change to keep mothers and their infants together and out of the NICU wherever possible. Similar program implementations are underway across the country within mother–baby and pediatric units.

2.5.5 Addressing Social Injustice

Social justice movements continue around the world where oppressive systems are now feeling the pressures and beginning to listen; these systems have caused the disparity of the social determinants of health and experiences within the healthcare system by certain races of peoples. In Canada, race-based data is rarely collected, and family experience is not systematically reported. Documents like the Truth and Reconciliation Commission Report (Truth and Reconciliation Commission of Canada 2012), the United Nations Declaration on the Rights of Indigenous Peoples (UNDRIP) (United Nations Declaration on the Rights of Indigenous Peoples 2015), and In Plain Sight Report (B.C. Government 2020) and programs like San'yas Indigenous Cultural Safety Training (Provincial Health Services Authority in BC n.d.) are a part of holding systems accountable to their responsibility to decolonize processes and services that continue to harm Indigenous peoples, and to provide trauma-informed, antiracist, and culturally safe care and learn from the historical atrocities caused by colonization which still exist today. Implementation of such initiatives is the responsibility of but remains at the discretion of each unit.

2.6 Conclusion

This chapter provides an overview of the current status of neonatal care in the context of neonatal nursing in Canada. While important advancements regarding neonatal nursing education, specialization and leadership, care delivery, and parent engagement have been made over the past decades, variation remains across Canadian NICUs, with a need for the development of additional national standards of neonatal care to guide consistent and equitable practice and care delivery.

References

B.C. Government (2020) In plain sight: addressing indigenous-specific racism and discrimination in B.C. Health Care. https://engage.gov.bc.ca/app/uploads/sites/613/2020/11/In-Plain-Sight-Summary-Report.pdf

B.C. Women's Hospital + Health Centre, Provincial Health Services Authority (2020) FIR model of care

Beveridge J, Bodnaryk K, Ramachandran C (2001) Family-centred care in the NICU. Can Nurse 97(3):14–18

Canadian Association of Neonatal Nurses (n.d.) https://neonatalcann.ca/

Canadian Nurses Association (2010) Canadian nurse practitioner core competency framework. Canadian Nurses Association. http://www.cna-aiic.ca/CNA/documents/pdf/publications/Competency_Framework_2010_e.pdf

Canadian Nurses Association (2017) Code of ethics for registered nurses. Canadian Nurses Association

Canadian Premature Babies Foundation (n.d.) CPBF. https://www.cpbf-fbpc.org

CNA Certification Program (2021) https://www.cna-aiic. ca/en/certification

EPIQ (n.d.) http://www.epiq.ca/

Franck LS, O'Brien K (2019) The evolution of family-centered care: from supporting parent-delivered interventions to a model of family integrated care. Birth Defects Research 111(15):1044–1059. https://doi. org/10.1002/bdr2.1521

Gibbins S, Stevens B, Yamada J, Dionne K, Campbell-Yeo M, Lee G, Caddell K, Johnston C, Taddio A (2014) Validation of the premature infant pain profile-revised (PIPP-R). Early Hum Dev 90(4):189–193. https://doi. org/10.1016/j.earlhumdev.2014.01.005

Grossman MR, Lipshaw MJ, Osborn RR, Berkwitt AK (2018) A novel approach to assessing infants with neonatal abstinence syndrome. Hosp Pediatr 8(1):1–6. https://doi.org/10.1542/hpeds.2017-0128

Grunau RE (2013) Neonatal pain in very preterm infants: long-term effects on brain, neurodevelopment and pain reactivity. Rambam Maimon Med J 4(4):e0025. https://doi.org/10.5041/RMMJ.10132

Johnston CC, Stevens B, Pinelli J, Gibbins S, Filion F, Jack A, Steele S, Boyer K, Veilleux A (2003) Kangaroo care is effective in diminishing pain response in preterm neonates. Arch Pediatr Adolesc Med 157(11):1084–1088

Johnston C, Campbell-Yeo M, Disher T, Benoit B, Fernandes A, Streiner D, Inglis D, Zee R (2017) Skin-to-skin care for procedural pain in neonates. Cochrane Database Syst Rev 2:CD008435. https://doi.org/10.1002/14651858.CD008435. pub3

O'Brien K, Robson K, Bracht M, Cruz M, Lui K, Alvaro R, da Silva O, Monterrosa L, Narvey M, Ng E, Soraisham A, Ye XY, Mirea L, Tarnow-Mordi W, Lee SK, FICare Study Group and FICare Parent Advisory Board (2018) Effectiveness of Family Integrated Care in neonatal intensive care units on infant and parent outcomes: a multicentre, multinational, cluster-randomised controlled trial. Lancet Child Adolesc Health 2(4):245–254. https://doi.org/10.1016/ S2352-4642(18)30039-7

Provincial Council for Maternal and Child Health (2013) Standardized maternal and newborn levels of care definitions, pp 1–13. https://www.pcmch.on.ca/wp-content/uploads/2015/07/Level-of-Care-Guidelines-2011-Updated-August1-20131.pdf

Provincial Health Services Authority in BC (n.d.) San'yas indigenous cultural safety training. https://www.san-yas.ca/

Shah PS, Herbozo C, Aliwalas LL, Shah VS (2012) Breastfeeding or breast milk for procedural pain in neonates. Cochrane Database Syst Rev 12:CD004950. https://doi.org/10.1002/14651858.CD004950.pub3

Shum J (2020) Maternal/fetal and neonatal services: tiers in brief to support system planning, p 21

Stevens B, Johnston C, Petryshen P, Taddio A (1996) Premature infant pain profile: development and initial validation. Clin J Pain 12(1):13–22. https://doi. org/10.1097/00002508-199603000-00004

Stevens B, Yamada J, Ohlsson A, Haliburton S, Shorkey A (2016) Sucrose for analgesia in newborn infants undergoing painful procedures. The. Cochrane Database Syst Rev 7:CD001069. https://doi. org/10.1002/14651858.CD001069.pub5

Taddio A, Lee C, Yip A, Parvez B, McNamara PJ, Shah V (2006) Intravenous morphine and topical tetracaine for treatment of pain in corrected neonates undergoing central line placement. JAMA 295(7):793–800

The Canadian Neonatal Follow-Up Network (n.d.) The Canadian neonatal follow-up network. https://cnfun. ca/

The Canadian Neonatal Network™ (n.d.) http://www. canadianneonatalnetwork.org/portal/

The State of Science and Technology in Canada (2012) https://cca-reports.ca/reports/the-state-of-science-and-technology-in-canada-2012/; https://cca-reports. ca/wp-content/uploads/2018/10/stateofst2012_fullre-porten.pdf

Truth and Reconciliation Commission of Canada (2012) Calls to action, pp 1–20. http://trc.ca/assets/pdf/Calls_ to_Action_English2.pdf

United Nations Declaration on the Rights of Indigenous Peoples (2015) https://www.un.org/development/ desa/indigenouspeoples/declaration-on-the-rights-of-indigenous-peoples.html/

van Veenendaal NR, van Kempen AAMW, Franck LS, O'Brien K, Limpens J, van der Lee JH, van Goudoever JB, van der Schoor SRD (2020) Hospitalising preterm infants in single family rooms versus open bay units: a systematic review and meta-analysis of impact on parents. EClinicalMedicine 23:100388. https://doi. org/10.1016/j.eclinm.2020.100388

von Baeyer CL, Stevens BJ, Chambers CT, Craig KD, Finley GA, Grunau RE, Johnston CC, Pillai Riddell R, Stinson JN, Dol J, Campbell-Yeo M, McGrath PJ (2014) Training highly qualified health research personnel: the pain in Child Health consortium. Pain Res Manag 19(5):267–274. https://doi. org/10.1155/2014/692857

South America

3

Andréia Cascaes Cruz, Flavia Simphronio Balbino,
and Ana Paula Dias França Guareschi

3.1 Introduction

The Brazilian Ministry of Health has instituted several programs, policies, and strategies focused on providing qualified assistance to newborns and women in the prenatal, childbirth, and puerperium period. Among the recommendations and actions contemplated for this assistance include: mandatory implementation of rooming-in settings in hospital institutions; nursing consultation within the first week after hospital discharge of the newborn and the woman who has given birth; newborn screening tests for early detection of congenital metabolic, ophthalmic, or cardiological diseases and congenital hearing loss; adherence to the Baby Friendly Hospital Initiative; regular monitoring of the child's growth and development up to 2 years of age; immunization; and an increase in the number of neonatal beds.

Neonatal hospital units are organized according to the complexity of the care offered to the newborn. The Neonatal Intensive Care Unit (NICU) provides services for the care of critically ill newborns or those at risk of death. According to Brazilian regulations, NICUs must have a specialized multidisciplinary team, its own specific equipment and appropriate technology for the diagnosis and treatment of newborns admitted to it. It should also adopt measures of ambience that provide the best development of the newborn and the participation of the parents during the entire hospitalization period. With regard to the nursing training, it is the Brazilian Ministry of Education that establishes the rules and guidelines for undergraduate, specialization, and residency programs for training neonatal nursing specialists. The title of neonatologist nurse is conferred by the Brazilian Society of Pediatric Nurses, upon fulfillment of minimum prerequisites and approval in a test prepared and applied by the corresponding society.

Although advances in neonatal care and improvements in neonatal health indicators have already been documented in scientific publications and technical reports, in a country with more than 200 million inhabitants and more than 8,511,000 km² of area, it is still a challenge guaranteeing access to quality and effective care on an equitable basis for all Brazilian newborns. The difference between the South/Southeast regions

A. C. Cruz (✉)
School of Nursing, Federal University of Sao Paulo, Sao Paulo, Brazil

Council of International Neonatal Nurses, Inc. (COINN), Yardley, PA, USA
e-mail: Andreia.Cruz@unifesp.br

F. S. Balbino · Ana Paula Dias França Guareschi
School of Nursing, Federal University of Sao Paulo, Sao Paulo, Brazil
e-mail: Balbino.Flavia@unifesp.br; Guareschi@unifesp.br

J. Petty et al. (eds.), *Neonatal Nursing: A Global Perspective*,
https://doi.org/10.1007/978-3-030-91339-7_3

when compared to the North/Northeast regions is enormous. This chapter will highlight the organization of neonatal care and the training/education of neonatal nurses.

Key "Think Points" for Learning

- There are different governmental public health policies and programs for neonatal care.
- Brazil's Federal Council of Nursing sets the standards for neonatal nursing practice.
- Neonatal care in hospital consists of different care levels that dictate what personnel and equipment must be available.
- The Brazilian Ministry of Education establishes rules and standards for neonatal nursing education/training at undergraduate, specialization, and residency programs.

3.2 Organization of Neonatal Care

3.2.1 Public Health Policies for Neonatal Care

In Brazil, since the 1970s, neonatal care is guided by public health policies and programs instituted by the Ministry of Health. The first program implemented was called "Maternal and Child Health Program" aimed at reducing morbidity and mortality among children and mothers. This program proposed actions to monitor prenatal care, to control home deliveries and the puerperium, and to promote children's health. Until the mid-1980s, this program had a limited scope, since it did not include important measures for neonatal care such as the guarantee of qualified hospital care. In the late 1990s, approximately 70% of infant mortality occurred in the neonatal period as the individuality and specificity of the neonatal population were neglected. Therefore,

several initiatives were developed and revised by the Ministry of Health to organize and improve perinatal care.

The first program that considered the newborn as a subject of nursing care, regardless of the care for women/mothers, was the Perinatal Health Care Program, developed in 1991. This program focused on five objectives: (1) organize perinatal care in a hierarchical and regionalized manner; (2) improve the quality of childbirth care and newborn care; (3) encourage breastfeeding; (4) provide guidance for family planning; and (5) supervise and evaluate the care provided to newborns. Among the various endeavors of the Brazilian Ministry of Health in this decade, it is important to highlight the mandatory implementation of rooming-in during the hospitalization period of both the woman who has given birth and the newborn. Rooming-in was implemented to encourage breastfeeding, favor the mother–child relationship, and to develop educational programs in maternal and newborn health.

Brazil was one of the UN member countries selected to start the baby-friendly Hospital Initiative, launched by the World Health Organization (WHO) in partnership with UNICEF. The first Brazilian unit was implemented in 1992, and by 2015, there were 326 institutions accredited according to the baby-friendly Hospital Initiative (Lamounier et al. 2019). Breastfeeding rates have increased from 1986 to 2006. The prevalence of exclusive breastfeeding at 6 months, in children under 2 years old, and continued up to 1 year of age increased rising from 4.7%, 37.4%, and 25.5% in 1986 to 37.1%, 56.3%, and 47.2% in 2006, respectively (Boccolini et al. 2017).

To provide humanized and qualified assistance to low birth weight newborns, in 2000 a public policy called "Standard of Humanized Care for Low Birth Weight Newborns—The Kangaroo Method (KM)" was developed. The KM was supported by four basic principles: welcoming the baby and the family, respecting the singularities, promoting skin-to-skin contact as early as possible, and increasing participation of parents and family in the care of the newborn. The KM recommended by this policy consists of three stages, the first two being carried out in hospitals and the last in the newborn's home, monitored by a primary healthcare team.

Considering the importance of carrying out an early diagnosis of some congenital diseases, such as phenylketonuria, congenital hypothyroidism, sickle cell disease or anemia and cystic fibrosis, the Brazilian Ministry of Health instituted the National Neonatal Screening Program in 2001, guaranteeing every newborn the right of accessing Neonatal Screening tests free of charge. In 2013, the program was reformulated to include clinical screenings to detect ophthalmic, auditory, and cardiological congenital changes.

Based on the finding that maternal and infant mortality remained high, with intense medicalization of childbirth and technology use without scientific evidence (e.g., cesarean sections and unnecessary interventions in childbirth), in 2011 the Brazilian Ministry of Health implemented the strategy called "Rede Cegonha" (Stork Network), emphasizing the urgency in reviewing the care processes in the Brazilian maternities (da Silva Cavalcanti et al. 2013).

Aiming at reducing child morbidity and mortality rates, in 2015 the National Policy for Comprehensive Child Health Care was instituted. This policy outlined several actions, among them the "5th Day of Integral Health" strategy: a nursing consultation with the mother and baby, from the third to the fifth day of life; and a home visit in the first week after hospital discharge, for mother/infants who did not show up for the consultation at the Primary Health Care Unit.

At-risk newborns who had prolonged hospitalizations received these follow-up visits more frequently than those with shorter lengths of stay. These visits coordinated by multidisciplinary and primary healthcare teams occurred from the first week after hospital discharge. Despite the reduction in neonatal mortality, which corresponded to 26 neonatal deaths for every 1000 live births in 1990 and decreased to eight neonatal deaths for every 1000 live births in 2016, the Brazilian neonatal mortality rate is still quite high and differs between the regions of the country, being worse in the north and northeast regions (Lansky et al. 2014; UNICEF et al. 2017).

3.3 Hospital Organization for Neonatal Care

The criteria for classification and qualification of beds in the neonatal units, recommended by the Brazilian Unified Health System for the care of critically or potentially critically ill newborns, are established according to the needs of the care, being divided in the following terms:

1. Neonatal Intensive Care Unit (NICU).
2. Neonatal Intermediate Care Units, with two typologies:
   (a) Conventional Neonatal Intermediate Care Unit;
   (b) Kangaroo Neonatal Intermediate Care Units. The number of beds in Neonatal Units will meet the following criteria according to the population need: for every 1000 (thousand) live births, there can be two NICU beds, two Conventional Neonatal Intermediate Care Unit beds, and one Kangaroo Neonatal Intermediate Care Unit bed. Neonatal Intensive Care Units (NICU) consist of hospital services aimed at the care of critically ill newborns or at risk of death, being considered in this classification:

- Newborns of any gestational age who require mechanical ventilation or newborns who present in an acute phase of respiratory failure requiring FiO_2 greater than 30%.
- Newborns under 30 weeks of gestational age or with birth weight below 1000 g.
- Newborns requiring major surgery or immediate postoperative surgery for small- and medium-sized surgeries.
- Newborns who need parenteral nutrition.
- Newborns requiring specialized care, such as the use of central venous catheters, vasoactive drugs, prostaglandin, antibiotics to treat severe infections, mechanical ventilation, and oxygen fraction (FiO_2) greater than 30%,

blood transfusion or blood products transfusion for acute hemolytic conditions, or coagulation disorders.

The NICU should have a specialized multidisciplinary team, its own specific equipment, and adequate technology (described in detail by the Brazilian Ministry of Health) for the diagnosis and treatment of critically ill newborns or those at risk of death. In addition, the NICU must comply with the following requirements: noise and lighting control; air conditioning; natural lighting for the new units; guarantee of free access to the mother and father, and permanence of the mother or father; guarantee of scheduled visits by family members; and guarantee of information on the evolution of patients to family members, by the medical team, at least once a day.

The multidisciplinary team to provide care at NICUs must be composed of at least:

Neonatologists or pediatricians: One physician, considered the technician responsible, with a minimum daily workload of 4 h; one physician with a minimum daily workload of 4 h for each ten beds or fraction; one physician staffing for each ten beds in each shift.

Nursing team: A nurse coordinator with neonatology specialization degree or at least 2 years of proven professional experience in pediatric or neonatal intensive care to fulfill a daily workload of 8 h; one registered nurse for each ten beds in each shift; a licensed practical nurse, at least one for each two beds in each shift.

Other team members: one exclusive physiotherapist for each ten beds in each shift; one physiotherapist coordinator with at least 2 years of proven professional experience in a pediatric or neonatal intensive care unit, with a minimum daily workload of 6 h; one speech therapist available for the unit.

Conventional Neonatal Intermediate Care Units are hospital units aimed for caring for newborns considered to be of medium risk and requiring continuous assistance, but of less complexity than at NICU.

Conventional Neonatal Intermediate Care Units are responsible for the care of newborns in the following conditions: newborns who, after discharge from the NICU, still need ancillary care; newborns

with mild respiratory distress that do not require mechanical ventilation assistance, CPAP, or Hood with high Oxygen Fraction (FiO2) (FiO_2 > 30%); newborns weighing more than 1000 g and less than 1500 g, when stable, without central venous access, in full enteral nutrition, for clinical monitoring and weight gain; newborns weighing more than 1500 g, requiring peripheral venous access for venous hydration, tube feeding, and/or antibiotics use with a stable infectious condition; newborns on phototherapy with bilirubin levels close to blood transfusion levels; newborns who underwent a blood transfusion procedure, after minimum observation time in NICU, with descending bilirubin levels and hemodynamic balance; newborns undergoing stable medium-sized surgery after the immediate postoperative period in the NICU.

Kangaroo Neonatal Intermediate Care Units are hospital units whose physical and material infrastructure allows mother and child to practice the kangaroo method (Kangaroo Mother Care), to rest and stay in the same environment for 24 h a day, up to hospital discharge. Newborns eligible for being hospitalized in these units are the ones weighing more than 1250 g, clinically stable, in full enteral nutrition, whose mothers express the desire to participate in the kangaroo method and have time available. The Kangaroo Neonatal Intermediate Care Unit provides mothers with support by an appropriately trained healthcare team, which allows the provision of care and guidance to the mother about both her and her newborn's health.

Private hospital institutions also organize neonatal units according to the complexity level of care. However, they are not obligated to follow the same nomenclature as described above, nor to have the Kangaroo Intermediate Care Units.

The Brazilian Ministry of Health's recommendations for interventions such as the "Breastfeeding within the first hour after birth" and "The Golden Minute after a child is born" are highlighted to improve the quality of neonatal care. In cases of births that take place in hospitals where there are no intermediate or intensive care units, but if the newborns need them, the newborn is transferred with appropriate equipment and qualified professionals to hospitals that have beds available in these units. The nursing team in

Brazil is organized into four categories: registered nurse, nursing technician, nursing assistant, and midwives. According to the rules of the Brazilian Ministry of Health and the Brazilian Professional Nursing Practice law established by the Federal Nursing Council, only licensed practical nurses and nurses can provide nursing care in Neonatal Intensive Care Units.

Registered Nurses are exclusively responsible for nursing management and direct care activities for critically ill patients with greater technical complexity, which require care based on adequate scientific knowledge and the ability to make immediate decisions.

The licensed practical nurse performs a mid-level activity, involving guidance and monitoring of nursing care at an assistant level. They participate in the planning of nursing care, with the responsibility of, among other tasks, carrying out nursing care activities under the supervision of the Registered Nurse, except those activities listed by law as exclusive to the Registered Nurse.

Registered Nurses who have a bachelor's degree in nursing can provide care in neonatal units, carrying out the planning and assistance to the newborn and their family. The recommendation of the Brazilian Federal Nursing Council is that only registered nurses, and not a licensed practical nurse, provide care to newborns that need highly complex care in the NICU. In Brazil however, this recommendation is not being met, except in some private institutions that have quality certifications, such as the one granted by the Joint Commission International. With regard to the work of specialist nurses in Neonatal Units, the Professional Exercise Law does not make it mandatory; it only recommends that critically ill patients should be treated by specialist nurses in neonatology. Brazil faces a shortage of both intensive care units and neonatology nurse specialists working in existing units around the country.

3.4 Role of Professional Associations

Most of the actions developed aimed at improving the neonatal technical-scientific and clinical practices based on scientific evidence were led by the Brazilian Society of Pediatrics. This is a medical society that offers improvement and qualification training, elaborates on and disseminates protocols and guidelines for neonatal care, such as the guidelines for resuscitation of full-term and preterm newborns in the delivery room. With regard to nursing associations, in Brazil there are two associations that bring together nurses in the neonatal area: the Brazilian Society of Pediatric Nurses (SOBEP in Portuguese) and the Association of Midwives and Obstetric Nurses (ABENFO in Portuguese). Both nursing associations promote courses, hold conferences, and disseminate recommendations related to maternal, child, and neonatal health and care.

The main difference between these associations regarding the neonatal area is the fact that the Association of Midwives and Obstetric Nurses links neonatal health to maternal health, with a focus on pregnancy and assistance to healthy newborns during childbirth and in rooming-in.

The Brazilian Society of Pediatric Nurses focuses on issues that go beyond the healthy newborn at the time of birth, delivery, and rooming-in, also including preterm newborns with congenital and/or acquired diseases in intermediate and intensive care units. The Brazilian Society of Pediatric Nurses holds the certification process to confer the title of Neonatologist Nurse, recognized by the Brazilian Federal Council of Nursing. The certification takes place every 2 years and includes the fulfillment of minimum criteria by the candidate nurses such as clinical experience in neonatal area of at least 5 years, analysis and completion of the curriculum, and a writing test.

3.5 Education and Training

In Brazil, the entire curriculum and course subjects are determined by the Brazilian Ministry of Education. There is an organization chart with the disciplines for each year during the undergraduate nursing course. The instruction in neonatology nursing during the undergraduate course varies in workload and content in the different curricula. In some universities, neonatology is seen as an autonomous discipline. In most curricula, it is inserted in the discipline of obstetric nursing or women's health. In others, it is offered within the pediatric nursing or public health disciplines.

The content related to neonatal health generally encompass policies and programs for newborn care in primary health care, their adaptation to extrauterine life, immediate care for newborns in the delivery room, characteristics and classification of newborns, physical examination and care for newborns at term, preterm, and post-term. Moreover, the neonatology discipline or specialization includes the kangaroo method, the assistance to the newborn in rooming-in, breastfeeding, the neonatal screening, neonatal emergencies, and the assistance to the newborn with metabolic and respiratory disorders.

After graduation, with the title of Bachelor of Nursing, nurses may or may not become specialists in a certain area. Therefore, they need to take specialization/graduate courses or residency programs offered by public or private institutions, previously approved by the Brazilian Ministry of Education. Although recommended, the specialization in neonatology is not mandatory training for nurses to work in neonatal care within hospitals or primary healthcare institutions.

For the specialization/graduate courses in Neonatal Nursing in Brazil, the minimum workload must be 360 h, distributed between theory and practice, at the discretion of higher education institutions. With regard to the practical part of the course, not all institutions include the provision of direct care to newborns admitted to neonatal units by nurses who have taken the specialization course. In some institutions, the practical part includes only the observation of care provided by the healthcare teams of the neonatal units, which weakens the training of neonatology nurse specialists. Nurses pay a monthly fee to take the graduate courses.

Residency courses last for 24 months and have a minimum workload of 5760 h, distributed in 80% of practical hours and 20% of theory. During the practical experience, the resident nurse joins the team of neonatal units, providing direct care to newborns hospitalized in low-, medium-, and high-risk units and in primary health care units. Residents receive financial assistance from the Brazilian Ministry of Education during the residency program in public institutions.

The institutions value and expect that the neonatology nurse specialist has training courses in neonatal resuscitation, transport of the newborn, insertion/maintenance of peripherally inserted central catheter (PICC), and breastfeeding. Nurses who wish to perform teaching and research activities take a master's (training in up to 2 years) and/or doctorate (training in up to 4 years) degree in public or private institutions of higher education. Nurses with only a master's degree (MSc) and/or doctorate degree (PhD) are not considered specialists in neonatology and are unable to work in clinical practice. Not all health institutions differ in salary in terms of nurses who work in direct care for newborns and who have a master's and/or doctoral degree.

3.6   Evidence-Based Practice

The conceptual foundations, decrees, and operational guidelines of programs and public policies enhanced the possibility of revising concepts and values in the way of caring for newborns. Moreover, they brought new perspectives for planning and programming the neonatal care in different areas of the Brazilian territory. Consequently, the offer of neonatal care expanded, accompanied by a necessary readjustment of models of care and reversal of care practices that are out of line with guidelines for humanized care for the newborn.

The growing articulation among university hospitals with the Brazilian Neonatal Research Network for joint actions in the qualification and humanization of neonatal care has been strengthening the adoption of recommended care practices. In recent years, the consolidation of "evidence-based neonatology," which is globally recognized and legitimized, has marked the formation of new generations of professionals who work in the care of the newborn.

Aspects valued in the context of health policies, such as the Kangaroo Method, since its formulation and implementation in Brazil, have been demonstrating its impact on immediate and medium-term neonatal results (psycho-affective, cognitive and neuromotor development). Therefore, neonatology services committed to good practices and clinical excellence have been incorporating physical changes and processes, all compatible with offering the best care to the newborn and family (de Amorim Almeida et al. 2016; Veronez et al. 2017).

Case Studies/Reflective Practice

Case Study 1: Clinical Care Example

Couto Family is composed of the couple Juca (22 years old) and Mariza (18 years old). They have been living in the south-eastern region of Brazil for 2 months. They are originally from the north of the country. Mariza had seven prenatal consultations at a primary healthcare unit before moving to the south-eastern region. According to data on the pregnant woman's card and Mariza's report, the pregnancy was uneventful.

The consultation within the first week of the newborn's life after hospital discharge, as recommended by the Brazilian Ministry of Health, did not happen. The couple took the newborn at 10 days of life to the first nursing consultation in the primary healthcare unit.

The nurse welcomed the family into the office and started the interview using the genogram and ecomap to understand the family system. After this initial approach, the nurse performed an evaluation of the pregnant woman's card and the child's health booklet, to collect data on the pregnancy and birth.

Delivery and birth data: full-term, female newborn, 38 weeks of gestational age, suitable for gestational age, Apgar 9 and 10, weight 3200 g, received immediate care and was placed to perform the first

feeding in the delivery room. The child's father participated in the delivery and cut the umbilical cord. While in the hospital, the newborn screening tests, vaccination against tuberculosis, and hepatitis B virus were performed.

On physical examination: the newborn is tearful when manipulated, the fontanelle slightly depressed, the suction reflex, search, Moro, prehension and Babinski are present, bilateral chest expansion, globose abdomen, with the presence of mummified umbilical stump in the process of falling. A Mongolian spot was noted in the dorsal region, hyperemic perineum, bladder, and intestinal elimination present.

Vital signs: weight 3100 g, HR 130 bpm, RR 45 rpm.

Data collected from the mother: Mariza reports feeling pain in the right nipple during breastfeeding; Mariza reports that her baby daughter is taking a 40-min break between feedings, even at dawn, which is making her feel very tired, as she has woken up several times. Faced with this tiredness, Mariza questions the introduction of artificial milk. During the interview, Mariza reports being afraid the newborn will choke, because a brother of hers died when he was a baby while sleeping. Due to this fear, the baby has been sleeping in the couple's bed.

Case Study 2: Vignette from Parent at NICU

[…] I went to see my baby, I was all happy, hoping to see him better. But when I lifted the cloth that covered the incubator, I swear: the shock was huge, looking at my little baby and seeing him with all those devices, all those tubes […] I left the NICU, aimless and unable to believe what was happening. A nurse came to me and explained […] (Mother at NICU).

Tuesday […] he was quiet, peaceful, the nurses were trying to find a vein in him for tests […] from that moment on, I started observing everything around me, I saw how well he was being treated by the entire team [...] I was more confident knowing he was in good hands. (Mother at NICU).

Case Study 3: Vignette from Neonatal Nurse at NICU

Suddenly, you end up doing things, sometimes fearfully heroic things, and perhaps all of that wasn't needed (...) Will these actions cause any trouble up ahead? To what extent should I do it? Just to allow this infant to become what" then? Does the family have conditions to be able to take care of his/her baby with special needs? (...) If you think of quality of life as one would imagine of a child ... playing in the street, being happy, doing everything, being healthy and happy... without having to leave the baby will be dependent all their lives... because that's what will happen!.

3.7   Conclusion

This chapter describes neonatal care, how it is organized, the role of professional associations in supporting nursing care, and the education and training needed for neonatal nurses. Brazil is a very large country with regional differences, but the commonalities have been presented.

References

Boccolini CS, de Moraes Mello Boccolini P, Monteiro FR, Venâncio SI, Giugliani ERJ (2017) Breastfeeding indicators trends in Brazil for three decades. Rev Saude Publica 51:108. https://doi.org/10.11606/S1518-8787.2017051000029

da Silva Cavalcanti PC, Gurgel Junior GD, de Vaconcelos ALR, Guerrero AVP (2013) A logical model of the Rede Cegonha network. Physis Rev Saúde Coletiva 23(4):1297–1316. https://doi.org/10.1590/S0103-73312013000400014

de Amorim Almeida F, de Moraes MS, da Rocha Cunha ML (2016) Taking care of the newborn dying and their families: nurses' experiences of neonatal intensive care. Rev da Esc Enferm da USP 50:22–129. https://doi.org/10.1590/S0080-623420160000300018

Lamounier JA, Chaves RG, Rego MAS, Bouzada MCF (2019) Baby friendly hospital initiative: 25 years of experience in Brazil. Rev Paul Pediatr 37(4):486–493. https://doi.org/10.1590/1984-0462/;2019;37;4;00004

Lansky S, de Lima Friche AA, Silva AAM et al (2014) Birth in Brazil survey: neonatal mortality, pregnancy and childbirth quality of care. Cad Saude Publica 30(Suppl 1):S192–S207. https://doi.org/10.1590/0102-311X00133213

UNICEF, WHO, The World Bank Group, UN Population Division (2017) Levels and trends in child mortality: report 2017. United Nations Inter-gr Child Mortal Estim. Published online

Veronez M, Borghesan NAB, Corrêa DAM, Higarashi IH (2017) Experience of mothers of premature babies from birth to discharge: notes of field journals. Rev Gaúcha Enferm 38(2). https://doi.org/10.1590/1983-1447.2017.02.60911

Australia

4

Karen Walker, Jennifer Dawson, Kylie Pussell, and Karen New

4.1 Introduction

This chapter begins by providing demographics, contemporary statistical data on the population and context of the healthcare system in Australia. This provides a framework to understand the evolution and integration of nursing and the specialty of neonatal nursing and neonatology within the Australian healthcare system, including the more recent development of the specialist roles within neonatal nursing. One of the most gratifying changes in neonatal care has been the involvement of parents, and this revolutionary process will be discussed from the Australian perspective.

K. Walker (✉)
University of Sydney, Sydney, Australia

Royal Prince Alfred Hospital, Sydney, Australia

Council of International Neonatal Nurses, Inc. (COINN), Yardley, PA, USA
e-mail: boardpresident@coinnurses.org; karen.walker@health.nsw.gov.au

J. Dawson
The Royal Women's Hospital, Melbourne, VIC, Australia

K. Pussell
CEO Miracle Babies Foundation, Sydney, NSW, Australia

K. New
School of Health and Behavioural Science, University of the Sunshine Coast, Sippy Downs, QLD, Australia

Key "Think Points" for Learning

- Neonatal nursing is a recognized specialty in Australia.
- The role of Australian neonatal nurses continues to evolve.
- The Australian College of Neonatal Nurses sets the standards for neonatal nurses.
- Neonatal care is available free of charge in public hospitals in Australia.
- Parents are integral as partners in care.

4.2 Australian Population Data

Australia is a very large country, with a land mass of 7.6 million km², with a population of approximately 25.6 million as of 2020, making up just 0.3% of the total world population (https://www.abs.gov.au/ accessed January 2021). The Commonwealth of Australia is made up of six states, New South Wales, Queensland, South Australia, Tasmania, Victoria and Western Australia, and two territories, Australian Capital Territory and the Northern Territory. There is a Commonwealth (National) Prime Minister and Health Minister; however, each state and territory are independently governed by a Premier/Chief Minister and Health Minister, and as a result,

J. Petty et al. (eds.), *Neonatal Nursing: A Global Perspective*,
https://doi.org/10.1007/978-3-030-91339-7_4

there are components of health care managed at the Commonwealth and State/Territory levels.

Australia has one of the world's oldest cultures, with the Indigenous Aboriginal and Torres Strait Islander peoples representing approximately 6.9% of the population. Australia is also a strong multicultural society, with approximately one in every four Australians born overseas and more than one fifth speaking a language other than English at home. The most common countries for those born overseas are the United Kingdom, New Zealand, China, and India, and the most common languages spoken other than English are Mandarin, Arabic, Cantonese, and Vietnamese (https://www.abs.gov.au/ accessed January 2021).

Australia is considered a high-income country with a current average life expectancy of approximately 83.9 years; however, as in many countries, there are inequalities. The life expectancy of Indigenous Aboriginal and Torres Strait Islander peoples is approximately 10 years less, with clear differences also in infant and child mortality. The latest data from the Closing the Gap Report 2020 shows that the Indigenous infant mortality rate was 1.8 times higher than for non-indigenous infants (5.1 compared with 2.9 per 1000 live births) (https://www.niaa.gov.au/sites/default/files/publications/closing-the-gap-report-2020.pdf). From a population growth perspective, over 300,000 babies were born in 2018, an increase of 1.9% from the previous year, with slightly more males born compared with females (51.4% versus 48.6%) (https://www.abs.gov.au/ accessed January 2021). Approximately 1 in 5 newborns (31,838) were admitted to a neonatal unit, and while there has been some closing of the gap in health disparities, for indigenous newborns, this was 1 in 4 newborns (https://www.aihw.gov.au/reports/mothers-babies).

4.3 Australian Neonatal Healthcare System

The Australian healthcare system is regarded as one of the best in the world and is based on a dual public–private system. The public system is funded under a Universal Health Insurance Scheme, called Medicare, providing Australians with free access to in-patient hospital and community health care, this includes pregnancy and neonatal care. Most public hospitals offer a degree of neonatal care; however, all public intensive care neonatal units are in large metropolitan public hospitals. The private system offers healthcare changes under private health insurance schemes for in-patient and outpatient care. Private hospitals are owned and operated by independent organizations/companies and many of the private hospitals provide neonatal care but only a small number provide intensive care. Many families opt for pregnancy care under the private system, but should their newborn require neonatal intensive care, families can transfer to the public system and receive all care at no change. Each State and Territory have a framework or service plan for all aspects of neonatal care which includes levels of care that each public and private hospital can provide. While there has been an effort to standardize the levels across the nation, this has not been fully achieved. The older system, which is still in use in some areas is from 1 (low level of care) to 3 (high level of care); which are very broad and do not adequately reflect differences in services offered within the same level. The newer system introduced additional levels to better distinguish the level of services offered at each hospital; Level 1 providing care to healthy term infants, to level 6, in which the highest level of care is provided (intensive care with specialist neonatal services). The hospital location (remote, rural, regional, metropolitan) and the number of people the hospital services are general indications of the level of care offered. That is, the more remote and rural the lower level of care increases to the highest level of care offered within the largest cities in each State and Territory. Thus within Australia, there is also a vast number of names used to describe neonatal units: well-baby nursery (WBN), special care baby unit (SCBU), special care unit (SCU), special care nursery (SCN), high dependency unit (HDU), and then, neonatal intensive care unit (NICU) is reserved for those units who provide intensive care services (ventilation, surgery, care of extreme preterm neonates). The larger hospitals have a combination of units, with neonates graduating from the highest to lowest levels of care in preparation of being discharged home and/or to a neonatal unit closer to home. Additionally, Australia has *National Safety and Quality Health Service Standards*, which provide a nationally consistent statement about the quality of care consumers can expect from health services (https://www.safetyandquality.gov.au/standards/nsqhs-standards).

Due to the vastness of Australia, and the centralized location of higher level of care units, many neonates cannot be cared for in a neonatal unit close to home and will have to be "retrieved" to receive care in a NICU. Dedicated retrieval services are available in all states and most territories and are managed with teams of medical and nursing staff with specialist training in stabilization and transportation of sick infants. Neonatal nurse practitioners and advanced practice neonatal nurses have been vital to the success of neonatal retrieval in Australia. Additionally, much research has been undertaken into looking at outcomes for those vulnerable neonates born outside a hospital with a NICU and retrieved, to those that have been inborn at a hospital with a NICU and specialist neonatal trained doctors and nurses. Inborn neonates have much better outcomes, and therefore, in Australia, an aim is that all women with an identified high-risk pregnancy are transferred to a facility appropriate for the birth.

4.4 Evolution of Neonatology and Neonatal Nursing

In Australia, neonatology is one of the "youngest" sub-specialties in pediatrics with the term neonatologist first used in 1960. Over the past 50 years, there has been incredible advances, including the use of surfactant and noninvasive ventilation techniques which has seen the survival rate of premature neonates less than 28 weeks increasing into the 90% range (Manley et al. 2015). Pre and up to the early 1990s, to work with neonates in neonatal units, a mid-

wifery qualification was required. As nursing and midwifery workforce shortages continued, this changed and registered nurses (without a midwifery qualification) were employed into neonatal units, undertaking "transition to neonatal nursing programs" and university-based specialist courses in neonatal care. Neonatal nursing is now a recognized specialty and is continuing to evolve with increasing specialization and development of advanced practice roles.

4.5 Education and Training

In Australia, as in many high-income countries, the minimum qualification for registration as a nurse is an undergraduate bachelor's degree. In the undergraduate role, there is little focus on neonates although some undergraduates may have the opportunity to rotate through a neonatal unit. Following completion of the undergraduate degree, this can then lead to the opportunity to specialize and undertake further studies with specialty postgraduate qualifications, graduate certificates, diplomas, master's, and PhD.

The career pathway for neonatal nurses is diverse, with specialist roles in clinical care, education, management and research. Clinical roles include registered nurses and clinical nurses (CNs)/clinical nurse specialists (CNSs). CNs/CNSs are experienced, senior, and are allocated leadership roles such as shift in charge and coordination. Respiratory therapists within neonatal units in Australia are uncommon. Instead, following consultation with a neonatal nurse practitioner or medical officer, it is the registered and/or CN/CNS that makes the required changes to ventilator settings and who are responsible for assisting with intubation/extubation, suctioning, and re-strapping endotracheal tubes.

Depending on the level of care provided by a neonatal unit, additional roles that do not involve a patient load include clinical facilitators (support new staff clinically), clinical nurse consultants (overall clinical management including aspects such as policy and procedure development), nurse unit managers (management of overall neonatal nursing workforce), and neonatal educators (support education requirements of all staff). These are advanced practice roles that involve expertise in all or most of the following five domains: clinical practice, education, research, clinical leadership, and clinical service planning and management. These strategic leadership roles are integral for advancement of clinical care and service delivery.

The newest advanced practice role in Australian neonatal units is that of the neonatal nurse practitioner, an experienced clinical nurse with advanced knowledge, skills, and qualifications. Nurse practitioner pilot projects began in Australia in the mid-1990s with the first two nurse practitioners authorized to practice in 2000. Several years later the first neonatal nurse practitioners were employed in a regional hospital in New South Wales before expanding to other regional areas that found it difficult to attract medical trainees and junior doctors (Forbes-Coe et al. 2020). To become a neonatal nurse practitioner, nurses must meet the minimum criteria of registration as a nurse in Australia, hold a graduate certificate in a specialty and have 3–5 years post registration experience to be able to enroll in a generic nurse practitioner master's course as a nurse practitioner candidate. At present there are 14 universities which offer the postgraduate master's course leading to nurse practitioner qualification with endorsement in a specialty area. In addition to successfully completing a master's degree in nursing/science, candidates must complete 500 h of supervised clinical practice to receive the qualification (Forbes-Coe et al. 2020).

Research and Academia are evolving as emerging roles for neonatal nurses, with some dedicated nurse research positions in neonatal units. Whilst initially nurses were employed as research nurses to work in clinical trials and coordinate research, increasingly they lead research.

There are various neonatal-specific courses available. A number of Australian universities offer postgraduate courses in neonatal nursing. The Australian College of Neonatal Nurses keeps an up-to-date list on their website https://www. acnn.org.au/neo-nursing/.

4.6   Professional Organizations

All nurses in Australia must be registered with The Australian Health Practitioner Regulation Agency (AHPRA) which is the organization responsible for implementing the National Registration and Accreditation Scheme across Australia. Registration must be renewed annually. The Nursing and Midwifery board of Australia (NMBA) works in partnership with AHPRA and is responsible for registration and registration requirements for nurses and midwives, educational standards and codes of practice, disciplinary matters, and, among others, the assessment of internationally qualified nurses (https://www.ahpra.gov.au/, https://www.nursingmidwiferyboard.gov.au/).

There are two primary professional organizations in Australia, one for nurses, the Australian College of Nursing (ACN), and the other for midwives, the Australian College of Midwives (ACM). In addition, there are many sub-specialty nursing and midwifery professional organizations, including the Congress of Aboriginal and Torres Strait Islander Nurses and Midwives (CATSINaM) and the Australian College of Neonatal Nurses (ACNN). However, it is not mandatory to belong to any organization.

ACNN is the professional body for neonatal nurses in Australia, with membership open to all registered nurses, midwives, and nurse practitioners who work with neonates and families; is a founding member of the Council of International Neonatal Nurses (COINN); and provides the voice of Australian neonatal nurses on the international forum. ACNN develops Standards for Practice for neonatal nurses (https://www.acnn. org.au/resources/acnn-standards/), to be used as a framework within the context of the Australian healthcare system to ensure nurses and midwives caring for neonates and their families provide safe, high-quality clinical care.

In 1995, the Australian and New Zealand Neonatal Network (ANZNN) was established as a collaborative network to collect a core data set on neonatal demographics and care, for the purpose of benchmarking to improve outcomes for neonates and their families. All Australian and

New Zealand neonatal units who provide intensive care contribute data and an increasing number of units providing high level, non NICU care now contribute data as part of the network. Reports are published annually, covering outcomes by year and 2- to 3-year follow-up outcomes. These reports are available at www.anznn.net and (Chow et al. 2019).

4.7 Parent Support Organizations

Like many countries, Australia has very well-established parent organizations, who operate nationally and/or locally, who provide many services to parents who experience having a newborn in a neonatal unit. These parent organizations raise awareness around many issues including preterm birth outcomes and needs. Additionally, they are strong advocates in the promotion of the importance of the role of parents, the concept of Family Integrated Care into Neonatal Units and recognition of the true value of parental involvement. Parent support organizations and "graduate" parents are increasingly involved as consumers in guiding development of research and quality improvement activities directed at improving care and experiences for neonates and their families.

The parent organizations are able to provide emotional support to parents who are in the midst of the hospital rollercoaster of a neonatal unit experience, as members have experienced this journey. Experienced "graduate" parents offer valuable insight and are able to give hope toward discharge and a future in which the baby is at home with the family.

4.8 Australian Nurses' Contribution

Australian neonatal nurses have been at the forefront of neonatal research and evidence-based clinical care, and this is evident by the many publications and impact on the international stage on a number of important topics. The recent textbook by Kain et al. included novice writers mentored by senior academic nurses writing in partnership and culminating in the first Australian and New Zealand neonatal textbook (Kain and Mannix 2018). From a research perspective, there are too many neonatal nurse researchers and studies to mention, but just one example is the contribution to the topic "*Babies feel pain.*" This statement might seem self-evident, but this has not always been the case. Research has provided evidence that all babies, irrespective of their age, feel pain even from short procedures such as a heel lance. Exposure to multiple painful procedures has been shown to have lasting effects and neonatal nurses have been at the forefront in testing strategies that reduce neonatal pain (Harrison et al. 2015). It is important for neonatal nurses to translate this high-quality evidence into practice. Strategies that have been shown to be effective in reducing neonatal pain include breastfeeding, skin-to-skin care, sometimes called kangaroo care, and small amounts of sweet solutions, either sucrose or glucose (Harrison et al. 2015).

4.9 2020 in Australia

The pandemic, as in the rest of the world, has impacted Australia, and while to a much lesser degree, this has still had an impact in the neonatal context. A major impact has been around hard lockdowns and border closures resulting in the restriction of family and extended family involvement in the care of their newborn. Restricted visiting was limited to parents, and in some instances, only one parent could visit at a time. Siblings and extended family members were unable to visit. Disruption to the family-centered care approach has been distressing for families, nurses, and doctors alike. Fortunately, positive COVID-19 cases in infants and children have been uncommon and only resulted in mild symptoms.

There have been many papers published about the impact of COVID-19 in the last year. Three recent papers from collaborations between neonatal nurses in Australia and the United Kingdom highlight the importance of keeping mothers and babies together unless there are clinical reasons for separating them. Continuing to promote breastfeeding to enhance the immune response and consideration of the developmental impact of facemasks for babies and young children are important aspects (Green et al. 2020a, b). How the pandemic ends and the long-term effects remain to be realized.

Case Studies/Reflective Practice
Case Study 1

Baby Anne, born at 26 weeks' gestation, weighing 660 g, was due for her first eye screen to check for signs of retinopathy of prematurity (ROP) as she was now 30 weeks postmenstrual age. Her parents Bob and Janet had been told that ROP is an eye disease that can affect babies born prematurely and the screening test, which takes about 10 min, was important as early detection allowed for early management and treatment. Anne would continue to have examinations every 1–2 weeks until she reached the equivalent of full term. The procedure was explained to Bob and Janet, being told that the examination is conducted by a team of two specially credentialed nurses. One nurse examines and takes pictures of the retinas while the second nurse assists and monitors the baby's condition during the examination. In preparation for the examination, Anne would be swaddled to provide comfort and containment and eye drops that dilate the pupils administered. She would also be given sucrose for pain management, before a tiny speculum is placed to hold the eyelids open, a scleral depressor used to allow the entire retina to be checked. An indirect ophthalmoscope, with a bright light, allows the nurse to see the back of the eye to take clear pictures of the retinas, which are sent electronically to be reviewed by a pediatric ophthalmologist.

Reflect on the diverse roles of neonatal nurses.

There are many clinical roles for neonatal nurses, reflecting on this case study, do neonatal nurses undertake eye examinations where you work? Are there other roles that they undertake in your work unit similar to this case study?

Case Study 2

Neonatal nurse Joanne was caring for baby George born at 25 weeks' gestation and weighing 600 g, receiving respiratory support via *nasal prongs with continuous positive airway pressure (CPAP) and 30% oxygen. George was very stable, and Rachel was keen to hold her baby for the first time but anxious that the experience might harm George. Joanne spent time talking with Rachel about how together they would carefully remove George from his incubator to place him on her chest. Joanne discussed the benefits to George and Rachel from skin-to-skin cuddles. Rachel was having trouble establishing lactation and was encouraged to hear that skin-to-skin cuddles will likely help her to produce more breastmilk. Together Joanne and Rachel worked together to prepare George and the equipment before transferring him to nestle on her chest between her breasts. Rachel told Joanne it took her a little while to relax and enjoy the experience however she also said that it was the first time she felt like a real mother. Joanne took photographs of Rachel and George for Rachel to have whilst expressing at home to help with lactation.*

Think point: Reflect on the importance of skin to skin contact for both mother and baby.

Case Study 1: A Parent's Journey

Growing up I always thought you just started your family and children when you were ready! Little did I know that at 22, newly married, the struggles and heartache we would endure to have our family. After an early devastating miscarriage, a diagnosis of Poly Cystic Ovarian Syndrome (PCOS) and an emotional journey with IVF, we were delighted to find out that we were having twins. However, at 16 weeks my membranes ruptured and yet again I "miscarried". Whilst it is called a miscarriage at 16 weeks, it is very different. I was having contractions, laboured and delivered a baby boy and baby girl, named David and Angel. Those days were dark and just to cut a little deeper my milk came in. It took a while for us to find the courage to try again.

I did fall pregnant and a scan at 6 weeks confirmed we had one healthy baby growing well. So, we were here again, all the fears and nerves were there again too! Would we be able to keep this baby? We had so many unanswered questions and we kept the pregnancy to ourselves and immediate family as mostly I didn't want to see the pity in my friend's eyes. At 22 weeks I required a cervical suture, was admitted to hospital for bedrest for 7 weeks and had been given the statistics on premature babies and visited the NICU so I felt a little prepared for what lay ahead. At almost 30 weeks gestation I went home, however 3 days later I woke up to ruptured membranes and while I was scared, I was also so excited. I was able to deliver naturally, a beautiful baby girl weighing 1585 g, who went to the NICU and was on CPAP. She was tiny and I was very scared to touch her at first as she had many lines and tubes, but I mainly remember how beautiful and perfect she was and after 6 weeks she came home with us.

This gave us confidence to try again and in preparation for this I had surgery to assist with cervical incompetence, but sadly miscarried at 5 weeks. Then we had wonderful news that I was pregnant with twins. My membranes ruptured at 25 weeks and I delivered my son weighing 785 g and my daughter weighing 640 g. Both babies were critical, and we were only able to touch their fingers though the humidicrib port hole. My son, Marcus, suffered major complications from his extreme prematurity and he was baptized before passing away 2 days after his birth.

A few weeks later Scarlet developed and recovered from Necrotizing Enterocolitis, and later at 32 weeks required surgical treatment for Retinopathy of Prematurity. While the surgery went well, she did not wake up from the anesthetic and was not showing any signs of movement. Remaining ventilated for the next 5 days, she was diagnosed with Central Anticholinergic Syndrome, and by stopping the eye drops, like a miracle within hours she started to wake up and by the end of the day she was breathing on her own. Bringing Scarlet home was an emotional day. The staff at the hospital had become like family, they had comforted me when I cried, held my hand when I was scared and shared in Scarlet's milestones.

Whilst it took a few more years we fell pregnant again and through a closely monitored but trouble-free pregnancy I carried my son to term. This was such an amazing experience. To actually be awake during his birth and to hold him once he was born was so precious. Through so many pregnancies this was the first time I had held a baby straight away. Through tears of happiness and maybe some of sadness for what we missed out on before, we just stared at his gorgeous big face. Weighing, for us, a massive 3.5 kg Liam was with me in my room and we went home as planned all together as a family. My children join the thousands of Australian newborns that are born early or unwell. An astounding 48,000 babies are born each year requiring specialized care. It is more than the amount of people diagnosed with breast cancer and prostate cancer combined. It is an issue that Miracle Babies Foundation brings awareness to. Kylie Pussell.

Think point: Reflect on how, as a nurse, you would support this family during each of their admissions to the neonatal unit.

4.10 Conclusion

Australian neonatal nursing is continuing to evolve with roles becoming more diverse, which makes this an exciting time to be a neonatal nurse. Neonatal nurses are integral to fostering family-centered care, engaging and providing support and education to parents and families. Neonatal nurses are not only recognized that they skillfully care for the smallest and sickest babies but that they are strategic leaders, integral to directing future research to improve the quality of care for neonates and their families, and decision-making at the highest level of health systems.

References

Australian Bureau of Statistics (2021) https://www.abs.gov.au

Australian College of Neonatal Nurses (2021) https://www.acnn.org.au/neo-nursing/

Australian Health Practitioners Registration Authority (2021) https://www.ahpra.gov.au/

Australian Institute of Health and Welfare (2021) https://www.aihw.gov.au/reports/mothers-babies

Chow SSW, Creighton P, Chambers GM, Lui K (2019) Report of the Australian and New Zealand neonatal network 2017. ANZNN, Sydney. www.anznn.net

Closing the Gap Report (2021) https://www.niaa.gov.au/sites/default/files/publications/closing-the-gap-report-2020.pdf

Forbes-Coe A, Dawson J, Flint A, Walker K (2020) The evolution of the neonatal nurse practitioner role in Australia: a discussion paper. J Neonatal Nurs 26(4):197–200

Green J, Petty J, Staff L, Bromley P, Jones L (2020a) The implications of face masks for babies and families during the COVID-19 pandemic: a discussion paper. J Neonatal Nurs 26(4):197–200

Green J, Petty J, Bromley P, Walker K, Jones L (2020b) COVID 19 in babies: knowledge for neonatal care. J Neonatal Nurs 26(5):239–246

Harrison D, Bueno M, Reszel J (2015) Prevention and management of pain and stress in the neonate. Res Rep Neonatol 7(5):9–16

Kain V, Mannix T (eds) (2018) Neonatal nursing in Australia and New Zealand: principles for practice. Elsevier, Chatswood

Manley BJ, Doyle LW, Davies MW, Davis PG (2015) Fifty years in neonatology. J Paediatr Child Health 51(1):118–121

Nursing and Midwifery Board (2021) https://www.nursingmidwiferyboard.gov.au/

Safety and Quality Standards (2021) https://www.safetyandquality.gov.au/standards/nsqhs-standards

New Zealand

5

Debbie O'Donoghue, Petra Harnett, and Joanne Clements

5.1 Introduction

Neonatal care from a New Zealand perspective represents a vital part of maternal child health. New Zealand honors the roots of the Indigenous people of Aotearoa—the Māori while upholding the rights of the Pakeha (non-Māori). One must understand the cultural context of care before examining the specialization of neonatal nursing.

Key "Think Points" for Learning

- Biculturalism is an important aspect of care.
- Cultural safety reflects the belief that self is a culture bearer.
- Neonatal care consists of different levels of care that outline personnel needs.
- Neonatal nursing education has standards for basic and advanced education.
- The Nursing Council of New Zealand sets the standards for practice and education.
- Professional neonatal nursing organizations help shape the standards for the practice and education.

D. O'Donoghue (✉)
Christchurch NICU, Canterbury District Health Board, Canterbury & West Coast, Christchurch, New Zealand

Council of International Neonatal Nurses, Inc. (COINN), Christchurch, New Zealand
e-mail: Debbie.ODonoghue@cdhb.health.nz

P. Harnett
Christchurch NICU, Canterbury District Health Board, Christchurch, New Zealand

J. Clements
Kidz First Children's Hospital, Middlemore Hospital, Counties Manukau District Health Board, Auckland, New Zealand

5.2 Cultural Awareness and Cultural Safety Within Nursing and Neonatal Nursing in New Zealand: Debbie O'Donoghue

Biculturalism is an indelible part of the social landscape and national discourse of Aotearoa, New Zealand. Biculturalism is a relationship in

J. Petty et al. (eds.), *Neonatal Nursing: A Global Perspective*,
https://doi.org/10.1007/978-3-030-91339-7_5

which the social and intellectual histories of two (or more) peoples are intertwined over many generations. The New Zealand population like the rest of the world is becoming more multicultural; however, there is an obligation under the Treaty of Waitangi (1840) to ensure the rights of both Māori (Indigenous people of Aotearoa) and Pakeha (non-Māori) are protected (Stewart 2021).

The Aotearoa, New Zealand health system is committed to Te Tiriti o Waitangi with the Treaty of Waitangi being the nation's founding document signed in 1840 by the British Crown and the Indigenous Māori people of New Zealand. This document acknowledges the rights of all peoples to their place in this land. Māori as Tāngata Whenua and others as Iwi kainga (those that have come to make a home for themselves in New Zealand). As a Registered Nurse in New Zealand under the Health Practitioners Competence Assurance Act (2003), the Nursing Council of New Zealand sets and monitors standards and competencies for nursing registration and ongoing practice which ensures safe and competent care for the public of New Zealand. Cultural Safety, the Treaty of Waitangi and Māori health are aspects of nursing practice that are reflected in the Council's standards and competencies for nursing (Nursing Council of New Zealand 2007).

Cultural safety education is broad in its application and extends beyond ethnic groups to include age, gender, sexual orientation, occupation and socioeconomic status, religious or spiritual beliefs, and disability. The content focuses upon the understanding of self as a cultural bearer, the historical, social, and political influences on health and the development of relationships that engender trust and respect. The Treaty of Waitangi provides nurses with the understanding of the Treaty and its principles within the context of Aotearoa, New Zealand and within nursing practice and health, its practical application of the three principles of partnership, participation, and protection as the basis of interactions between nurses and Māori consumers of the services they provide.

- Partnership—working together with iwi and whanau and Māori communities to develop strategies and appropriate services for Māori health gain and appropriate health and disability services.
- Participation–involving Māori at all levels including decision making, planning, development, and delivery of health and disability services.
- Protection—working to ensure Māori have at least the same level of health as non-Maori and safeguarding Māori cultural concepts, values, and practice.

Thirdly Māori health and nursing practice "Kawa Whakaruruhau" focuses upon cultural safety and its contribution to the achievement of positive health outcomes for Māori through nursing education and cultural awareness that enables safe service to be defined by those who receive the service (Nursing Council of New Zealand 2011). The New Zealand Nursing workforce should reflect Aotearoa's population with cultural safety embedded in practice and a Te Ao Māori lens embedded in its health structures, policies, and processes. Health professionals care about people; they work in the healthcare profession because they respect people and they respect life. And, above all, they want people to have the best life possible. Like medical and nursing protocols, Māori protocol has evolved over centuries (Tikanga Māori) and the customs and protocol aim to be caring, non-threatening, and minimal in fuss and complication (New Zealand Nurses Organisation 2005).

Improvements in Māori health are critical, given that Māori, on average, have the poorest health status of any other group in New Zealand and widening disparities and inequalities in health care delivery and services and health outcomes (Ministry of Health 2019b). Within neonatal nursing, research, and statistics demonstrate that having a premature or low birth weight baby increases the risk of mortality, morbidity, sudden infant death (SIDS), child abuse, and neglect compounded by the stress on families due to a long hospital stay of a sick baby. The indigenous people of New Zealand are disproportionally over represented in poverty statistics, child abuse, hospitalization rates, and neonatal mortality and morbidity. Neonatal death rates are higher in Māori compared to the rates in European and other (Ministry of Health 2019b).

Fig. 5.1 Illustration of The Te Whare Tapa Whā. Source: Re-drawn/ Adapted from a model, attributed to Sir Mason Durie (1994)

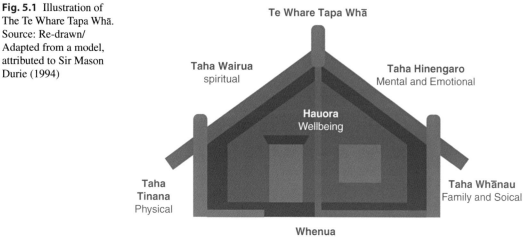

To guide the healthcare system and personnel delivering the care and services, there are a number of frameworks that provide tools and understanding for those people to fulfill their stewardship obligations and care for those individuals and their families (whanau) who identify as Māori. Hauora is the Māori philosophy of health and well-being, and The Te Whare Tapa Wha (The four cornerstones) model of care compares the four walls of the Whare (Māori meeting house) to four different dimensions providing strength and stability (Fig. 5.1). They are;

- Physical.
- Emotional/mental.
- Social.
- Spiritual.

These values and well-being beliefs determine the way people view life and what they identify with and the healthcare system needs to reflect the values of

- Whanaungatanga "everyone belongs".
- Manaakitanga "respect for all".
- Tino Rangatiratanga "empowering whanau/family".
- Aroha "Love and empathy".
- Oranga Tonutanga "health and well-being".
- Mana Taurite "Equity".

An example of these principles, values, and competencies in neonatal nursing practice can be found within the Neonatal Nurses College Aotearoa Neonatal Palliative Care for New Zealand Neonatal Units "Comfort as a Model of Care"—"Whakamarietia rite kit e tauira o te tiaki" guiding resource (2015). The document and resource package include a clear set of principles for staff to assist in providing palliative care in partnership with families/whanau both within neonatal intensive care and special care units within the hospital and at home. It provides guidance for the care of any baby within the neonatal setting for whom a decision has been made to introduce palliative care. The vision for neonatal palliative care in New Zealand is that, when needed, all babies have access to appropriate, high quality, coordinated, and culturally appropriate palliative care that meets their physical, psychological, social and spiritual needs, and their family/whanau are involved in partnership from the time of diagnosis through the course of illness and continue after the death of their baby. In Māori culture, events surrounding times of illness, dying,,death and grieving are among the most sacred and important. They are steeped in Tapu (sanctity), Kawa (protocol) and include Karakia (prayers) and Waiata (chants and oral literature) (Herbert 2001).

The development and use of this care document are to enhance practice and designed to be used as an educational tool that may be used to develop individual approaches in consideration to the resources available, with the parents being the best people to make decisions for their baby. The resource provides information on the principles of neonatal palliative care, the planning of palliative care with families/whanau, the management of care, supports available and caring for the carers possible support and advice. Templates are provided in English for personnel adaption and to assist the parents with decisions and approaches to palliation (Neonatal Nurses College Aotearoa 2015). The document elaborates on wider supports that are available to parents and staff from a range of professionals such as clinical psychologists, counselors, social work, and community organizations such as Sands NZ (2011) who have a "three-point model of care" to support health professionals working with parents into the practicalities of perinatal death.

1. Slow down.
2. Assist in active parenting.
3. Help to create memories.

These resources have been specifically developed for practice in New Zealand and supporting cultural best practice; however, the underpinning principles are relevant globally. Nursing staff are guided to be respectful of each family/whanau's beliefs and rituals, asking the family/whanau about their individual spiritual and religious beliefs including important rituals and procedures and how these can be incorporated into the care within the hospital setting. A parent's spirituality/faith may influence their emotional, psychological and physical response to bereavement, and the staff should be in a place to provide or seek the necessary supports such as interpreters for those families where English is not their first language and for those that identify as Māori the support of the hospital Hauora Māori team which works across the hospital providing awhi/support to turoro/patients and their whānau/family as they journey through the hospital.

The intended scope of this "Comfort as a Model of Care" is primarily for neonatal nurses and aims to complement other resources that are available within New Zealand and within local hospitals. The Paediatric Palliative Care Clinical Network in association with the Paediatric Society of New Zealand and the Ministry of Health (2015) have also completed national guidelines for end of life care as a valuable evidenced-based resource.

5.3 Nursing Education and Training: Petra Harnett

In Aotearoa, New Zealand, to practice as a registered nurse, the student will have to obtain a New Zealand Nursing Council approved Bachelor of Nursing degree. The New Zealand government has made a commitment to improve educational outcomes among their indigenous Maori population. Educational nursing programs are designed to foster inclusive, ethical, and professional relationships that acknowledge Aotearoa, New Zealand's cultural diversity within its population (Calman 2015).

Hauora, Maori's world view, is embraced in Mason Durie's holistic model of health, Te Whare Tapa Wha. The model, designed for the healthcare sector, has now also been integrated in the educational sector. When Maori learners can learn as Maori, their educational success improves.

Applying the Durie's model into an educational setting interprets the first dimension, Te Taha hinengaro (psychological health) as the student's mental and emotional well-being. The students whose Te Taha hinengaro is healthy will be effective learners. They will have the necessary coping strategies and resilience to enjoy the learning process and celebrate their successes. The second pillar is a dimension of the model that symbolizes Te Taha wairua (spiritual well-being). Being an effective learner in this dimension means that the learner is cognizant of who they are and their personal value system, their goals, and career aspirations. An example of applying indigenous epistemologies such as Taha Wairua in nursing programmes includes presenting the study subject with enthusiasm and passion (Open Polytechnic (2020). This inspires and motivates learners to further explore the subject in their own time. The third dimension, Te taha tinana (physical health), represents a learner who is physically fit and healthy. Healthy students in this dimension are attentive and able to access necessary resources to allow them to learn effectively. The last dimension is Te taha whanua (family health). This dimension symbolizes the learner who is part of a strong whanau (family). They are able to be effective learners as a result of enjoying a strong identity and support networks, and they have the ability to work collaboratively with others. Integrating aspects of Taha Whanau can be achieved through careful scheduling of the study days. Professional development study days are scheduled in a way that considers external commitments such as family and non-work-related commitments of the learners. The learning environment reflects a family-like environment and is warm and welcoming to all attending learners. Seating is arranged in a manner that is inclusive and stimulates discussion. The concept of connectedness and family is particularly important from a cultural context when teaching Maori learners to minimize feeling culturally isolated (Māori into Tertiary Education 2011).

At the end of the 3-year degree programme, nursing students complete a "transition to practice" placement which offers a further 360 h of clinical experience in an area of their choice. Nursing students receive minimal nursing education that is relevant to the neonatal setting during their training. The clinical placement offers nursing students an opportunity to consider the specialty as an area for employment once registered.

Until the beginning of the millennium, neonatal units required nurses to have at least 2 years of acute postgraduate experience, preferably in an acute clinical setting. However, at this time, it became evident that the nursing population in the New Zealand healthcare sector was aging so significantly that the profession was on a trajectory toward a dramatic and serious nursing shortage. In response to an impending forecast of significant nursing shortages, tertiary institutions increased the number of nursing students, and neonatal units began employing new graduate nurses. A shift in nursing culture has seen many graduate nurses adopt a specialist area early on in their career, and many new graduate nurses remain in specialist areas such as neonatal units and have now adopted senior and advanced positions within the specialty which is bridging the gap in experienced neonatal nurses.

Another strategy, neonatal units adopted to secure a balanced future workforce, was the implementation of the Nurse Entry to Practice programme (NetP) offered to graduate nurses as part of the recruitment process. Nurse graduates are offered a 1-year position under the programme. The programme is endorsed by the nursing council, local tertiary education providers and the district health boards. It offers the new graduate nurse a supportive environment in their first year and incorporates an ongoing educational programme. When the programme has been successfully completed, it fulfills the requirements for a Professional Development and Recognition Programme (PDRP) portfolio at competent level as set out by the New Zealand Nursing Council framework (www.health.govt.co.nz).

Providing quality educational nursing programmes for registered nurses is integral to nurses being able to continue practicing and provide competent nursing care to the New Zealand public. The public's safety is protected under the 2003 Health Practitioners Competence Assurance Act (Nursing Council New Zealand n.d.-b). Nurses are required to produce evidence that they have completed a minimum number of hours of nursing practice and professional development. They have to satisfy the nursing council that their practice meets the competencies as set out in their scope of practice to a satisfactory standard. Provided the conditions set out by the council are met, nurses will be eligible to apply for an annual practicing certificate (Nursing Council New Zealand n.d.-a, -b).

The nursing council introduced a PDRP. The PDRP programme is optional and recognizes three different levels of nursing practice: competent, proficient, and expert. Nurses compile a portfolio that assesses their practice against a set of criteria for each level. The PDRP recognizes ongoing professional development and the nurses' contribution to their workplace. Nurses who do not participate in the PDRP programme may be subject to being audited by the council.

Clinically based nursing education in Aotearoa, New Zealand is dynamic and challenging. To maintain registration, registered nurses are required to submit evidence of 60 h of ongoing professional development over a 3-year period, which includes 20 h of lactation education for neonatal nurses (Nursing Council New Zealand n.d.-a). The role of the clinical (hospital based) nurse educator is to facilitate educational programmes that enable the development of excellence in clinical nursing practice and fulfill council requirements.

Under the 2003 Health Practitioner Competence Assurance Act, nurses are required to maintain the conditions provided by the nursing council to maintain their practicing certificate. Nurses who have not practiced for 5 years or more and want to return to nursing will have to complete a competency assessment programme (CAP) before they are eligible to apply for a practicing certificate. The CAP programme is an educational pathway that is supported by the employer and is offered by tertiary institutions who engage in council approved nursing education programmes.

The career pathway of nursing in New Zealand now includes the role of nurse practitioners. Positions in advanced neonatal nursing practice are offered to neonatal nurses who have obtained advanced education and have completed postgraduate neonatal nursing papers. The pathway to becoming a neonatal nurse practitioner starts with the successful completion of approved postgraduate nursing papers which includes specialist neonatal and child health papers, advanced pharmacology, pathophysiology and an introduction to research paper. Once completed, the nurse is eligible to apply for a position on the nurse practitioner pathway with the District Health Boards (DHBs). The neonatal practicum is a compulsory paper which provides the nurse with clinical teaching and supervision of specialist advanced skills and knowledge beyond the level of a registered nurse. Once all the educational requirements are completed, the nurse will qualify with a master's degree.

Once employed on the nurse practitioner pathway, the scope of the nurse changes to that of an advanced practice/ nurse specialist. The scope for NPs includes the provision of a wide range of assessment and treatment interventions, including the prescribing of medicines as it pertains to the neonatal specialty. They are specialist, clinical leaders and directly influence the care delivery provided to one of our most vulnerable populations in the healthcare setting. The combination of advanced nursing skills, diagnostic reasoning and advanced therapeutic knowledge provides neonates and their whanau (family) with an unsurpassed excellence in patient- and family-centered care. Following the completion of the nurse practitioner portfolio that showcases advanced practice, the neonatal nurse can apply for nurse practitioner registration. Registration is provided to those nurses who have successfully completed the requirements laid out by the assessment panel. The panel evaluates candidates for their assessment, diagnosing, planning, implementation and evaluation of care and triangulates the evidence.

New Zealand universities offer a doctoral degree to those nurses who wish to advance their academic knowledge to the highest level. The doctoral degree is offered as a Doctor of Philosophy (Ph.D.). The degree enables nurses to advance nursing research in specialist areas embedded in an Aotearoa, New Zealand context.

5.4   Organization of Neonatal Care

5.4.1   Neonatal Transportation: Petra Harnett

Aotearoa, New Zealand's team of five million is distributed over a relatively vast and geographically complex area. To make a comparison, New Zealand compares well in land area to the United Kingdom. However, New Zealand's population density is low at 18 people per square kilometer compared to approximately 243 people per square kilometer in the United Kingdom (www.stats.govt.nz 2020). As a result, not all district health boards (DHBs) are able to provide intensive care, surgical care or complex care cots to their local neonatal population. The New Zealand Ministry of Health (2020) explains that "Level 3 units are geographically located to service the largest populations. However, the geographical locations of the highest levels of care do not align with areas with the highest proportion of the population needing NICU care." This necessitates the transfer of sick or premature neonates to a unit that is able to provide the necessary level of care. It drives the requirement for the transfer of neonates between DHBs including up to a one-quarter of babies needing L3 care to neonatal units away from where they lived (MOH 2020).

The neonatal emergency transport services are coordinated and provided by the level 3 units who deliver a highly specialized and dedicated state of the art service. New Zealand extends its health-care service to the South Pacific island nations as well as the retrieval of infants in the South Pacific requiring urgent care is coordinated by the Auckland District Health Board (NZAAS 2020).

The transport team consists of experienced registered neonatal nurses with a minimum of 5 years' experience in the intensive care area and a neonatal registrar or a neonatal nurse practitioner. Teams are large enough to ensure 24/7 nursing and medical cover for retrievals and back transports. The team is led by a clinical nurse manager and a senior medical officer. In some DHBs, neonatal transport teams also provide retrieval services for the "pediatric neonate," an under-resourced area in some areas of Aotearoa, New Zealand. The neonatal transport nurse needs to be adaptable in their role as the nurse takes on the role of transport nurse only when the need arises and functions as part of the daily clinical nursing team with an allocated workload. This means that when a job for the transport team arrives, the nurse has to re-allocate her workload for the duration of the retrieval.

Modes of transportation used in New Zealand are fixed wing (Figs. 5.2 and 5.3), helicopter (Fig. 5.4) and ambulance services (Fig. 5.5). Neonatal nurses complete an aeromedical retrieval course to support the delivery of best practice. Maintain relevant annual competencies and hold a personal level of physical and mental fitness that enables the nurse to cope with the demands and stressors of the transport environment. Transport nurses have sound knowledge of the physiological effects of altitude and the stressors related to the aviation environment.

Back transports make up a significant part of the service the transport team provides. Reasons for back transports can be repatriating "outlying" infants when space was not available at the time of delivery and in utero transfer enabled the safe delivery to take place at another DHB.

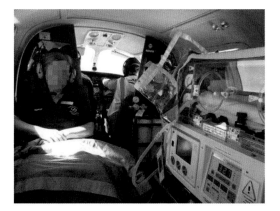

Fig. 5.2 Inside a fixed-wing plane

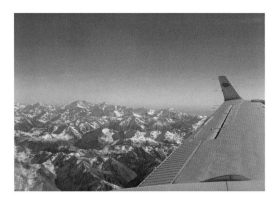

Fig. 5.3 View from a fixed-wing plane

An infant who no longer requires an intensive care environment may be transferred to a step-down facility. An infant within the same DHB who required more care than the home facility was able to deliver may be repatriated when the neonatal care required can be provided by the infant's home facility. Depending on the level of care required during the transport, the infant may be transferred back as a nurse only transfer or alternatively a nurse/doctor team transfers the infant back.

Distances between referral and receiving hospitals can be large (hundreds of kilometres) in New Zealand, and it can take many hours before the retrieval team arrives at the referring hospital. The choice of mode of transport is determined by the urgency of the retrieval, clinical diagnosis, weather, availability, and destination. Retrieval teams may be required to use a combination of road and air travel before arriving at their destination. Telemedicine is proving to be a valuable tool in the

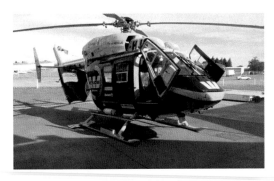

Fig. 5.4 Transport helicopter

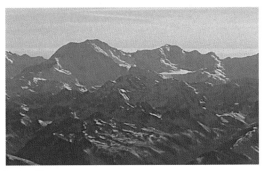

Fig. 5.6 Mount Cook

The transport team travels from Invercargill Hospital to Te Nikau Hospital in Greymouth and captures a glimpse of Aoraki Mount Cook (Fig. 5.6).

In Aotearoa, New Zealand, parents remain present (if they choose to) during the stabilization process. During the stabilization process, the team communicates regularly and keeps the parents informed of the baby's condition and the care the baby requires. Factors that determine whether a parent(s) accompanies the retrieval team back are space and medical fitness to travel. The obstetrician or midwife has to clear the baby's mother is fit for travel and does not require obstetric or midwifery care. The mode of transport will dictate whether there is room for an accompanying parent. At times parents decide to travel in their own private car, so that they have their own transport at the receiving destination. If, for any reason, parents do not accompany the retrieval team, informed consent is obtained for the transportation of the infant and the delivery of ongoing treatment and management of the infant. With a nurse-led back transport, a parent usually accompanies the infant back to their home-based hospital. Out of town families are provided accommodation funded by the government during the infant's hospital stay.

Infants are retrieved from either well-equipped tertiary units or birthing centers that carry only the basics. Therefore, the team carries equipment that enables them to deliver care that is equivalent to what the infant would receive if cared for at the receiving center. Equipment includes a portable incubator fixed on a Mansell which is fitted with hoses for humidified gases, including NO, for

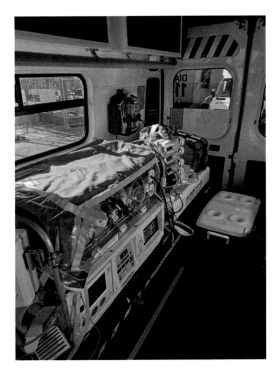

Fig. 5.5 Inside an ambulance

delivery of expert remote neonatal medicine. When an unexpected premature delivery occurs, or neonates become acutely unwell, healthcare providers can use telemedicine to gain clinical support and expertise from neonatologists during the stabilization process while the retrieval team is on route. Telemedicine can also provide support to the retrieval team. With the use of a camera at the referral facility and a large screen TV with audio-visual telecommunication capabilities at the receiving facility, the neonatologist is able to provide support and direction of clinically complex situations.

invasive conventional ventilation and non-invasive ventilation equipment (see picture). Suctioning equipment and syringe pumps are available for use. The transport nurse must have operational knowledge of all equipment and is able to trouble-shoot problems on route. The transport incubators are fitted with an interface that is compatible with a variety of transport modalities and environments and adaptors are carried for use depending on the referral centers' unique fitting requirements. Most centers operate with remote backup engineering support, however, technical problems that arise outside of office hours are often solved by the team themselves or with the assistance of support gleaned from the team back home.

Other essential pieces of equipment are distrib-uted around the Mansell in pouches. A large retrieval pack is taken which contains a limited number of all pieces of equipment that can be found in the intensive care area. The incubator has the capacity to fully monitor the infant; invasive monitoring equipment is also available. UV light is available to treat jaundice. A broad range of medications are carried to cover a broad range of critical clinical conditions. A cool bag is used to carry refrigerated drugs in. An i-stat enables the nurse to analyze blood gases, electrolytes, blood sugar levels and hemoglobin. An I-pad is taken that stores relevant documentation such as drug protocols, neonatal handbook, infusion sheets, intubation drug calculator.

Infants retrieved include:

- Premature and extremely premature infants.
- Surgical infants such as abdominal wall defects.
- Congenital heart disease.
- Medical conditions including jaundice, sei-zures, hypoglycemia, respiratory distress.
- Suspected infections/sepsis.
- Bowel obstructions, esophageal atresia, and tracheoesophageal fistulas.
- HIE.
  (Lynn and Moore 2020)

In Aotearoa, New Zealand, parents remain pres-ent during the stabilization process. The team com-municates regularly and keeps the parents informed of the baby's condition and the care the baby requires. Factors that determine whether a parent(s) accompanies the retrieval team back are space and be medically fit to travel. The obstetrician or mid-wife has to clear the baby's mother is fit for travel and does not require obstetric or midwifery care. The mode of transport will dictate whether there is room for an accompanying parent. At times parents decide to travel in their own private car so that they have their own transport at the receiving destina-tion. The team will seek consent to provide care during the transport. With a nurse led back trans-port, a parent usually accompanies the infant back to their home-based hospital.

Case Study: Baby P

History

    37/40, female, NVD.

    Age 26 days, weight 3.8 kg.

    Two days of cough, fever, and poor feed-ing, cyanosed on arrival to rural medical facil-ity. Transferred to secondary hospital facility on nasal prong O_2. Further deterioration 8 h later with increasing oxygen requirement and moderate respiratory acidosis and tertiary facility asked to retrieve the infant.

    The retrieval took place during night-time hours which ruled out a direct flight to the base hospital as there are no landing lights. The team flew to an alternative nearby coastal airport. A

volunteer paramedic drove the team 30 min down the road to the referral hospital and offered to stay while the team stabilized the infant. The pilots waited at the airport and we kept in touch with an approximate ETA by phone.

Stabilization

    To retrieve the infant, the team took an ambu-lance from the hospital to the airport, followed by a flight over the Southern Alps to the West Coast, followed by an ambulance trip from the airport to the base hospital. The infant was cared for in the emergency department and handed over care to the retrieval team. On arrival, baby girl P. was on 3 L O_2 via nasal prongs, appeared pale, febrile, capillary refill time was 4 s, and she was very cold peripherally.

She was hypotensive, tachycardic, tachypneic with significant subcostal recession and grunting. A peripheral IV was in situ. A CBG revealed severe respiratory acidosis with a pH 7.0, pCO_2 81 mmHg, HCO_3 22. Baby P. was having frequent bradycardias and desaturations that required stimulation to correct.

Plan of Care

Commence CPAP via neopuff mask with a PEEP of 6, FiO_2 of 0.40—increasing to 0.50.

Suctioned nasal secretions.

Commenced IV antibiotics.

2× saline boluses at 10 ml/kg.

Repeat CBG revealed no improvement.

Following a phone consultation with the neonatologist, the infant was intubated and ventilated.

A nasogastric tube was placed and vented.

On-call radiographer was called, and an X-ray confirmed the correct endotracheal tube and nasogastric tube placements.

An attempt was made to place second PIV but was unsuccessful.

Maintenance fluids as well as a morphine infusion were commenced.

The baby was transferred to the transport incubator, full monitoring (heart rate, non-invasive blood pressure, respiratory rate, oxygen saturations, and servo skin temperature) was applied to the baby, she was securely buckled in and ventilated on assist control mode with PIP/PEEP-24/5, FiO_2: 0.50–0.55 to maintain saturations in target range.

In New Zealand, time spent in transit back to the receiving hospital can be substantial, and it is routine practice that the team does not leave the referral destination until such time that the baby is stabilized and is ready for transfer.

Where Can We Provide Appropriate Care for This Very Sick Baby Girl?

Prior to leaving, it took many phone calls to determine where the infant should be cared for as the initial plan to transfer to pediatric HDU was now inappropriate.

Options for the safe delivery of care for baby P. were:

1. Transfer the infant to NICU, Christchurch—however, the unit was over capacity and the isolation room was not available.
2. Starship Hospital (Auckland PICU) to retrieve the infant and the retrieval team continues to care for the infant until Starship's retrieval team arrives. Starship's team was out on a retrieval at the time of the call.
3. Transfer infant to ICU in Christchurch and ICU to care for infant until such time Starship retrieval team available for pick up (ICU can provide short term care for ventilated infants).

The latter option was chosen to be the most appropriate option and provided the team with a place to transfer the infant to and later that day Starship retrieved the infant where she was cared for in PICU for 5 days before being discharged to the ward. The next day the NICU team back transported the infant from Auckland to the Christchurch children's ward before she was discharged home a couple of days later.

The Team Arrives at the Airport in Christchurch

Baby P's oxygen and ventilation requirements continued to increase with a maximum requirement of 90% when the team landed at Christchurch airport. Consultation with the neonatologist and ventilation pressures were adjusted to enable the infant to make the trip by road between the airport and the hospital. On arrival at Christchurch's hospital's ICU, a CBG result revealed a much-improved respiratory acidosis. The infant's temperature was normo-thermic. Her blood pressure was within the normal range, and she appeared comfortable. A thorough handover was provided to the nursing and medical intensive care team as well as the pediatrician who was in charge of coordinating ongoing care with Starship hospital. The infant was transferred to Starship hospital later that day and remained in intensive care for a further 5 days. Upon discharge from the PICU, she was transferred back to the pediatric ward at Christchurch Hospital for ongoing care. She was discharged home 2 days later after a full recovery.

5.5 Evidence-Based Practice: Joanne Clements

The profession of nursing is built on the evaluation and implementation of evidence-based practice. Neonatology is a highly researched field of medicine ensuring that nursing care is constantly changing to keep aligned with current research outcomes. Topical areas of research include but are not limited to: delayed cord clamping at birth, minimally invasive surfactant therapy (MIST), nutrition and growth, microbiome of the gut, use of probiotics for gut health, neonatal hypoglycemia, ethical issues within neonatology, developmental care, family centered care and cultural practices, breast feeding practices, and discharge pathways. All of the above impact on how nurses deliver care to the neonate.

> **Reflective Practice**
>
> *When I started working in neonatal advanced nursing practice the care of the infant at birth was very different from today's practice. Infants were suctioned on the perineum; there was no delayed cord clamping and minimal opportunity for families to provide their cultural practice for the newborn. Infants were resuscitated using 100% oxygen, naloxone was regularly used for newly born respiratory depressed infants and sodium bicarbonate was a mainstay of resuscitation drugs. Today we know that there is no evidence to recommend suctioning on the perineum; delayed cord clamping is part of regular practice with research reporting clinical benefits and commencing resuscitation in 100% oxygen is no longer recommended and can delay time to the newborn's first breath. There is no evidence for the use of naloxone and no improvement in survival or neurological outcomes in infants where sodium bicarbonate was used as a resuscitation drug (Wyckoff et al. 2015; Perlman et al. 2010). It is accepted that cultural practices at the time of birth can impact the wellbeing of the mother and infant. Today*

> *cultural practice during the pregnancy and birth of the infant are part of regular care. In pregnancy Māori women can make a muka pito (NZ flax umbilical tie) and ipu whenua (placental burial) box for the newborn infant. The whānau (family) will tie the umbilical cord using the muka pito (Fig. 5.7) instead of a plastic umbilical clamp and place the placenta in the ipu whenua to take home.*

On-going recognition of cultural practice can be experienced throughout the newborn's journey in neonatal care with the integration of whānau hui's (family meetings) to discuss infant care with extended family members, cultural support experts within the neonatal unit and pathways to discharge which include cultural support strategies and community cultural agencies. As a Nurse Practitioner, an integral part of my discharge planning is to ensure whānau are aware of safe sleep practices for their newborn and are offered a Pēpi-Pod (Fig. 5.8) or Wahakura (Fig. 5.9) to support a safer sleeping environment.

Hayman et al. (2015) reported that between the years of 2002 and 2009 New Zealand had the highest rate of death due to suffocation in the place of sleep, in the developed world, with two-thirds of these deaths attributed to bed-sharing. Māori rates were eight times higher than European, with the most common age at death being less than 1 month (Abel and Tipene-Leach 2013). As part of Māori culture, it is not unusual

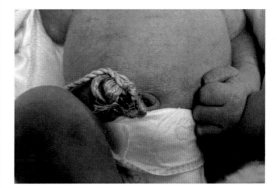

Fig. 5.7 The Muka Pito (NZ Flax Umbilical tie)

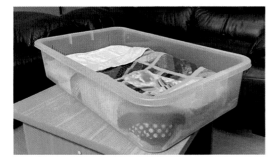

Fig. 5.8 Pēpi-Pod

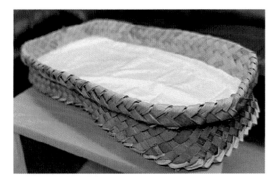

Fig. 5.9 Wahakura

to bed share with the pēpi (baby); therefore, it was important to work in partnership with whānau (family) to support those who chose to bed-share with their pēpi, to provide a safe sleep environment. This led to the introduction of the Wahakura and the Pēpi-Pod as safe sleep devices (Abel and Tipene-Leach 2013). Over the period from 2009 to 2015 post-perinatal mortality fell by 29%, with the majority of this reduction seen with Māori in areas where Wahakura and Pēpi-Pods along with safe sleep education was provided (Tipene-Leach and Abel 2019).

Traditionally preterm infants requiring respiratory support in a neonatal intensive care unit (NICU) were intubated and ventilated. These days we know that mechanical ventilation can be associated with adverse outcomes; therefore, the majority of preterm infants are now managed primarily with non-invasive respiratory support devices such as continuous positive airway pressure (CPAP) or high flow. However, an obstacle for placement on non-invasive respiratory support is the instillation of exogenous surfactant for those infants with respiratory distress syndrome. These infants needed intubation to enable surfactant delivery and as a consequence of this could remain ventilated for a period of time (Aguar et al. 2014). For these infants born in hospitals with special care baby units (SCBU), this would require transfer of both the mother and infant to an alternative hospital where there was an NICU available to provide care for the ventilated infant. This practice-imposed barriers to families, particularly for the most vulnerable communities, which include our Māori population.

In 2013, Dargaville et al. conducted a feasibility study exploring instillation of exogenous surfactant using a MIST technique. With the infant continuing on non-invasive respiratory support, a semi-rigid vascular catheter was passed into the trachea (the Hobart technique), and the surfactant instilled. The researchers found that the procedure was generally well tolerated by the infants with nil requirements for premedication or the use of narcotic agents. Following the procedure, the researchers noted a reduction in both FiO_2 requirement and need for intubation. This is now a procedure which is regularly used throughout New Zealand and has reduced the need for transfer from a SCBU to a NICU.

Case Study

A male infant, of Māori ethnicity was born at 32 weeks gestation and admitted to a SCBU. The mother had received limited antenatal care and the infant was born via a precipitous vaginal delivery. Due to the precipitous nature of the delivery antenatal steroids were unable to be administered. The infant was assessed by the Nurse Practitioner and placed on Hudson CPAP. He was noted to have a respiratory grunt, subcostal recession and a FiO$_2$ requirement of 0.52 to maintain SpO$_2$ 93%. He was transferred from the delivery room to SCBU where a clinical management plan was formulated. A blood gas was taken which reported a pH 7.16, PCO$_2$ 9.0 kPa, Bicarbonate 23 mmol/L, followed by a chest X-ray which showed low volume lungs, air bronchograms and a fine granular lung pattern. A diagnosis was made of respiratory distress syndrome. A decision to administer exogenous surfactant using MIST technique was made. In following the Hobart technique, a narrow bore venous catheter was inserted into the trachea and a dose of surfactant administered, while the infant remained on CPAP support. There was noted to be a rapid decrease in work of breathing and over the following 2 h he was weaned to FiO$_2$ 0.23. The infant did not require any further instillation of surfactant. He remained on non-invasive respiratory support for a further 10 days at which time he successfully trialled off. The ability to instil surfactant using a MIST technique enabled the infant to remain on CPAP support ensuring his on-going care could be continued in the SCBU. This small change in how we can instil surfactant has far-reaching benefits particularly for our most vulnerable communities. Nursing practice in New Zealand is shaped by our founding document Te Tiriti o Waitangi (Treaty of Waitangi), which contain the principles of Kawanatanga (Crown governance) and Tino Rangatiratanga (Māori self-determination). An important part of our role as nurses is to improve service delivery to Māori and work in partnership with Māori to improve health outcomes (Nursing Council of New Zealand 2011). For this infant and his whānau the nearest NICU was 35 km away, therefore being able to remain in the SCBU near the whānau's place of domicile reduced barriers to the infant's on-going care. Whānau had easier access to the infant enabling attendance at ward rounds, discussions around the care of the infant, facilitation of kangaroo cares, mother crafting, and the establishment of breastfeeding.

5.6   Conclusion

This chapter illustrates how culture plays an important role in neonatal care. Practice and education for nurses including neonatal nurses are regulated, and there are clear standards and competencies for different levels of nursing education. High standards of care promote very good outcomes for the small and sick newborns.

References

Abel S, Tipene-Leach D (2013) SUDI prevention: a review of Maori safe sleep innovations for infants. N Z Med J 126(1379):86

Aguar M, Vento M, Dargaville PA (2014) Minimally invasive surfactant therapy: an update. NeoReviews 15(7):e275–e285

Calman R (2015) Māori education – mātauranga - Māori education policy. Te Ara - the encyclopaedia of New Zealand. http://www.TeAra.govt.nz/en/maori-education-matauranga/page-7

Dargaville PA, Aiyappan A, De Paoli AG, Kuschel CA, Kamlin COF, Carlin JB, Davis PG (2013) Minimally invasive surfactant therapy in preterm infants on continuous positive airway pressure. Arch Dis Child Fetal Neonatal Ed 98(2):F122–F126

Durie M (1994) Whaiora: Maori health development. Oxford University Press, Auckland

Hayman RM, McDonald G, de C Baker NJ, Mitchell EA, Dalziel SR (2015) Infant suffocation in place of sleep: New Zealand national data 2002–2009. Arch Dis Child 100(7):610–614

Herbert A (2001) Protocols and Custom at time of a Maori death. http://www.whakawhetu.co.nz/sites/default/files/Protocols

Lynn A, Moore S (2020) Transport Nursing Team/CNS-ANP/NNP. In: Christchurch Neonatal Emergency Transport Team handbook. http://www.edu.cdhb.health.nz/Hospitals-Services/Specialist-Care/Canterbury-Neonatal-Service/Pages/Transport-Team.aspx

Māori into Tertiary Education (2011) Maori into tertiary education [Video file]. https://www.youtube.com/watch?v=JxRc8CA1WG4

Ministry of Health (2019b) Wai 2575 Māori health trends report. Wellington. https://www.health.govt.nz/publications/report-MāoriHealthTrends-2019

Ministry of Health (2020) Fetal and infants' deaths webtool. Wellington. https://www.health.govt.nz/publication/fetal-and-infant-deaths-web-tool

Ministry of Health (MOH) (2020) https://www.health.govt.nz/publication/review-neonatal-care-new-zealand

National Paediatric Palliative Care Clinical Network (2015) National Paediatric Palliative Care clinical guidelines. https://www.starship.org.nz/for-health-professionals/national-paediatric-palliative-care-clinical-guidelines

Neonatal Nurses College Aotearoa (2015) Neonatal palliative care for New Zealand neonatal units. Comfort as a model of care. Wellington. https://www.nzno.org.nz

New Zealand Air Ambulance Service (NZAAS) (2020) Paediatric & newborn transportation. https://www.nzaas.co.nz/what-we-do/paediatric-and-newborn-transport/

New Zealand Nurses Organisation (2005) Tikanga Maori for Aotearoa-New Zealand Health Settings. Wellington www.nzno.org/publications

Nursing Council New Zealand (n.d.-a) Continuing competence. https://www.nursingcouncil.org.nz/Public/Nursing/Competence_assessment/NCNZ/nursing-section/Competence_assessment.aspx

Nursing Council New Zealand (n.d.-b) Standards and guidelines for nurses. https://www.nursingcouncil.org.nz/Public/Nursing/Standards_and_guidelines/NCNZ/nursing-section/Standards_and_guidelines_for_nurses.aspx

Nursing Council of New Zealand (2007) Competencies for registered nurses. https://www.nursingcouncil.org.nz/competenciesforRegisterednurses

Nursing Council of New Zealand (2011) Guidelines for cultural safety, the Treaty of Waitangi and Maori health in nursing education and practice. http://pro.healthmentoronline.com/assets/Uploads/refract/pdf/Nursing_Council_cultural-safety11.pdf

Open Polytechnic (2020) ATT501 an introduction to the Maori Worldview of Education. https://openpolytechnic.iqualify.com/course/-LyBr4vgkqv7IWUWRoJL/#/page/p19; https://openpolytechnic.iqualify.com/course/-LyBr4vgkqv7IWUWRoJL/#/page/p56; https://openpolytechnic.iqualify.com/course/-LyBr4vgkqv7IWUWRoJL/#/page/p59

Perlman JM, Wyllie J, Kattwinkel J, Atkins DL, Chameides L, Goldsmith JP, Guinsburg R, Hazinski MF, Morley C, Richmond S, Simon WM (2010) Part 11: neonatal resuscitation: 2010 international consensus on cardiopulmonary resuscitation and emergency cardiovascular care science with treatment recommendations. Circulation 122(16_suppl_2):S516–S538

SANDS New Zealand (2011) www.sands.org.nz

Stewart G (2021) Rebooting biculturalism in Aotearoa-New Zealand. https://briefingpapers.co.nz/rebooting-biculturilism

Tipene-Leach D, Abel S (2019) Innovation to prevent sudden infant death: the wahakura as an indigenous vision for a safe sleep environment. Aust J Prim Health 25(5):406–409

Wyckoff MH, Aziz K, Escobedo MB, Kapadia VS, Kattwinkel J, Perlman JM, Simon WM, Weiner GM, Zaichkin JG (2015) Part 13: neonatal resuscitation: 2015 American Heart Association guidelines update for cardiopulmonary resuscitation and emergency cardiovascular care. Circulation 132(18_suppl_2):S543–S560

UK

6

Tracey Jones, Jennifer Lowe, and Kirstin Webster

6.1 Introduction

This chapter aims to offer an overview of neonatal healthcare provision in the United Kingdom (UK). The UK, located in Western Europe, is unique in its formation of devolved nations, England, Wales, Scotland, and Northern Ireland (NI), with specialist neonatal care available in each. The UK population of 67 million people is diverse, with 28.7% of live births in 2019 in England and Wales recorded to mothers born outside of the UK (Office for National Statistics 2020a). In 2018 the average age of mothers and fathers increased for the tenth consecutive year, and there were more live births and stillbirths to mothers living in the most deprived areas than the least deprived areas (Office for National Statistics 2019). The chapter will help you understand the four nations that make up the UK and how the National Health Service (NHS) provides care that is free of charge to all at the point of need, functions to provide neonatal care, and more specifically how neonatal nursing is arranged. The structure of neonatal nursing education will be examined to offer an understanding of the educational opportunities and career structure for nurses who choose to work in neonatal care in the UK. The influences and national directives that guide neonatal provision will be explained in detail to allow the reader to have a transparent exposure to the beneficial way in which both charities and the government can work together to support both parents and nurse staffing numbers.

On July 5, 1948, an historic moment occurred in UK history, the culmination of a bold and pioneering plan to make healthcare no longer exclusive to those who could afford it but to make it accessible to everyone irrespective of wealth or privilege. The NHS was born. The brainchild of the Welsh politician Aneurin Bevan, as parliamentary cabinet minister for health, housing, and local authorities he saw the National Health Service Act through parliament to law, this allowed people to receive a medical diagnosis and treatment either in a hospital or at home, free to all at the point of delivery and provided

T. Jones (✉)
Division of Nursing, Midwifery and Social Work, School of Health Sciences, University of Manchester, Manchester, UK

Council of International Neonatal Nurses, Inc. (COINN), Yardley, PA, USA
e-mail: tracey.m.jones@manchester.ac.uk

J. Lowe
North West Neonatal Operational Delivery Network, Manchester, UK

K. Webster
ANNP Lead for the Scottish Neonatal Nurses Group (SNNG), Fife, Scotland, UK

National Maternity and Perinatal Audit (NMPA), Royal College of Obstetricians, London, UK according to need, not the ability to pay. The NHS has evolved to become one of the world's largest healthcare systems and is seen as a benchmark for healthcare provision around the world, often viewed as an attractive organization for many nurses to train and progress within their careers.

Healthcare and health policy for England is centrally funded and the responsibility of the Department of Health. A national body NHS England oversees the commissioning of budgets. Whereas in Scotland, Wales, and NI, it is the responsibility of the respective devolved governments. Funding is based on a set tariff per patient and is channeled down through clinical commissioning groups to individual hospitals or groups of hospitals that make up NHS Trusts in England and NI, and Health Boards in Wales and Scotland. Due to disparity in the budget systems in each devolved nation, the total UK NHS budget for 2020/2021 is an estimated £226 billion (Wales Government 2019; Northern Ireland Assembly 2020; Office for National Statistics 2020b; Scottish Government 2020). The NHS is one of the largest employers in the world, employing 1.9 million staff, of which 724,516 are qualified nursing and midwifery staff (Nursing and Midwifery Council 2020; The King's Fund 2020).

Neonatal services in the UK sit under the remit of the Royal College of Paediatrics and Child Health (RCPCH) with input from the Royal College of Obstetricians and Gynaecologists (RCOG). An inaugural meeting of the British Paediatric Association (BPA) took place in 1928 before receiving Royal College status to become the Royal College of Paediatrics and Child Health in 1996. The first neonatal unit in the UK was established in Birmingham in 1929 by doctors Ethel Cassie and Victoria Mary Crosse (Dunn 2007), the number now sits at 196 units across the UK. UK neonatal clinicians work closely with colleagues from Europe, Australia, New Zealand, the USA, and Canada to share knowledge and experience to provide the most up-to-date, evidence-based practice when caring for the 1 in 7 babies born in the UK that require neonatal unit admission.

Notable UK contributions to worldwide neonatal care, among others, include the direct antibody test (DAT), often referred to eponymously as the "Coombs Test" (Mollison and Cutbush 1949). The test is used worldwide to diagnose hemolytic disease of the newborn, to identify those at risk of significant hyperbilirubinemia. The use of phototherapy to treat neonatal jaundice was implemented following an accidental discovery of the effects of sunlight on a jaundiced infant in 1956 by Sister Ward at Rochford Hospital, Essex and a few weeks later in the hospital laboratory when a blood sample was left for some hours on the windowsill before analysis (Dobbs and Cremer 1975). This treatment is now offered worldwide to prevent excessive hyperbilirubinemia which, if left untreated, can cause irreversible brain damage, kernicterus, and even death. The 1960s saw John Inkster pioneer maintenance of functional residual capacity during respiratory support, giving positive end expiratory pressure (PEEP) ventilation to both neonatal and adult medicine, and Douglas Maynard develop cerebral function monitoring (CFM) (Shah et al. 2008; Neonatal Research 2021). In the 1980s, Peter Cooke introduced cranial ultrasound and Peter Fleming's research into sudden infant death syndrome informed the "Back-to-sleep" campaign of the 1990s, which saw a dramatic reduction in global deaths (Imperial College London 2020). The act of providing stabilization at birth of the neonate prior to the cord being clamped has been supported by use of a specially designed trolley that houses all the equipment found on a neonatal resuscitaire. In a format that allows it to be positioned close enough to the mother's bed or an operating table to allow the neonatal team to provide the support the neonate requires while facilitating optimized cord clamping (Thomas et al. 2014; Weeks et al. 2015; Inspiration Healthcare 2021).

The following sections in this chapter will detail the organization of neonatal care within the NHS, offer some insight into the structure of education and training that supports neonatal nursing in the UK and provide some detail of the evidence-based practice that underpins UK neonatal care provision.

Key "Think Points" for Learning

- Neonatology sits within pediatric and obstetric care within the NHS, with numerous stakeholders, charities, and agencies involved.
- A robust education and career progression exists for neonatal nurses, driven by national, regional, and local directives.
- Parents as partners in care are central to the entire team contributing to care of the neonate.

6.2 Organization of Neonatal Care

Neonatal services across the devolved nations of the UK are provided by 196 neonatal units (NNU) grouped into 14 neonatal networks across England, Wales, Scotland, and Northern Ireland. Three levels of neonatal care are available; level 1 is used to describe a special care baby unit (SCBU) where care is provided for neonates born ≥32 weeks gestation with an anticipated birth weight of >1000 g, SCBUs may also provide stabilization of babies prior to transfer to higher level units. Level 2 is used to identify a local neonatal unit (LNU) where care may be provided for singleton neonates born after 26 + 6 weeks gestation for singleton babies or multiple births after 27 + 6, providing the expected birth weight is greater than 800 g, short-term intensive care can be provided, as can high dependency care for babies born 27–31 weeks gestation. Level 3 denotes a neonatal intensive care unit (NICU) that provides care for the sickest and most immature neonates, born at <27 weeks gestation or <800 g, or those requiring ongoing intensive care and support of more than one organ (British Association of Perinatal Medicine 2011). Specialist neonatal units provide cardiac support, surgery, neurology, and extracorporeal membrane oxygenation (ECMO). Depending on the size and level of the unit, the medical staff may be made up of pediatricians, neonatologists or a mix.

Transitional care (TC) is offered in conjunction with postnatal maternity services to accommodate mothers and babies together, where a baby's level of care need is defined as "special care," TC units are staffed by either postnatal ward (PNW) midwives and nursery nurses or by NNU staff in either a standalone unit or as part of a PNW. Both these units are cost effective as they avoid NNU admission or prolonged stay for establishing feeding or phototherapy, and they reduce instances of mother–baby separation. Neonatal outreach support is provided in the community following discharge, by either standalone community neonatal nursing teams or by nurses from neonatal units. The level of support varies between teams and geographical location from home oxygen for babies with chronic lung disease or those with a stoma to babies requiring a heated mattress to aid weight gain, some teams are able to support parents with gastric tube feeding their baby and home phototherapy for physiological neonatal jaundice. Neonatal transport services are provided by either specialist neonatal teams or as part of pediatric transport services, with transport available by road, helicopter or airplane to facilitate emergency transfers and scheduled repatriations to home units.

6.3 Neonatal Structure in the Devolved Nations

Neonatal networks in England are termed operational delivery networks (ODN), of which there are 11, each covering a defined geographical area. Neonatal networks first introduced in 2003 were reconfigured to ODNs in 2013 with the express purpose of delivering a level of service that is standardized across the network, ensuring continuity of care between units within the network and coordinating patient pathways to improve productivity, consistency, and patient outcomes (British Association of Perinatal Medicine 2020).

Welsh neonatal services are coordinated by the Wales Neonatal Network with the primary aim of establishing sustainable neonatal services by implementing All Wales Standards, to ensure

Welsh mothers and babies receive safe, effective patient and family-centered care delivered by skilled, trained staff by developing consistent pathways of care across the nation. With the standardization of neonatal nursing education, all nurses in neonatal units in Wales are trained to the same high standard (Wales Maternity and Neonatal Network 2020).

Scottish neonatal services are arranged between three Managed Clinical Networks (MCN), North of Scotland (NoS), South East and Tayside (SEAT), and West of Scotland (WoS) with each working inter-regionally to provide high-quality services across the networks and to agree pathways of care and clinical guidelines. Scottish Government's redesign of neonatal services, named The Best Start, aims to establish three NICUs from 15 sites offering neonatal care, to ensure the smallest, sickest, and most vulnerable neonates are cared for in centers with the most expertise, to create a single MCN across the nation and to standardize education for all neonatal nurses (Scottish Government 2017).

Neonatal Network for Northern Ireland (NNNI) prioritizes a family-centered approach, to standardize practice across the region and a co-production approach to care with stakeholders and a Parental Engagement Group (Health and Social Care Board 2020).

6.4   The Multidisciplinary Team

Throughout the UK, care is provided collaboratively with a multidisciplinary team of consultant neonatologists, pediatricians, obstetricians, junior doctors, advanced neonatal nurse practitioners (ANNP), enhanced neonatal nurse practitioners (ENNP), consultant nurses, midwives, nurses with varying experience including those who have undertaken further neonatal training to become qualified in specialty (QIS), nursery nurses, healthcare assistants, nursing associates, physicians assistants, phlebotomists, radiologists, physiologists, dieticians, physiotherapists, pharmacists, feeding advisors, neuro-developmental care practitioners, clinical psychologists, chaplains, researchers, speech, and language

practitioners, occupational therapists, social workers, safeguarding leads, and, most importantly, parents. Great emphasis is placed on working with parents as partners in care for their child. Parents are actively encouraged to participate in clinical decision-making, during ward rounds and in all aspects of their child's care where appropriate. Parent Advisory (or Engagement) Groups (PAG/PEG) exist to involve parents in peer parent-to-parent support, and to work with neonatal units and networks, representing parents to ensure issues that affect families are addressed at a strategic level.

NNUs may be staffed by nurses, who have undertaken either adult or pediatrics nurse training, or midwives, both must hold professional registration with the Nursing and Midwifery Council (NMC). Medical trainees wishing to pursue a career in pediatrics and/or neonatology must sit exams for membership of RCPCH, who oversee the specialist neonatal grid training required to become a qualified consultant neonatologist.

Professional groups exist to facilitate networking between neonatal nursing colleagues, promoting education through conferences and organized study days in collaboration with other professional groups. The British Paediatric Perinatal Group was founded in 1976, registered as a charity in 1981 under the name British Association for Perinatal Paediatrics before changing to its current moniker British Association of Perinatal Medicine (BAPM) in 1985 (British Association of Perinatal Medicine 2019). BAPM is a professional association that supports staff working in perinatal care to develop their skills and knowledge as well as promoting research, quality improvement, and innovation in practice through collaborative working to produce frameworks for practice, quality improvement toolkits, and a programme of training and education and distribute infant journal to their members. Guidelines, standards, and frameworks for perinatal care are produced by BAPM working groups of multidisciplinary membership, in collaboration with the Royal Colleges and the National Institute for Health and Care Excellence (NICE). Each UK nation has also developed their own neonatal guidelines specific to their region, with individual units adjusting these guidelines to their own population demographic and local hospital policies and procedures. The standards expected of neonatal care are defined in the Neonatal Critical Care Service Specification (NHS England 2015). This document outlines 11 key outcomes covering a multitude of aspects of neonatal care (ensuring babies are kept within networks, retinopathy screening, recording blood infections, early surgery, transfer of extremely preterm babies, and much more) that ODNs must ensure are achieved. ODNs must produce an annual report that includes neonatal activity (where care was provided, when, and how), quality measures, and evidence that parent experience has been evaluated and actioned. A National Neonatal Programme Board meets twice a year to bring together neonatal stakeholders, policy makers, and commissioning bodies to share and update on advances in their own area of practice. The Neonatal Nursing Association (NNA) was established in 1977 with the intention of improving communication between neonatal units and to share advances within the specialty as well as to produce an official neonatal journal, the *Journal of Neonatal Nursing* (JNN). The Scottish Neonatal Nurses Group (SNNG), championing the work of neonatal nurses across Scotland, also has a dedicated ANNP group. These agencies regularly partake in working groups and on steering committees to drive forward national policies and frameworks for practice.

Numerous charities and organizations support neonatal care throughout the UK at local and national levels, providing support and information to parents, families, and healthcare professionals. Individual units may look to achieve UNICEF Baby Friendly Initiative (BFI) status (UNICEF UK 2019). Standards apply to both maternity and neonatal units, serving to signify that staff have undertaken extra training and pledge to uphold the standards that promote family integrated care, to support breastfeeding and abide by UK legislation that forbids the advertising or promotion of first formula milks (Baby Milk Action 2021). Bliss is a charity that sup-

ports families of babies in neonatal care while working with health professionals to improve resources, training and care across the whole of the UK with the aim to give every baby in neonatal care the best chance of survival and quality of life (Bliss 2020). They provide support and information for families of, and for healthcare professionals caring for, premature or sick babies. At an individual unit level, Bliss Champions are volunteers who visit neonatal units to offer their support to parents and families of babies admitted. The Bliss Baby Charter aims to standardize care across the UK by providing guidance and running training courses with more than 80% of units signed up. They run regular campaigns on behalf of premature or sick babies and their families at local, national and parliamentary level, working with Government and politicians on behalf of premature and sick babies. Most recently, Bliss was involved in the passing of a Bill to provide parents with extra paid leave on the death of a child and are now campaigning for paid leave for parents with a baby in an NNU. Bliss is heavily involved in national policy writing, offers support and funding for research, and call upon their Insight and Involvement Group made up of around 300 members with lived experience of neonatal care. The number of professionals involved in the care of neonates is vast; therefore, inter-disciplinary working is essential, while ensuring the infant and their family remains central to all decision-making.

6.5 Education and Training

The career structure for neonatal nurses in the UK follows a similar pathway whichever nation the nurse works in. All nurse education in the UK is taught at degree level and is directed by higher education universities in partnership with NHS Trusts and Health Boards. Student nurses, like other university students, pay for their degree education. They do however receive a training grant of at least £5000 a year, with up to £3000 further funding available for eligible students as part of the government's pledge to increase nurse numbers by 50,000 over the next 5 years. The government has also pledged an extra £33.9 billion by 2023–2024 to achieve a programme of improvements as set out in the NHS Long-Term Plan, which aims to guide the NHS forward providing high-quality lifesaving treatment and care for patients and their families, alongside reducing pressure on NHS staff and investing in new technologies (NHS 2019).

carrying out work on nursing standards, education, and practice. As the only trade union solely representing nursing and midwifery staff, they work to represent nursing staff working in the public, private and voluntary sectors, providing advice and support to individuals, government, and other UK bodies (Royal College of Nursing 2021).

6.6   Professional Registration

The NMC is the professional regulator for UK nurses and sets the standards framework for nursing and midwifery education, last updated in January 2019 (The Nursing and Midwifery Council 2018). Universities in the UK have to align their nursing education programmes to meet these standards, and representatives from the NMC will assess the course curriculum. Once a nurse is registered with the NMC and assures a position in a neonatal unit, the pathway for continuing education commences. Each nurse who joins the team of an NNU will undergo a period of orientation and a local unit induction, they may then continue on to a programme of university-based modules or in some parts of the UK a unit of study known as the induction to neonatal nursing programme all of which cover various aspects of neonatal care, from developmental/special care leading to intensive care and stabilization, upon successful completion a neonatal nurse will be considered qualified in specialty. This qualification assures the employing trust that the nurse has met a level of academic study and clinical competence to care for the sickest babies. Many trusts align their competence to the Council of International Neonatal Nurses (COINN) neonatal nursing competencies, these can be found on the COINN website. The Royal College of Nursing (RCN), which is the world's largest nursing union and professional body, produced a career framework of education and competence for neonatal nursing in the UK (Crawford and Teasdale 2011). The RCN is a membership organization representing over 450,000 registered nurses, midwives, nursing support workers, and nursing students. It is a professional body,

6.7   Neonatal Nursing Career Progression

Once qualified in neonatal specialty, there are further roles and education that can be accessed, commonly those of Practice Educator, ENNP, and ANNP roles, as well as community support and leading on areas of strategic development such as patient safety groups, guidelines review groups, and management. ENNP is a role that sits between that of QIS nurse and ANNP, ENNPs have undergone further training to enhance their clinical practice and the role may be similar to that of a junior doctor but without prescribing rights (Mitra and Bramwells 2017). The role of the ANNP was introduced in the United Kingdom in the late 1980s having first been seen in the United States in the 1970s. However, the first UK academic course was not established until 1992. ANNPs are now an integral part of the neonatal workforce and found the majority of NNUs throughout the UK. ANNPs provide flexible solutions to workforce pressures and are often said to be the professionals bridging the gap in a hybrid role between medical and nursing teams. ANNPs exercise professional clinical judgment in diagnosis and complex decision-making and non-medical prescribing, utilizing their extensive neonatal experience and acquired knowledge of pathophysiology and pharmacology. Offering support at high-risk births in the delivery room, ANNPs are often the point of medical contact for midwives and health visitors working in all areas of maternity including the community. ANNPs offer a vital contribution to workforce arrangements, often incorporated into the medical junior or middle grade rota. Progression of the ANNP role is guided by the four pillars of advanced practice. These are management and leadership, education, research, and advanced clinical practice devised by NHS Education Scotland (NES) in 2007 (NHS Education for Scotland 2018). A career framework for ANNPs has been published by BAPM to guide an ANNP from newly qualified through to Consultant level. The structure of the ANNP course varies significantly in content and duration between institutions of higher education, with trainees often deemed competent to work as independent ANNPs following successful completion of a postgraduate diploma which includes a non-medical prescribing qualification and subsequent entry of this on the NMC register; although it is now anticipated that the ANNP will continue to complete a higher degree resulting in a Master of Science (MSc) in advanced nursing practice.

6.8 Continuing Professional Development

All nurses are expected to maintain their competence with continuing professional development, they must provide evidence of this to the NMC every 4 years in order to maintain their professional registration. A programme of mandatory training is required to be completed, for neonatal nursing staff this includes adult basic life support as well as neonatal life support (NLS). The UK Resuscitation Council runs a programme of NLS courses that must be attended every 4 years, individuals may be invited by the faculty to undertake an instructor course to teach on future NLS courses. There is also an Advanced Resuscitation of the Newborn course (ARNI) that provides enhanced emergency situation training with an emphasis on communication with parents. Many NNUs run a programme of simulation training, intended to provide practice of real-life situational scenarios to identify areas of good practice and areas for development.

Nurses and midwives caring for newborns may wish to develop their practice by undertaking a routine examination of the newborn course entitled the Newborn and Infant Physical Examination (NIPE) to enable them to carry out

the routine screening of the newborn. In England the course is delivered by higher education institutions, in Scotland the Scottish Multiprofessional Maternity Development Programme (SMMDP) runs regular training courses, and courses remain in development in Wales and NI.

Bliss runs a Family and Infant Neurodevelopmental Education (FINE) course to provide education to neonatal healthcare professionals on aspects of neurodevelopmental care, to gain an understanding of infant behaviors, recognizing signs of stress and pain and offers skills to reduce noxious experiences that may impact upon the infant's development (Bliss 2021).

Neonatal nurses are encouraged to undertake regular training and continuing professional development to fulfill their potential and provide the best, up-to-date, evidence-based, family-centered care to the infants and families they are supporting.

6.9 Evidence-Based Practice

The UK is active in neonatal research within Europe and worldwide, collaborating with international colleagues on the boards such as European Foundation for the Care of Newborn Infants (EFCNI) and International Society for Evidence-Based Neonatology (EBNEO). Cochrane, an organization inspired by, and named in honor of, British epidemiologist Archie Cochrane was founded by Iain Chalmers in 1993. Cochrane has expanded worldwide and to include specialist interest groups such as the Cochrane Neonatal group, with the intention of disseminating evidence-based, regularly updated reviews of neonatal-perinatal medicine. The National Perinatal Epidemiology Unit (NPEU), a multidisciplinary research unit, conducts several programmes of research, one of which is MBRRACE-UK. A group appointed by the Health Quality Improvement Partnership (HQIP), to run a programme of confidential enquiry surveillance collecting information about mothers and babies who die either during pregnancy or soon after birth, with the intention of making recommendations to improve practice.

6.10 Data Collection and National Audit

All neonatal units across the UK use an electronic patient record (EPR), BadgerNet Neonatal (Clevermed 2020). This provides a platform for continuity of patient data if infants are transferred between units. Some centers also use the BadgerNet Maternity system where each baby has a record embedded within their mother's EPR entry, if a baby is admitted to NNU, the systems are able to link together to ensure continuity of recording of care. Data is transferred to the neonatal data analysis unit (NDAU) and held in a national neonatal research database (NNRD) as a national resource for neonatal researchers (Imperial College London 2020). The HQIP-commissioned National Neonatal Audit Programme (NNAP) and National Maternity and Perinatal Audit (NMPA) are programmes of continuous clinical audit, utilizing routinely collected data to produce a report of results on a number of neonatal and maternity measures at a national, Trust/Health Board and individual hospital level, where each site can benchmark their own level of practice against a national average or other units within Great Britain. Sprint audits and research papers utilizing data linkage between these databases and those held by other agencies such as Hospital Episode Statistics (HES), Second-Generation Surveillance System (SGSS), National Population Database (NPD) and Department for Education offer the chance to analyze aspects of perinatal care with optimal data quality and completeness.

In Northern Ireland, the Neonatal Intensive Care Outcomes Research and Evaluation (NICORE), a joint initiative between the Public Health Agency and Queen's University Belfast to improve outcomes for neonates and their families, is overseen by the NNNI (HSC Public Health Agency 2020). Routinely collecting data on key quality markers from neonatal units in NI since 1994 and allowing teams to reflect on standards of care, accurately inform parents regarding short/long-term outcomes, share good practice and compare performance with other units.

Aiding the Health Service Commission (HSC) to make informed decisions about future needs of sick babies in NI (HSC Public Health Agency 2020).

6.11 Dissemination of Evidence-Based Practice

Annual conferences are held by many of the neonatal organizations, including BAPM, NNA, SNNG, National Transport Group (NTG), RCPCH, RCOG, and REaSoN, drawing national and international speakers, audiences and research poster/oral submissions. The Covid-19 pandemic has influenced a shift to online learning and networking with neonatal colleagues around the world. A multitude of meetings, webinars and learning opportunities that are now available online have resulted in neonatal education and research becoming accessible to a wider range of the neonatal community.

6.12 Emerging Evidence into Practice

Supporting transition at the threshold of viability varies around the world and across Europe. BAPM released a framework for practice offering guidance of perinatal considerations and pre-term delivery decision-making prior to and/or at the time of birth at 26 weeks and 6 days or less (Bates et al. 2019b). The document offers a risk-based approach for decision-making to be made jointly between healthcare providers and parents. If a birth occurs at less than 22 + 0 weeks of gestation, active management is not appropriate, but there are increasing reports of neonates born from 22 + 0 onwards who survive (Smith et al. 2017; Wilkinson et al. 2018).

Many units are adopting practices to support transition to extrauterine life while delivering optimized cord clamping with the aim of delaying clamping the umbilical cord for at least 60 s. Approaches include use of the LifeStart™ trolley to facilitate neonatal interventions at the mother's bedside, either in the delivery room or in obstetric theater (Inspiration Healthcare 2021). An approach is proposed utilizing resuscitaire equipment commonly found in delivery suites and obstetric theaters to provide a low-cost alternative to the specialist trolley that is also potentially transferable to low- and middle-income settings (Bates et al. 2019a).

Emphasis is placed on family-integrated care (FICare), an evidence-based model to guide quality improvement programmes in supporting parents as partners in care, integrating parents into the neonatal team and to empower them as primary caregivers for their baby. Initiatives include parents performing cares (nappy changes, skin cleansing/bathing, mouth care), gastric tube feeding, taking temperatures, re-siting saturation probes and monitoring leads, and in some units, presenting their baby during ward round (PaediatricFOAM 2018; UNICEF 2019). Parental perinatal mental health is a key area for support and improvement in many NNUs, a few units are fortunate enough to have in-house clinical psychology services, but many parents are left without the support they need. Bliss published data in 2018 reporting that 80% of parents said their mental health suffered following their neonatal experience, just over a third reported their mental health was "significantly worse," a quarter of parents were diagnosed with anxiety, with 45% reporting no access to formal psychological support (Bliss 2018). Perinatal mental health for fathers receives less attention in comparison to that of mothers but the effect of having a baby admitted to NNU on fathers should not be underestimated. Overall rate of postnatal depression is 1 in 10 fathers, compared to 1 in 7 mothers, for parents with babies admitted to an NNU the rates of psychological distress are between 7.5% and 16.8% for fathers and 9.4% and 21.7% for mothers, with rates decreasing as gestational age at birth increases (Carson et al. 2015; Hanley and Williams 2020).

An age-old issue for families with a baby in the neonatal unit is the separation when parents are unable to stay. While unrestricted access is the norm for parents and the assurance that parents are not seen as "visitors," but as integral members of their baby's care team is a key component of FICare, this can still present a dilemma for parents when they have to leave the unit. This has been exacerbated during the Covid-19 pandemic. Many units were forced to implement enhanced restrictions to parental and family access to ensure the safety of all the babies in the unit and their families until more could be learned about this novel virus. Developed in 2017, the original vCreate Diaries platform was born out of a suggestion from a neonatal dad in Glasgow. The father had approached the neonatal unit his baby was being treated in to ask why there was not a secure way for him to receive video updates of his infant when the technology was available and being used by everything from car garages to retailers.

Galvanized by this feedback, a Consultant Neonatologist at the Royal Hospital for Children, Glasgow, began working with the vCreate team on a system that would help keep families connected with their baby when they could not be with them at the unit. The resulting innovation, vCreate Diaries, is a secure system that allows neonatal professionals to record and upload short video clips and photos of the babies on approved devices which are then shared directly with parents.

The service was trialed in Glasgow's unit in Spring 2017 and since then the service has advanced to facilitate patient to clinician video pathways and helped to support thousands of families. Live video calling platforms are available, but these present their own set of problems regarding network connections, confidentiality, patient privacy, and staff availability to assist patients. vCreate is a secure messaging platform where nursing staff can take photographs and record videos for parents and families to access. The technology is now in use across the UK, Ireland, France, North America, Australia, and New Zealand (Kirolos et al. 2021; vCreate 2021). Research, audit, and quality improvement projects are all routinely undertaken to ensure UK NNUs are providing the best up-to-date evidence-based care to their patients and families.

Case Studies/Reflective Vignettes

Case Study 1: Parent-to-Parent Peer Support

Parent Advisory Group members are parents and carers who have experience of a child who has been cared for in an NNU. They play a vital role in ensuring the views and experiences of parents, carers, and families drive improvements and changes in neonatal care. Parental involvement is essential and PAGs are widely used at an individual hospital, network, and national level across the UK, advising on projects, service design, and quality improvement initiatives. Within networks, PAGs have provided guidance to ensure standardization of care and facilities for parents and families in an attempt to alleviate some of the anxiety that parents encounter when their baby is moved from one unit to another, often from a local neonatal unit to an NICU for specialist care or on the reverse when repatriated to a unit closer to home is required. Many parents have often built up relationships with the neonatal team and become familiar with the surroundings so the difficulties of not only having the risk of transport but also having to rebuild both relationships and trust can be stressful. PAG members are often asked to provide a parent's perspective at study days and conferences, offering a unique insight into their lived experience to complement that of the professional's experience to enhance the learning and understanding across the multidisciplinary team. PAG perspective is also represented when producing parent information leaflets and resources.

> We are all really proud to be part of the […] Parent Advisory Group. It is a fantastic opportunity to be able use our own neonatal experiences and perspectives collectively to help facilitate co-design and improvements to neonatal services. There is something cathartic about being able to do this for other families and we feel very well supported by the network.

Case Study 2: Prematurity Across the Life Course

More babies born extremely premature are surviving to adulthood than ever before, but there is a paucity of evidence on the long-term outcomes for these premature infants into adulthood. Adult Preemies Advocacy Network is a group dedicated to championing the voice of the adults who were born premature (Adult Preemie Advocacy Network 2020).

> We are a group of like-minded adults born premature that strive to connect with and advocate for other adults born early, regardless of gestation at birth or outcome.
>
> Each of our own stories is unique to us, but we also found that there were common themes and understandings with the adult preemie community.

The group's strategy plan is not only to increase knowledge and awareness of the potential life-long effects of prematurity but also to establish and strengthen a support network for adults who were born premature.

> Our hope for the future is to be able to build a community for the growing number of adults born premature, so that the growing voices of adults born premature can be heard.

Collaborating with clinicians and researchers in the neonatal community, the Adult Preemies Advocacy Network has links with UK and international research projects. neoWONDER, a UK-based group of health professionals, researchers, parents, and adults born preterm, whose aim is to use data linkage between health, education, and environmental data to investigate interventions on the long-term health and educational outcomes in very preterm babies (neoWONDER 2020).

Many adults born premature will have participated in research during their stay in NICU, or during childhood. However, long term research is often sparse. It is expensive and time consuming; often taking years, or decades to complete. As the number of babies born premature has increased, there is a growing interest in long term outcomes of premature birth. As an adult your outcomes and experiences are still of interest to researchers and can help shape and improve the future for today's premature babies.

Case Study 3: Novel Coronavirus SARS-CoV-2

The novel Coronavirus SARS-CoV-2 sent the UK into a nationwide lockdown on 23 March 2020, bringing with it unprecedented challenges and changes to working practices for the entire NHS. NNUs swiftly examined their family visiting and parental access policies, putting in place strict measures to maintain the safety of the babies, their parents and the staff caring for them. As information about this virus poured in thick and fast, neonatal stakeholders, and policy makers were updating their guidance regularly, with some units initially issuing daily updates. Almost immediately units restricted access, regulations vary slightly between units, but the majority have restricted access to parents/partners only, one just one parent at a time, some have considered a designated person to support single parent families. Siblings and wider family members have not been allowed to visit. Risk stratification in national guidelines support the unit in where to position babies within the unit, whether it isolates or cohorts according to risk. Parents are asked to wear masks when moving around the units, some units allow them to be removed at the cot-side, while others request parents continue to wear masks at all times (British Association of Perinatal Medicine 021). Reports have appeared in the press voicing concerns

over babies not experiencing smiling faces of their parents and neonatal staff due to the wearing of masks, there is no research as yet to investigate the longer-term implications of this.

Staff felt the effects as many found themselves redeployed to adult areas, or staff shortages due to sickness or shielding. Final year nursing and medical students were offered the opportunity to enter the workforce early in an attempt to bolster staffing levels. Numerous clinical staff returned from retirement or non-clinical roles to bolster their colleagues directly caring for patients. Many nurses reported anxieties surrounding personal protective equipment supply shortages, contracting the virus themselves, or acting as vectors between their home life, family, and loved ones, and the babies and families in their care. Nurses expressed feelings of posing a greater risk of themselves to the babies rather than the other way around. Social distancing impacted upon meeting spaces, break rooms, training, and education.

> *My daughter had spent a short time in NICU and as a neonatal nurse with the knowledge and understanding it was difficult as a mum. The impact this has on parents in so many ways has been huge, not only is having a baby in the neonatal unit incredibly stressful and emotional, these parents were at times having to undergo this experience without their closest loved ones. It has had an impact on siblings, extended family members and also staff themselves especially in times of bereavement and palliative care*

> *As a nurse one of the things I have found difficult was the conflicting views of my own colleagues, their thoughts on restrictions, family support, the impact on themselves over the impact of parents. I have witnessed increasing anxieties from parents regarding infection control and Covid and having more of a 'not wanting to touch' their own baby which has been incredibly sad, and I wonder what impacts this has had on bonding.*

The impact of novel Coronavirus SARS-CoV-2 will undoubtedly have effects for many years to come, these quotes are from neonatal nurses working in the midst of a global pandemic.

I feel this has affected our nursing more due to increased stress on staffing and it is making FiCare and maternal/paternal bonding even more difficult. Isolating from your new baby is something we only ever imagined in nightmares before this pandemic and now it's a true reality and this barrier needs work, because it's causing our families to suffer.

As a neonatal nurse I find it hard not being able to be a literal shoulder to cry on. Being unable to give a devastated parent a hug or and even just a hand on the shoulder has been one of the hardest things to get used to. Being a paediatric nurse for over 20 years I also miss hearing the excited footsteps and chatter from young siblings keen to meet their new brother or sister.

6.13   Conclusion

This chapter outlines the unique construct of the NHS and neonatal care provision within it. The UK neonatal community has offered many innovations to the world of neonatology and continues to strive ahead in research and evidence-based practice. UK neonatal nurses are highly trained and committed to ongoing education to provide the best care possible for babies and offer support to their parents as partners in care. UK healthcare continues to evolve and change alongside new challenges and developments, this results in the publication of further guidance. The neonatal professional community is an area of healthcare that is significantly placed to embrace new research and treatments to support the best outcomes possible. This chapter has offered an understanding of the many facets and stakeholders that drive and underpin neonatal nursing in the UK.

References

Adult Preemie Advocacy Network (2020) Home. https://adultpreemies.com/

Baby Milk Action (2021) Guide to UK formula marketing rules—the rules that apply. http://www.babymilkaction.org/ukrules-pt1

Bates SE, Isaac TCW et al (2019a) Delayed cord clamping with stabilisation at all preterm births—feasibility and efficacy of a low-cost technique. Eur J Obstet Gynecol Reprod Biol 236:109–115. https://doi.org/10.1016/j.ejogrb.2019.03.012

Bates SE, Everett E et al (2019b) Perinatal management of extreme preterm birth before 27 weeks of gestation. A framework for practice, British Association of Perinatal Medicine. https://www.bapm.org/resources/80-perinatal-management-of-extreme-preterm-birth-before-27-weeks-of-gestation-2019

Bliss (2018) Bliss releases new research on mental health. https://www.bliss.org.uk/news/bliss-releases-new-research-on-mental-health

Bliss (2020) For babies born premature or sick. https://www.bliss.org.uk/

Bliss (2021) The FINE programme. https://www.bliss.org.uk/health-professionals/training-and-events/fine

British Association of Perinatal Medicine (2011) Categories of Care 2011. https://hubble-live-assets.s3.amazonaws.com/bapm/attachment/file/43/CatsofcarereportAug11.pdf

British Association of Perinatal Medicine (2019) History of BAPM. https://www.bapm.org/history-bapm

British Association of Perinatal Medicine (2020) Neonatal networks. https://www.bapm.org/pages/19-neonatal-networks

British Association of Perinatal Medicine (2021) Covid-19 pandemic frequently asked questions within neonatal services. https://hubble-live-assets.s3.amazonaws.com/bapm/redactor2_assets/files/824/COVID_FAQ_10.1.21-final.pdf

Carson C et al (2015) Risk of psychological distress in parents of preterm children in the first year: evidence from the UK millennium cohort study. BMJ Open 5(12):e007942. https://doi.org/10.1136/bmjopen-2015

Clevermed (2020) BadgerNet. https://www.clevermed.com/badgernet/

Crawford D, Teasdale D (2011) Competence, education and careers in neonatal nursing: RCN guidance. https://create.canterbury.ac.uk/10918/1/RCN_presentation.ppt

Dobbs RH, Cremer RJ (1975) Phototherapy. Arch Dis Child 50:833–836. https://doi.org/10.1136/adc.50.11.833

Dunn PM (2007) Dr Mary Crosse, OBE, MD (1900–1972) and the premature baby. Arch Dis Child Fetal Neonatal Ed 92(2):F151. https://doi.org/10.1136/adc.2005.077529

Hanley J, Williams M (2020) Fathers' perinatal mental health. Br J Midwifery 28(2):84–85. https://doi.org/10.12968/bjom.2020.28.2.84

Health and Social Care Board (2020) Neonatal Network Northern Ireland. http://www.hscboard.hscni.net/neonatalni/

HSC Public Health Agency (2020) NICORE. https://www.publichealth.hscni.net/directorate-public-health/service-development-and-screening/nicore

Imperial College London (2020) Neonatal Medicine Research Group. https://www.imperial.ac.uk/neonatal-data-analysis-unit

Inspiration Healthcare (2021) Neonatal resuscitation LifeStartTM. https://www.inspiration-healthcare.com/products/neonatal-intensive-care/resuscitation/lifestart

Kirolos S et al (2021) Asynchronous video messaging promotes family involvement and mitigates separation in neonatal care. Arch Dis Child Fetal Neonatal Ed 106(2):172–177. https://doi.org/10.1136/archdischild-2020-319353

Mitra T, Bramwells L (2017) Exploring new ways of working in the neonatal unit. http://www.londonneonatalnetwork.org.uk/wp-content/uploads/2015/11/Exploring-New-Ways-of-Working-in-the-Neonatal-Unit-LODN.pdf

Mollison PL, Cutbush M (1949) Haemolytic disease of the newborn: criteria of severity. Br Med J 1(4594):123–130. https://doi.org/10.1136/bmj.1.4594.123

Neonatal Research (2021) History of Neonatal Medicine & Research. https://www.neonatalresearch.net/history-of-neonatal-medicine%2D%2Dresearch.html#

neoWONDER (2020) neoWONDER. https://www.neowonder.org.uk/

NHS (2019) The NHS Long Term Plan. https://www.longtermplan.nhs.uk/wp-content/uploads/2019/08/nhs-long-term-plan-version-1.2.pdf

NHS Education for Scotland (2018) Advanced nurse practitioner—National Competencies, Advanced Practice Toolkit. http://www.advancedpractice.scot.nhs.uk/education/advanced-nurse-practitioner-national-competencies.aspx

NHS England (2015) Service specifications neonatal critical care. https://www.england.nhs.uk/commissioning/wp-content/uploads/sites/12/2015/01/e08-serv-spec-neonatal-critical.pdf

Northern Ireland Assembly (2020) Northern Ireland Executive Budget 2020–21. https://www.assemblyresearchmatters.org/2020/04/02/northern-ireland-executive-budget-2020-21-initial-allocations-with-more-to-come-later/

Nursing and Midwifery Council (2020) Mid-year update. https://www.nmc.org.uk/globalassets/sitedocuments/nmc-register/september-2020/nmc-register-september-2020.pdf

Office for National Statistics (2019) Birth characteristics in England and Wales: 2018. https://www.ons.gov.uk/peoplepopulationandcommunity/birthsdeathsandmarriages/livebirths/bulletins/birthcharacteristicsinenglandandwales/2018#the-average-age-of-mothers-and-fathers-increased-for-the-10th-consecutive-year-in-2018

Office for National Statistics (2020a) Births by parents' country of birth, England and Wales: 2019. https://www.ons.gov.uk/peoplepopulationandcommunity/birthsdeathsandmarriages/livebirths/bulletins/parentscountryofbirthenglandandwales/2019

Office for National Statistics (2020b) Healthcare expenditure, UK Health Accounts. https://www.ons.gov.uk/peoplepopulationandcommunity/healthandsocialcare/healthcaresystem/bulletins/ukhealthaccounts/2018

PaediatricFOAM (2018) Parent led ward rounds on a neonatal unit. https://www.paediatricfoam.com/2019/07/parent-led-ward-rounds-on-a-neonatal-unit/

Royal College of Nursing (2021) Royal College of Nursing. https://www.rcn.org.uk/

Scottish Government (2017) The best start: five-year plan for maternity and neonatal care. https://www.gov.scot/publications/best-start-five-year-forward-plan-maternity-neonatal-care-scotland/pages/9/

Scottish Government (2020) Record investment in health and care. https://www.gov.scot/news/record-investment-in-health-and-care/

Shah DK et al (2008) Accuracy of bedside electroencephalographic monitoring in comparison with simultaneous continuous conventional electroencephalography for seizure detection in term infants. Pediatrics 121(6):1146–1154. https://doi.org/10.1542/peds.2007-1839

Smith LK et al (2017) Variability in the management and outcomes of extremely preterm births across five European countries: a population-based cohort study. Arch Dis Child Fetal Neonatal Ed 102(5):F400–F408. https://doi.org/10.1136/archdischild-2016-312100

The King's Fund (2020) NHS workforce. https://www.kingsfund.org.uk/projects/nhs-in-a-nutshell/nhs-workforce

The Nursing and Midwifery Council (2018) Realising professionalism: standards for education and training. Part 1: Standards framework for nursing and midwifery education. https://www.nmc.org.uk/globalassets/sitedocuments/education-standards/education-framework.pdf

Thomas MR et al (2014) Providing newborn resuscitation at the mother's bedside: assessing the safety, usability and acceptability of a mobile trolley. BMC Pediatr 14(1):135. https://doi.org/10.1186/1471-2431-14-135

UNICEF (2019) Parents as partners in care, 2019. https://www.unicef.org.uk/babyfriendly/parents-as-partners-in-care/

UNICEF UK (2019) The Baby Friendly Initiative. https://www.unicef.org.uk/babyfriendly/

vCreate (2021) vCreate. https://www.vcreate.tv/

Wales Government (2019) Wales Budget 2020–21. https://gov.wales/sites/default/files/publications/2019-12/2020-2021-draft-budget-childrens-leaflet.pdf

Wales Maternity and Neonatal Network (2020) Welcome to the Wales Maternity and Neonatal Network. http://www.walesneonatalnetwork.wales.nhs.uk/home

Weeks AD et al (2015) Innovation in immediate neonatal care: development of the bedside assessment, stabilisation and initial cardiorespiratory support (BASICS) trolley. BMJ Innov 1(2):53–58. https://doi.org/10.1136/bmjinnov-2014-000017

Wilkinson D, Verhagen E, Johansson S (2018) Thresholds for resuscitation of extremely preterm infants in the UK, Sweden, and Netherlands. Pediatrics 142(Suppl 1):S574–S584. https://doi.org/10.1542/peds.2018-0478I

Western Europe

7

Agnes van den Hoogen, Ingrid Hankes Drielsma, Ellis Eshuis, and Joke Wielenga

7.1 Introduction

Neonatal care is in Western Europe, as in other countries, a small specialization. Within Europe, there are disparities in the care of newborn, preterm, and ill babies. Europe has no specific society covering all neonatal nurses, but neonatal nurses are included in the network of pediatric nursing societies of Europe (PNAE). In many European countries, neonatal nurses are seen as a specialized group within pediatric nursing. Others do not have any specialized groups of nurses and societies. The European Foundation for the Care of Newborn Infants (EFCNI) now sets the standards for neonatal nursing care and

A. van den Hoogen (✉)
University Medical Centre of Utrecht (UMCU),
Wilhelmina Children's Hospital,
Utrecht, The Netherlands

Council of International Neonatal Nurses, Inc.
(COINN), Yardley, PA, USA
e-mail: ahoogen@umcutrecht.nl

I. H. Drielsma
Workplace Bureau TOPZ and Path Project,
Amsterdam, The Netherlands

E. Eshuis
Leids Universitair Medisch Centrum,
Leiden, The Netherlands

J. Wielenga
IC Neonatology, Emma Children's Hospital/
Amsterdam University Medical Center,
Amsterdam, The Netherlands

education. The European Standards of Care for Newborn Health project provides European reference standards for this healthcare area (European Foundation for the care of the Newborn Infant (EFCNI) 2021). These standards have a transdisciplinary focus developed by international working groups. They can serve as a role model not only for European countries but countries worldwide. The perspective of parents, healthcare professionals, and relevant third parties were equally considered, aiming at identifying the current best practices. On a political level, addressing European Standards of Care for Newborn Health will stimulate a new debate that can help question existing structures, identify gaps and deficiencies, and advance national healthcare systems. Strengthening healthcare systems ultimately will lead to better neonatal health outcomes.

Within Western Europe, cultural and religious differences exist. Western Europe is formed by countries including those which are considered part of Central Europe now: Austria, Belgium, Croatia, Czech Republic, Denmark, Estonia, Finland, France, Germany, Hungary, Iceland, Ireland, Italy, Latvia, Liechtenstein, Lithuania, Luxembourg, Malta, Netherlands, Norway, Poland, Portugal, Slovakia, Slovenia, Spain, Sweden, Switzerland, and the United Kingdom. Depending on which country care is given, cultural and religious differences exist whether it is related to existing practices or beliefs. Nowadays with open European Union borders and a large number of refugees, accounting for cultural differences is challenging. This situation results in differences between and within countries.

The Dutch healthcare system, for example, is highly accessible. Healthcare resources provide a well-balanced geographical coverage: a general practitioner, physiotherapist, or midwife can generally be reached by car within a few minutes. In the Dutch obstetric and perinatal care system, there is a clear division between primary, secondary, and tertiary care. Within primary care, midwives assist women during a healthy pregnancy and childbirth often in home settings. In case of (expected) complications, midwives refer pregnant women to secondary care. Obstetricians in secondary and tertiary care help pregnant women at increased risk, sometimes from the beginning of pregnancy. In many cases it is after referral by the midwife. In the Netherlands, it is policy by law, which sets limits of viability in infants from 24 weeks gestational age (GA) onwards. Parents participate in decision-making whether to start treatment or not in the age group of 24 weeks of gestation and thereafter. In the Netherlands, infants below 24 weeks are officially not actively treated.

Neonatal mortality differs among European countries. The European Peristat project defined neonatal mortality as the number of deaths during the neonatal period, up to 28 days after birth, after live birth, or after 22 completed weeks of gestation (EURO Peristat 2018). Neonatal mortality in the Netherlands declined dramatically in the period 2004–2010, but it is still relatively high compared to the 12 other Western European countries. Only Spain (Valencia region) had a higher rate, while Finland had the lowest rate. Advanced maternal age and the related risk of multiple pregnancies, the large proportion of non-western migrant women giving birth, and smoking by expectant mothers may contribute to the Netherlands' high neonatal mortality rate. Also, the effects of the Dutch screening policy, the extent to which mothers have an abortion because of anomalies found through prenatal screening, the policy regarding early preterm

babies at the limit of viability and overall care at birth remain largely unexplained (National Institute for Public Health and the Environment (RIVM) 2015). In addition, in the Netherlands, it is accepted practice that once treatment is started, it is an ongoing process of decision-making as to whether to continue, withhold, or withdraw care. This decision-making is always undertaken in close collaboration with the parents.

This chapter will describe neonatal nursing practice/care and education and give exemplars to illustrate the Western European perspective. Family Integrated Care (FIC) is the standard in the Netherlands and integrated to a certain extent in all Neonatal Intensive Care units (NICUs) and neonatal care wards.

Key "Think Points" for Learning

- Europe has no specific society covering all neonatal nurses, but neonatal nurses are included in the network of pediatric nursing societies of Europe (PNAE).
- Neonatal nursing care and standards for neonatal nursing education are now set by the European Foundation for the Care of Newborn Infants (EFCNI).
- In the Dutch system of obstetric and perinatal care, there is a clear division between primary, secondary, and tertiary care. Within primary care, midwives assist women during a healthy pregnancy and childbirth often in home settings.

7.2 Education and Training

A survey under ESPNIC (European Society of Pediatric and Neonatal Intensive Care) authorization in 2019, among NICU members in 14 Western European countries ($N = 85$), showed that almost all Western European countries have stand-alone NICUs but in 5 out of 14 countries, NICU-PICU combined units exist (Wielenga et al. 2020). The level of education, to be allowed to work on a NICU, differs, varying from a hospital certificate to master's level. To start NICU nursing specialization, a basic level of nurse education (2–4 years) is necessary in all countries. A few countries (Ireland, Netherlands, Switzerland, Italy) require extra training to nurse children; in some other countries some hospitals have the same demands, but it is not nationwide (Belgium, Denmark, Sweden), but pediatric expertise is often enough. In some Western European countries (adult) intensive care training or expertise is required to start NICU nursing training.

The duration of NICU nursing training varies from 0 to 365 days of theoretical training and 0–365 days of training on the job. During the training period, the nurses are included in unit staffing in almost all units, and they are also allocated patients.

The curriculum in all countries show similarities; anatomy, advanced life support, mechanical ventilation, noninvasive ventilation, monitoring, gastrointestinal issues, fluid management, clinical skills, care for specific groups, and psychosocial aspects are part of the curriculum in all countries. Analgesia and sedation, breastfeeding, Family Integrated Care and developmental care, clinical decision-making, ethical decision-making, transport, contributing to quality improvement, contributing to evidence-based practice are also part of the curriculum in most countries. In a few countries, leadership management, research (performing, reading, applying, and/or understanding), the professional aspect of the nursing role, clinical assessment, counseling, renal failure, and extracorporeal membrane oxygenation (ECMO) may also be part of the curriculum. However, education varies not only between countries but also within countries. NICU training is not formally recognized in half of the Western European countries.

Most countries have specialty courses such as Advanced Pediatric Life Support (APLS) (64%), ECMO (29%), or Advanced Nursing Practice (36%). Most countries do provide master courses. These are clinical or generic, but also education and research master's courses are provided in most countries. All countries do have a PhD program for nurses. Most nurse responders of the

European Society of Paediatric and Neonatal Intensive Care (ESPNIC) survey do see benefits of a set of minimum standards for the Western European countries.

In the Netherlands, all students complete a basic training of 3½ years before being registered and able to work as a general nurse. There are two training levels to become a general nurse. One is level 4 and is the equivalent of a practical nurse. The other is the bachelor training program at level 6. This meets the European qualification framework (EQF). During the basic training, students receive very basic training in child development and basic maternal, newborn, and pediatric care but may lack some experience during nursing school clinically. After graduation, every nurse wanting to work in a specific field has to follow a postgraduate course. All postgraduate education courses have to meet the national qualification standards within the specialized field of expertise.

In the Netherlands, there is a national institute, the college of quality and control of postgraduate training (CZO). They are the regulatory bodies that control the duration of the given courses, the quality of the given curriculum, and whether training hospitals meet the clinical requirements needed for the postgraduate students to become skilled in the specific field of expertise. Only then, nurses receive a national diploma in a specific field of expertise. The neonatal as well as the pediatric intensive care courses are only given by educational departments of the university hospitals that have a level 3 and 4 NICU or PICU.

As the Dutch government has stated, every nurse working with children and families in all settings has to have specific skills to meet the quality of care needed for children and their families inside and outside the hospitals. Therefore, all pediatric intensive care and neonatal intensive care nurses first follow a basic part of the postgraduate pediatric nursing course. The pediatric intensive care nurses follow the curriculum that covers pediatrics in the clinical setting for children from 0 to 12 years. Neonatal nurses follow the course from 0 to 1 year and together with the obstetric nurses, they participate in the curriculum on newborn and infant care. After completion of the first part of the pediatric course, pediatric and neonatal intensive care nurses follow a part of the intensive care course together. The final part of the curriculum is specifically geared toward pediatric or neonatal intensive care. This part of the course is given on a national level. This means universities rotate in organizing the lessons and students must follow placements in all NICU's of university clinics. If a neonatal nurse works in a level 2 or level 3 hospital, they follow part of the neonatal intensive care course but do not receive the national diploma. These neonatal nurses receive a certificate and then follow with the theoretical course at the university hospital. They receive a diploma in neonatology from their own hospital. If a neonatal nurse wants to become a neonatal intensive care nurse and work in a NICU, the nurse will have to do the final part of the neonatal intensive care course and work as a student in an NICU before getting the national diploma. Right now, all the postgraduate courses are changing their programs and are moving toward entrustable professional activities (EPAs). The aim is to make it easier for nurses to move from one specialized field to the next, if competencies are demonstrated.

7.3   Evidence-Based Practice

Different working groups nationwide in the Netherlands exist where all NICUs are represented in order to enhance evidence-based neonatal care in line with key national reports and research (EURO Peristat 2018; National Institute for Public Health and the Environment (RIVM) 2015; Picciolini et al. 2015). These working groups provide sources where every neonatal ward, including NICUs, can ask questions or obtain knowledge. New knowledge is formed based on scientific evidence in literature or practice-based consensus in these working groups. Subsequently, new research can be initiated. Every nursing head of existing NICUs in the Netherlands support the different groups. The following groups exist: (1) innovation and

research, (2) pain, (3) extreme premature, and (4) devices and materials.

There is no neonatal nursing organization in the Netherlands; however, general nurses are organized in V&VN (Dutch Society for Nurses and Caregivers) including an intensive care nursing group and a scientific nursing research group. There is a close cooperation with the Dutch parent organization (VOC), as well as the European Foundation for the care of the Newborn Infant (EFCNI 2021). In addition, with the National Association of Neonatal Nurses (NANN), the AAP (American Academy of Pediatrics), and the Association of Women's Health, Obstetric and Neonatal Nurses (AWHONN) guidelines are used in the Netherlands as well (see Chap. 1, USA).

Case Report and Lessons Learned

Umbilical venous catheters (UVCs) are commonly used in neonatal care. Although the insertion is a relatively safe procedure, complications of UVCs have been reported including infection, hemorrhage, thrombosis, malposition, and cardiac tamponade. Air embolism through an UVC is rarely reported but serious, sometimes a life-threatening, complication. In this case report, a brief description is given of a premature girl with systemic air embolism, resulting in temporary respiratory problems, circulatory skin changes, small intestinal necrosis, and cerebral air embolism, due to a disconnected UVC.

Lessons learned from this case report and the aim are to illustrate and create awareness of a case of air embolism with serious complications. In addition, it is to alert clinicians and other healthcare professionals of the cause of this disastrous event.

A girl, part of a bichorial twin, was born at 31 + 3 weeks gestation. Apgar scores were 6, 8, and 9 at 1, 5, and 10 min, respectively. Birth weight was 1885 grammes.

After admission at the neonatal intensive care unit (NICU), an umbilical venous catheter (UVC) was placed to administer nutrition and medication. An X-ray confirmed that the position of the catheter tip was correct. Continuous positive airway pressure (CPAP) and one dose of surfactant via the intubation, surfactant, then extubation (INSURE) technique were given because of idiopathic respiratory distress syndrome (IRDS). CPAP was continued until day 4, after which respiratory support with low flow nasal cannula was started. On day 7, a nurse was asked to remove the UVC. After accidently disconnecting the line, the patient started gasping and oxygen saturation dropped to 42%. She was not reacting to stimulation and the administration of extra oxygen. Resuscitation with 100% oxygen was started successfully. The skin of the left foot went from pale to marbled purple, extending to both legs and the left part of the body. Inspection of the UVC showed an open lumen of the UVC. Therefore, aspiration of blood from the inserted catheter was collected, which was without air bubbles, and the UVC was removed. After 45 min, the skin color became normal.

After a few hours, the abdomen became dilated and gastric feeding was not well tolerated. An X-ray showed portal air; however, no signs of free abdominal gas were shown. After 10 hours, the X-ray was repeated and showed free abdominal gas. A laparotomy was performed and showed patchy necrosis of the small intestine without signs of enterocolitis. One necrotic part showed a perforation. A total of 45 cm of small intestine was resected, and eight connections were made. Pathology examination showed multiple jejunal resections with the histological picture of disturbed circulation, focal transmural necrosis, and pseudomembranous colitis with multiple perforations.

Cranial ultrasonography performed before the laparotomy showed evidence of cerebral air embolism, as a number of echogenic densities were created an acoustic shadow with no through transmission, mainly on the left hemisphere. Cranial ultrasonography was repeated after 1 day and showed inhomogeneous white matter and an intraventricular hemorrhage grade 1 on the left. Magnetic resonance imaging (MRI) of the brain, performed shortly after the incident, showed two small white matter lesions on the left hemisphere, which fully recovered on an MRI after 2 months with a good neurologic prognosis.

Outcome and follow-up: The girl showed good recovery after the surgery with no intestinal complications. She had normal Griffiths neurodevelopmental assessment scores at the corrected age of 1.5 years (Picciolini et al. 2015). At the time of this incident, an official incident statement was made with the board of the hospital and an investigation was performed. The parents were informed, and psychological support was provided for parents and staff.

It was concluded that air embolism from the open UVC must be the explanation of the clinical deterioration of this infant. Medical and nursing protocols were revised to prevent such a serious complication in the future.

7.4 Conclusion

This chapter outlines neonatal nursing education and training practices in Western Europe. The organization of neonatal care in this region of the world is described. Evidence-based practices and standards have been developed and care outcomes are improving. Neonatal nurses who are well trained are key to improving health outcomes.

References

EURO Peristat (2018) European perinatal health report. https://www.europeristat.com/images/EPHR2015_web_hyperlinked_Euro-Peristat.pdf

European Foundation for the care of the Newborn Infant (EFCNI) (2021) https://newborn-health-standards.org/

National Institute for Public Health and the Environment (RIVM) (2015) Dutch health care performance report 2014. https://www.rivm.nl/bibliotheek/rapporten/2015-0050.pdf

Picciolini O, Squarza C, Fontana C, Giannì ML, Cortinovis I, Gangi S, Gardon L, Presezzi G, Fumagalli M, Mosca F (2015) Neurodevelopmental outcome of extremely low birth weight infants at 24 months corrected age: a comparison between Griffiths and Bayley Scales. BMC Pediatr 15(1):1–9. https://doi.org/10.1186/s12887-01

Wielenga JM, NICU nursing standards. The 8th Congress of the European Academy of Paediatric Societies (EAPS 2020) virtual congress 16-18 October, 2020. Abstract Publication - EAPS 2020 (kenes.com)

Eastern Europe

8

Marina Boykova

8.1 Introduction

Neonatal care in Europe varies from the eastern and western perspectives. I will use Russia, or Russian Federation, as the example for Eastern Europe, realizing there are large variations in other eastern European countries. Russia is the largest country in the world, and it spans from Europe to Japan, having 11 time zones, with the population totaling approximately 143 million people and birth rate around 13.2 births per 1000 (Baranov et al. 2016). There are about 12 million people living in Moscow (the capital city) and about 5.5 million people residing in the second-largest city of Saint Petersburg; almost ¾ of Russia's population lives in the European portion of the country (Baranov et al. 2016). Russia underwent a period of transition during perestroika (1985–1991) moving from the Soviet Union socialist model of healthcare (that was free to citizens) to one that offers the free services as well as one of privatized care at present. This chapter describes personal perspectives on neonatal nursing education and practice using the author's own exemplars to illustrate the Russian

M. Boykova (✉)
School of Nursing and Health Sciences, Holy Family University, Philadelphia, PA, USA

Council of International Neonatal Nurses, Inc. (COINN), Yardley, PA, USA

neonatal care and the impact of the international collaborations in helping infants to survive.

> **Key "Think Points" for Learning**
>
> - Neonatal nursing education/training is part of general and pediatric specialties.
> - Professional nursing education standards are set by the Ministry of Education.
> - Professional nursing practice standards are set by Ministry of Health Care.
> - International collaboration is the key for improving neonatal care/policies in countries where nurses have little autonomy.

8.2 Organization of Neonatal Care

Neonatal nursing care in Russia is a subspecialty of pediatric and general nursing care. Under the Soviet Union healthcare system, maternity houses were set up to provide care for the mother during labor, delivery, and immediate period after the birth (first days and weeks). Care was free, and there was an emphasis on health promotion/disease prevention; care was centralized according to the Semashko Health Care Model named

J. Petty et al. (eds.), *Neonatal Nursing: A Global Perspective*,
https://doi.org/10.1007/978-3-030-91339-7_8

after the Minister of Health from 1918 to 1930 (Baranov et al. 2016). According to UNICEF (2020), the infant mortality rate and neonatal mortality rate were 4.9 and 2.6 per 1000 live births in 2019, respectively. The national healthcare system established during the Soviet Union era is still working effectively at present. During the last few decades, there were several large perinatal centers established throughout the country. At present, almost all citizens have state-based health insurance; they can also use private health insurance and pay for private care if they so desire.

Almost 99% of babies are delivered in the maternity houses, where they usually stay 3–5 days (as well as mothers) before being discharged to home. While some maternity houses have the ability to provide advanced neonatal care, in most cases when an infant is born sick or prematurely, the baby is transported to a specialized neonatal unit housed within a children's hospital. Home births are almost nonexistent. All citizens have access to the regionalized system of health care and free transportation to a hospital as the system retains a socialized medical perspective. Distances between a rural hospital and a tertiary center often result in delays; at present, air transports are being used more often than decades ago.

8.3 Nursing Education and Competencies

Nursing basic education in Russia is a part of the country's mid-level education and does not belong to the higher education system (such as one existing for medical professionals). There are different types of nursing schools in Russia that provide education and training, with the programs that usually last about 3–4 years (similar to the bachelor's degree in western countries). There are (1) nursing schools that prepare nurses for general practice, (2) nursing schools that prepare pediatric nurses specifically, and (3) there are schools for midwives. Some schools have extended programs/tracks to train advanced practice nurses (called "feldshers") who often serve

on ambulances and provide care in remote, rural areas (delivering babies, managing minor traumas, and so on).

According to the Russian Nurses Association (RNA) (2013), nurses can specialize in many aspects of nursing care: operating room, anesthesia, pediatric and psychiatric care, massage and dentistry, nutrition, and diet, to name a few. The advanced nursing practice role (such as in the USA, for instance) does not exist in its fullest extent (for instance, nurses cannot prescribe medications). There are several departments of higher nursing education (in universities) that provide education and training in leadership and management (such as University of the Great Novgorod, the Pavlov Institute in Saint-Petersburg, I.M. Sechenov First Moscow State Medical University). All nursing education programs and its content are regulated by the Ministry of Higher Education and the Ministry of Health Care of the Russian Federation. The RNA in conjunction with the International Council of Nurses (ICN) established nursing standards and the title of Bachelor of Nursing to be used by those nurses who have experience and received education at the bachelor level (RNA 2013). In addition to the diploma in nursing received upon finishing a nursing school, nurses have to have a certificate (similar to a license) in order to work as a nurse. Recertification occurs every 5 years (Difazio et al. 2004); the RNA sets standards for professional nursing, in line with the recommendations, guidelines, and decrees from the Ministry of Health Care and the Ministry of Education.

Many practicing neonatal nurses receive their basic education/training as general or pediatric nurses. The basic aspects of neonatal care are well covered in the nursing schools (such as umbilical cord care, neonatal jaundice, thermoregulation, physiological transitions, aspects of breastfeeding and immunizations, for instance), but not the advanced neonatal care. Extra training/specialization is done on the neonatal unit itself during orientation programs where nurses, in most cases, are taught by physicians who provide information on more advanced topics in neonatal care (e.g., artificial lung ventilation, tracheoesophageal fistulas, heart defects, malrotations, short bowel syndrome). Orientation programs for novice neonatal nurses usually last for several weeks (up to 2 months); also, novice nurses work with a preceptor for a few first shifts. There are also professional development/refresher courses (called "enhancing qualification courses") that are repeated periodically and where examinations are required (and used for the certificate renewal). Neonatal nursing care competencies are not described/present. Nurses who have at least 3 years' experience can also participate in a professional advancement system. This system is similar to a clinical ladder system for promotion in other countries.

8.4 Challenges and Opportunities

One of the first challenges is the hierarchy in medicine and nursing: nursing is considered a subservient profession and nurses do not have full autonomy when caring for their patients. Prescriptions/permissions from medical doctors/physicians are always required for the care to be provided by a nurse. Funding for nurses and nursing education still lags behind medicine. Due to low salaries and just the mere size of the Russian Federation, nurses often cannot afford traveling long distances to conferences to share experiences. Nurses often cannot afford attending international conferences abroad as well, due to financial reasons. There are no Russian-language neonatal care textbooks written specifically for nurses by nurses; there are no neonatal nursing journals at present. Language barriers and insufficient funds also prevent nurses from paying a subscription for English-language neonatal care journals or paying membership fees for international neonatal nursing organizations. Nurses are often tasked with non-health-related work (such as mopping floors, cleaning equipment, and other tasks) that take them away from the bedside. This situation is slowly changing. The Russian government made great strides to decrease neonatal and infant mortality rates in recent decades (perinatal centers, appropriate, and contemporary equipment), but there is still a way to go.

8.5 Research and Evidence-Based Practice

Nurses still lack as many opportunities for advanced education as found in medical education, research methods are rarely taught, and nursing research is in its beginning stage. At present, few nurses have an experience with conducting research as a research degree (Doctor of Philosophy or PhD) is still not available for nurses in Russia. Evidence to support many neonatal nursing care protocols reside in medicine that do not always address the importance of the core element of nursing—human caring. Often, evidence is coming from studies conducted in foreign countries. However, Russian nursing research and evidence-based practice are slowly growing and developing.

8.6 Professional Associations

There are approximately 1.24 million employed nurses in Russia (data as of 2018) (Statista Research and Analysis 2020). The Russian Nurses Association, founded in 1992, represents Russian nurses to the International Council of Nurses (ICN), sets professional standards for nursing and defines nursing specializations. Most nurses belong to this organization. The organization recognizes a lack of legislative recognition for nursing and a growing need for higher level nursing education and practice guidelines/standards. The RNA supports the development of evidence-based practice guidelines as well as the development of neonatal nursing networks.

Neonatal nurses have a chapter under the RNA. The RNA's Neonatal Chapter sets a goal of improving neonatal nursing practice by setting standards of care that are evidence-based. Some Russian neonatal nurses belong to the Council of International Neonatal Nurses, Inc. (COINN). Because of the lack of voice for our specialization until recently, neonatal nursing care has not progressed as quickly as neonatal medicine. However, collaborations with colleagues from abroad, educational exchange programs with other countries—for instance, Sweden, Finland,

United Kingdom, and United States—have helped boost the development of the nursing role as well as nursing education.

Reflective Practice

My first education was at the small village school (called 'srednya schola' in Soviet Union). This was general education similar to a high school education in other countries (Difazio et al. 2004); the course of study was 10 years, starting at the age of 7 years old; it was free for all citizens. Upon finishing my high school, at the age of 17, I wanted to explore the world and I moved to the city of Leningrad (later renamed Saint Petersburg, the second largest city in Russia), which was about 400 miles (660 km) from my home. My mom worried about me, but she let me go—I was stubborn and a determined child. I was then accepted into a nursing school #3 (called 'medizinskoe uchulishe') in Leningrad to study nursing. My basic nursing education was completely free—there was no tuition to be paid and all the textbooks were provided in the school's library. Also, as a student in good standing, I received a stipend that helped with my living expenses in a big city while being a student. My nursing school did not specialize in paediatric nursing care—it was a general nursing practice program where nursing students were mostly taught by physicians and only occasionally by nurses (usually those who were practising clinically adjunct clinical faculty). The basic neonatal care (care for healthy newborn babies) was completely covered in my course of study, but not advanced neonatal care. This education resulted in the title "medical sister" upon my graduation ('medizinskaya sestra' in Russian language, an equivalent to a 'nurse' in western and westernized countries). My basic nursing education, by western standards, was

at the diploma level—just a little bit longer than 2 years of nursing education following high school—but it served me very well all my life. I believe the program for nurses at that time was very strong, despite the fact that it was medically oriented and lasted for only about 2 years. In those times, there was no certification or license requirement to practice as a nurse—my diploma was my license and my certificate.

Upon finishing my nursing program, I was hired by the neonatal intensive care unit (NICU) at the Children's Hospital #1 of Saint Petersburg, with the 12-bed capacity department for sick newborns. The regular shifts for nurses at that time were 24, 12, and 8 h. I started working 24-h shifts (as a novice). For the first few weeks, I worked with a preceptor to gain more knowledge and experience in neonatal care, which was required by the rules of the Soviet healthcare system at these times. The guidance from an experienced nurse was really helpful. Also, every Autumn there was an in-service/orientation program lasting a few weeks where novice nurses/staff nurses were given more education in neonatal care, usually by neonatologists because in the 1990s nurses could/ were not allowed to teach neonatal care.

Everything was extremely foreign to me during my first days in the neonatal intensive care unit—everything there was well above the basic newborn care! I was scared to touch babies (who were blueish and hardly breathing because they had respiratory distress syndrome), I could not read their signs, I had a little knowledge about respiratory equipment etc.—and I was a very good student all my life, but I did not study all of 'this' at my nursing school! The first months and years of being a neonatal intensive care nurse were really stressful. I remember myself coming home after my 24-h shift and just falling asleep while sitting on the couch—I was so tired. But I loved working with babies and my job was so rewarding—and so, I worked as a staff nurse in my unit for almost 20 years.

My unit was small (12 beds). We had very limited equipment and supplies (many of those were not disposable, such as syringes, endotracheal tubes (ETT), catheters for suctioning ETT); we had only a limited number of incubators and ventilators. As we had only three cardiac/blood pressure monitors, we mostly had to rely on our own patient assessment skills. The unit's mortality rate was high (around 30%); nurses had to perform many non-nursing tasks (cleaning used syringes before sterilization, mopping floors, dusting cabinets, taking trash to the garbage bins outside, etc.). Nurses in my unit usually had to care for 3 to 4 babies every shift (including preterm and surgical patients); most nurses worked ten or eleven 24-h shifts per month. All neonatal patients were transported from maternity facilities outside our paediatric hospital. Parents could only visit babies at certain hours during the day; they were allowed to just see their baby from behind the wall glass window.

As nursing is subservient to the medical profession, staff nurses were not involved in daily medical rounds; asking nurses' opinions regarding their patient status was rare. Use of nursing process and nursing documentation of a patient's status was absent; we only recorded heart and respiratory rates, blood pressure (when a monitor was available), input/output/temperature, number of ETT suctioning and parameters of lung ventilation set up by physicians. Most nursing care was about recording vital signs, mixing and administering intravenous (IV) solutions, administering medications by physician's prescription, suctioning ETT, collecting urine for tests/sputum for culturing, oral feedings and skin/umbilical cord care. At that time, in the 1990s, staff nurses were not allowed to draw blood for tests or put peripheral IV catheters. In my unit we had only one nurse who could do it as she was more experienced. Such a nurse was called a 'procedure nurse'. In addition to taking venous blood for tests/putting peripheral IV catheters, she would also perform wound dressing changes for all surgical patients on the unit and assist physicians/surgeons during procedures (e.g., exchange blood transfusion, lumbar puncture). A procedure nurse was on the day-hours shift schedules from 9 am to 5 pm. Every morning she drew venous blood to send to the laboratory (for electrolytes and culture). During night hours or weekends, when there was no procedure nurse, a physician on duty would draw blood for testing, but not staff nurses. There were a lot of challenges those days, but despite all the difficulties and hierarchical structure, we had a very good team of nurses and doctors—there were not so many of us and we all knew each other very well (even celebrated holidays together such as New Year).

As we did not have any neonatal nursing care books or journals, I had to use medical literature to educate myself about advanced care for neonates. In the beginning of 1990s, we did not have Internet; there was only one book in our hospital library that was translated into Russian—the book written by American neonatologist, Sheldon B. Korones, "High-risk newborn infants: The basis for intensive nursing care" in 1972. Following recommendation by a neonatologist in my unit, I read this book—and it was very helpful for me. I also read other materials—anything I could find, mostly medical textbooks that I borrowed from my unit's physicians. Then I became lucky—as perestroika evolved and more people had travelled to Russia after the period of the 'iron curtain', American nurses and doctors visited my unit from Children's Hospital Oakland, California.

I only had about 1 year of experience as a NICU nurse when the first visit of the American team occurred. The collaboration between two children's hospitals continued for almost 15 years; visits occurred approximately once a year, for about 2 weeks. The American team usually consisted of neonatologists, nurses, respiratory therapists, biomedical engineers, and sometimes other specialists (such as surgeon, neurosurgeon, nurse practitioner, infection control nurse). During these visits, the American nurses and doctors were making clinical rounds, discussing difficult cases, lecturing on specific advanced care management in neonatal practice. During the first visit, the American neonatal team brought us some equipment (such as incubators, ventilators, humidifiers, pulse oximeters, suctioning equipment) and helped to provide direct care to preterm twins, the first extremely preterm infants admitted to our unit. Later on, they were bringing educational materials as well—medical and nursing neonatal textbooks, hospital's care protocols, medical and nursing journals. I remember how excited I was when my American nurse colleague brought me a neonatal nursing care textbook in 1995 (the first edition of Comprehensive neonatal nursing care of 1993 by Carole Kenner, Ann Brueggemeyer, and Laurie Porter Gunderson)—the huge (more than 1200 pages) and heavy (almost 7 lb) book was all about neonates and caring for them! It was the knowledge that I really needed and wanted to have.

These visits were eye-opening experiences: I was able to observe who nurses could be and what nurses could do! It was amazing to see the advanced skills, knowledge, teamwork and autonomy nurses had while providing care and advocating for the patient. Nurses were involved in the rounds, nurses were lecturing, nurses were putting percutaneous central lines in, taking blood samples from the arteries—some of the things that we, Russian nurses, were not permitted to perform. But we learned from our American colleagues, whose levels of neonatal knowledge and experiences were very high. Gradually, we changed practices in our unit: nurses stopped performing non-nursing tasks (cleaning/dusting), domestic/technician personnel were hired, and the respiratory care nurse role was developed. Procedure nurses' roles were expanded by my unit: we started putting peripheral and central lines around the clock, as well as put arterial peripheral catheters in. Nurse-patient ratio was decreased from one nurse to two patients. The unit was expanded, more beds were created, and more nurses were hired. Nurses began to spend more time with the patients. Some Russian nurses and doctors were able to visit the NICU Children's Hospital Oakland and shared their knowledge gained abroad with the Russian team upon return from the U.S.A.

Of course, these changes did not happen overnight. It took quite a long time and a lot of effort from nurses, neonatologists as well as support from the unit/hospital and city administration. Also, in my case, the professional collaboration grew into real friendship with my American colleagues— people who broke my mind, whom I have known over 30 years now, and who showed me what nurses can do and who nurses can be. I would like to acknowledge at least some of them here, my dearest friends: nurses Carolyn Lund, Beryl Epstein, and Susie Adams, doctors David Durand and Art D'Harlingue.

As a result of this long-lasting collaboration and changes, I am proud to say that the mortality rate in my unit was reduced to 3–5%. My unit became the largest unit in the city, with the lowest mortality rates in critically ill neonates. My unit became an exemplar for the highest quality of neona-

tal care in my country, and we started to share our experience with nurses and doctors from other hospitals, regions of Russia and former Soviet Union republics. My unit became a well-known neonatal teaching centre. City's neonatal mortality rate (NMR) was also reduced—it became the lowest NMR in the country, and my unit's medical director was nationally recognised for his and our work. All this happened because of the following: (1) the collaboration was not a 1-day project, it was a continuous programme, (2) the key people in both teams, American and Russian, were the same through the years which provided better understanding of needs and needed consistency in exchange of information/knowledge and experiences, and (3) support from hospital and city leadership/administration was present. And of course, passion from people involved in this international collaboration.

There was also one another critically important factor that helped my unit to become the best in the country—educating neonatal nurses. After about 4 years working as a staff NICU nurse, I became a student again—I was admitted to the collaborative project between nursing school in Chester, England, and Russian nursing school, the Medical College #1 (aka nursing school #1) in 1994. It was the time of perestroika and international programs/collaborations were blooming. My unit's chief of neonatology, Dr. Vjacheslav (Slava) Lubimenko, was very innovative and supportive physician who strongly believed that nurses should teach nurses—we had very good working relationships and we talked a lot about it in our unit—nurses (including me) needed to know more about neonatal advanced care (and not just basic neonatal care). When he heard a radio announcement that there was a course/program to be developed between Russian college and nursing school in England, he phoned me immediately (I was on my vacation in my hometown, about 6 h by train from Saint-Petersburg) and said that I would have an interview tomorrow afternoon for the program that would prepare me to teach our nurses. I jumped on the train, and the next morning I was interviewed by British professors—and admitted to the collaborative programme. At that time, it was a certificate programme—a certificate in teaching nursing. Me and five other Russian nurses stayed at Chester College for 2–4 weeks of study twice per year. This certificate program lasted approximately 1.5 years and was sponsored by Chester College, with Ms. Dorothy Marriss, the Dean of the School of Nursing and Social Work, and Reverend Binks, the President, being extremely supportive to us. Everything was free for Russian nurses—we only paid for our airline tickets and visas (which was really expensive because of very low nursing salaries in my country). This education and trips to England opened my mind, thanks to the wonderful teachers we had there as well to the support received from Russian nursing school administration, Drs. Irina Bublikova and Zoya Gaponova.

After receiving my teaching certificate in 1995, I continued to work in the NICU as a staff nurse and I began teaching nurses at my unit using textbooks and materials brought to my unit by our American colleagues. The collaboration between Medical College #1 and Chester College continued: later on, I earned my BSc and MS degrees from Chester College. Each program was about 2 years of study, kind of distance learning, with about 2-weeks stays in England twice a year. I also attended the Great Novgorod University Department of Higher Nursing Education (about 3 h drive from Saint Petersburg) to obtain a diploma in nursing management (Difazio et al. 2004). This took about 4 years to complete *and it was not easy as I was a student at two universities (England and Russia) simultaneously and worked full time as well. My trips to England usually took place during my vacation time; Novgorod trips were my paid leave of absence as my neonatal medical director, Dr. Slava Lubimenko, and my hospital chief, Dr. Anatoly Kagan, were very supportive as well. We developed a program for teaching neonatal nursing care in our unit that we shared with all our visitors from other regions of Russia. In 2008, 1 year following my graduation with a master's degree from Chester, I went to the United States of America to pursue a doctoral degree (Doctor of Philosophy, PhD). I wanted to continue my education—at that time there were no research degree programs for nurses in Russia and even now, to my knowledge there is still no comparable program for doctoral studies in Russia. I successfully completed my PhD course of study and defended my dissertation in 2015. At present, I am teaching at a university and involved in international work with the Council of International Neonatal Nurses, Inc. (COINN).*

8.7 Conclusion

Russia is changing as is neonatal nursing. The visibility of neonatal nursing should grow. This chapter has highlighted the organization of neonatal care, training and education of neonatal nurses, and some of the challenges and opportunities. Providing appropriate/advanced education for nurses who take care of neonates, affording neonatal nurses the opportunity to be involved into the international projects/collaborations, to attend conferences, to meet nurse researchers, and to establish new networks is vitally important for reducing neonatal and infant mortality— locally, nationally, and internationally. These activities along with the support from professional nursing organizations will also advance professional neonatal nursing.

References

Baranov A, Namazova-Baranov L, Albitskiy V, Ustinova N, Tertetskaya R, Komarova O (2016) The Russian child health care system. J Pediatr 177S:S148–S155

Difazio R, Lang D, Boykova M (2004) Nursing in Russia: a "Travelogue". J Pediatr Nurs 19(2):150–156. https://www.academia.edu/23478783/Nursing_in_Russia_a_travelogue_

Russian Nurses Association (RNA) (2013) Advanced practice nursing in the Russian Federation (Russia). Int Adv Pract Nurs. https://internationalapn.org/2013/11/06/russia/

Statista Research and Analysis (2020) Number of practicing nurses employed in Russia from 2000 to 2018. https://www.statista.com/statistics/463479/practising-nurses-employment-in-russia/

UNICEF (2020) Monitoring the situation of children and women. https://data.unicef.org/resources/data_explorer/unicef_f/?ag=UNICEF&df=GLOBAL_DATAFLOW&ver=1.0&dq=RUS.CME_MRM0.&startPeriod=1970&endPeriod=2020

South Africa

9

Carin Maree

9.1 Introduction

South Africa is a developing country, part of the Sub-Saharan region and a land characterized by diversity, and this applies to neonatal care as well. Healthcare is provided in a two-tier system divided between public healthcare funded by government and private healthcare. Public healthcare is available to all citizens, while private healthcare is available to those who can afford private health insurance or to pay for private care. The care is further diversified amongst urban, semi-urban, and rural areas, while healthcare consumers are characterized by a variety of cultures, languages, religions, as well as socioeconomic backgrounds (Young 2016).

State-of-the-art neonatal intensive care units can be found in private hospitals in larger towns and cities, as well as in some tertiary or academic hospitals associated with universities. Unfortunately, neonatal intensive care units can also be found in old and dilapidated facilities with lack of working equipment and with a much higher demand for care than what can be provided for.

The staffing situation reflects the same picture and varies from units being staffed with sufficient and trained staff to units being understaffed and often with staff with limited neonatal experience. The categories and training of nurses in South Africa is regulated by the South African Nursing Council (SANC) and will be explained later in the chapter.

The neonatal mortality rate is reported as being between 12 and 21 deaths per 1000 live births in 2016 (Rhoda et al. 2018). The variance might be alluded to the different settings being reported on by the different databases being used to monitor and report on the neonatal mortality rate. The District Health Information System (DHIS) is mainly used in the public sector. The Perinatal Problem Identification Programme (PPIP) and Child Problem Identification Programme (Child PIP) report on information from the public and private health sectors, but only on facilities that participate voluntarily. Vital Statistics of South Africa (StatsSA) report on official deaths reported by the public and private sectors (Department of Statistics, RSA (STATSSA) 2019). The South African Demographic Health Survey (SADHS) and Rapid Mortality Surveillance (RMS) reports are attempts to collate the data from the different databases. The Medical Research Council (MRC), the National Perinatal Morbidity and Mortality Committee (NaPemmCo), and the

C. Maree (✉)
Department of Nursing Science, University of Pretoria, Pretoria, South Africa

Council of International Neonatal Nurses, Inc. (COINN), Yardley, PA, USA
e-mail: carin.maree@up.ac.za

National Department of Health (NDoH) collaborate to provide the reports on the South African neonatal mortality (Rhoda et al. 2018).

The Neonatal Nurses' Association of Southern Africa (NNASA) is a nonprofit organization with the aim of improving neonatal care, especially through creating informal training opportunities and collaboration. Any nurse with an interest in neonatal nursing can become a member of the association.

> **Key "Think Points" for Learning**
>
> - Neonatal care in South Africa is clarified in terms of different care levels and the related equipment, skills, and personnel.
> - Training of nurses in South Africa is complicated, especially specialization in neonatal nursing.
> - Neonatal care advanced as knowledge and technology improved.

9.2   Education and Training

Nurse training of all categories are regulated by the SANC under the Nursing Act (Act no. 33 of 2005). Changes in South African legislation related to higher education to move towards a national qualification framework (Minister of Higher Education and Training 2013) had a ripple effect on nursing education. Nursing education is therefore currently in a phase of transition. Auxiliary nurses previously followed a 1-year course, and this category of nurses will remain—they will now obtain a higher certificate in nursing after successful completion of a 1-year programme. The 2-year programme for enrolled nurses will now be replaced by a 3-year diploma programme, and successful candidates will register as a general nurse. A general nurse will be able to enroll for a 1-year advanced diploma to register as a midwife (https://www.sanc.co.za/wp-content/uploads/2021/04/SANC-Study-brochure.pdf). These programmes could and still can be presented by nursing colleges or nursing schools in the public and private sectors

(South African Nursing Council (SANC) 2015, 2016).

Professional nurses could previously follow a 4-year bachelor's degree, or a 4-year diploma programme to register as general, community, and psychiatric nurse and midwife. They could also follow the 2-year programme for enrolled nurses plus a bridging programme to be registered as a general nurse. Of these programmes, the bachelor's degree was presented by universities, and the other programmes were presented by nursing colleges or nursing schools from the public and private sectors. With the changed curricula, professional nurses can follow only a Bachelor of Nursing degree at a university to be registered with SANC as a professional nurse and midwife (https://www.sanc.co.za/wp-content/uploads/2021/04/SANC-Study-brochure.pdf).

During the system which is being phased out (commonly referred to as legacy qualifications), specialization in a variety of nursing disciplines could be done through successful completion of a 1- or 2-year programme at a college or university. From 2001 until 2012, specialization in neonatal nursing was acknowledged by the SANC, and they were registered with an additional qualification in neonatal nursing. The qualification was discontinued as an independent specialization from 2012. There were only 334 specialized neonatal nurses reflected in 2020 on the SANC website who obtained registration between 2001 and 2012. Specialized programmes that include at least a component of neonatal nursing are child critical care nursing (6), child/pediatric nursing (3101), advanced/post basic midwifery and neonatal nursing (5104), advanced pediatric and neonatal nursing (13), of which the numbers registered in brackets were relevant in 2020 (http://ncsacoms.co.za/wp-content/uploads/2021/04/Stats-2020-2-Registrations-and-Listed-Qualifications.pdf). Some specialized neonatal nurses who possessed a bachelor's degree continued to obtain a master's and even doctoral degree in neonatal nursing. As these qualifications are not acknowledged by the SANC and there is not another body to capture the information, it is not known how neonatal nurses have obtained postgraduate degrees in neonatal nursing. The legacy qualifications will be replaced by one-year postgraduate diplomas presented by universities in a range of specializations. Unfortunately, specialization in neonatal nursing is not included in the range for acknowledgement by the SANC. Specializations with a component of neonatal nursing will be child nursing, child critical care nursing, and midwifery (https://www.sanc.co.za/education-and-training/).

As the regulatory body of nursing, the SANC is responsible for the regulations, competency frameworks, and scope of practice of the various categories of nurses (Nursing Act no 33 of 2005). There is currently not a specific competency framework for neonatal nurses in South Africa. A competency framework was proposed by the Neonatal Nurses Association of South Africa to the SANC as part of a motivation for recognition of neonatal nursing as a specialization, but as the specialization will not be acknowledged, the competency framework will also not be formally accepted (Maree et al. 2021; Scheepers et al. 2020). The current scope of practice for registered nurses is relevant (SANC Reg. 786 of 2013), while a new scope of practice is expected to be published in the near future for public comment (SANC Press Release 4/2020, 2020a, b).

The standards for neonatal care are adopted from a variety of sources, but it is left to the respective settings which ones are applied. Commonly used guidelines to support unit-specific standards include the Bettercare Programmes (https://bettercare.co.za/), the World Health Organization's guidelines for newborn care (https://www.who.int/maternal_child_adolescent/newborns/care_at_birth/en/) and guidelines provided by the National Department of Health as part of South Africa's national strategic plan for a Campaign on Accelerated Reduction of Maternal and Child Mortality in Africa (CARMMA) (Department of Health 2015).

9.3 The Organization of Neonatal Care

Adequately trained staff is needed to provide neonatal care in public and private settings. Neonatal care is catered for in the public sector on different levels in 251 district hospitals (level I services), 48 regional hospitals (level II services), and 27 tertiary hospitals (level III services) (Health Systems Trust 2012). Level I services refer to basic care of the healthy newborn and stabilization and transfer of a sick baby. Level II services include basic care, stabilization of a sick baby, and a receiving facility for sick babies with common illnesses, who might need noninvasive ventilation or invasive ventilation for a relatively short period of time. Level III services imply care of babies born from high-risk pregnancies, sick babies, and babies in need of specialized intensive care. Level III services serve as receiving hospitals for referrals and transfers from regional hospitals and are often associated with universities that provide healthcare training.

Neonatal care in the private sector is provided by approximately 230 private hospitals (Health Systems Trust 2012). The private healthcare facilities are not specifically classified according to levels of service, and the same facility might provide level I service in some disciplines and level II or III in other disciplines. There is also a more fluid referral system between the facilities.

The total number of facilities that accommodate high-risk and sick neonates are therefore a minimum of 556, with the number of beds per facility varying from 4 to 40. Although the ideal would be for all shift leaders to be specialists, there is a severe shortage. When possible, the shift leaders are specialized in neonatal nursing, child nursing, advanced midwifery or critical care (adult) nursing, but they are often registered nurses with neonatal nursing experience only and no specialization. The shift leaders are supported by registered nurses and enrolled nurses, and in some units, they might even employ auxiliary nurses to manage despite the staff shortage. According to SANC (Nursing Act no 33 of 2005), the enrolled and auxiliary nurses are supposed to work under the direct supervision of a registered nurse.

The nursing staff forms part of the multidisciplinary teams in the neonatal intensive care units, which might include medical practitioners, physiotherapists, occupational therapists, speech therapists, dieticians, breastfeeding consultants, psychologists, and counsellors. In limited settings, the team might include a neonatal/pediatric surgeon, geneticist, pediatric neurologist, cardiologist, nephrologist, or endocrinologist. In the public sector, they are employees of the government, while in the private sector, they tend to be self-employed or be in partnerships.

The medical practitioners form a crucial part of the team and are found in all NICUs. The medical practitioners in the tertiary hospitals are commonly working in groups or firms headed by a pediatrician or neonatologist. The other members of the groups or firms might include registrars who are in the process of specialization as a pediatrician or neonatologist, and medical officers with various levels of experience as medical practitioners. The secondary hospitals follow a similar structure, but without registrars. District hospitals might employ pediatricians or not. There should always be one or more medical practitioners on the premises of a hospital available to the NICU. There is also a staff shortage of medical practitioners in South Africa, especially of specialists, which negatively impacts on public sector NICUs.

In the private sector mainly, pediatricians are involved in NICUs. The individual pediatricians or partnerships usually have agreements with the private hospitals to admit critically ill or at-risk neonates to the NICUs. They then do hospital visits to see their patients and are the rest of the time available telephonically for consultation. If necessary, they will return to the NICU for example for cases of emergency, very unstable patients or new admissions. The implication is that there is not necessarily a medical practitioner available to the NICU on the premises, and if they are on the premises, they do not attend to other practitioners' patients. The nursing staff in the NICU is expected to cope with emergency cases until the pediatrician arrives, or to continue with care following telephonic requests.

The situation is very similar with the other multidisciplinary team members in the public and private sectors, except that physiotherapists, occupational therapists, speech therapists, and dieticians are not always available at all the NICUs in either public or private sector. In the public sector, they are mainly available at the last tertiary facilities and to various degrees in the regional and district hospitals, where they would be employees. It is common practice for them to do ward rounds on a daily basis and see all neonates who need to be seen.

The team members in the private sector are usually private practitioners either on their own or as part of group practices. They are commonly only located in urban areas. There might be slight variations on how they are recruited to consult patients, but usually they receive formal referral invitations. There is a fee related to their services which is paid by the parents' medical insurance or the parents need to fit the bill. This has an impact on availability of services in the private sector.

9.4 Evidence-Based Practice

Neonatal care over the last few decades was characterized by leaps and bounces in advances in knowledge, technology, and innovation (Cuttini et al. 2020). This is also true in the South African context (Rhoda et al. 2018). Areas where significant change took place include respiratory support with training of the Helping Babies Breathe® in all kinds of settings, and Advanced Neonatal Life Support® for staff in NICUs, as well as advances in the use of mechanical ventilation and oscillation in high-tech NICUs, and the use of CPAP in low-resource settings as well as high-tech NICUs. Significant progress was also made with neurological monitoring and support with the use of aEEG and head cooling, neonatal surgery, and prevention of mother-to-child transmission (PMTCT) of HIV. Further strategies contributed to a reduction of neonatal mortality such as the Neonatal Baby Friendly Hospital Initiative (Neo-BHFI), (Nordic and Quebec Working Group 2015), Campaign on Accelerated Reduction of Maternal and Child Mortality in Africa (CARMMA) (Department of Health 2015), Limpopo Initiative for Newborn Care (LINC) (http://www.lincare.co.za), and the Road to Health Booklet (Department of Health 2018).

Some of the most important advances in neonatal care that were introduced were the roll-out of Kangaroo Mother Care (KMC) (Feucht et al. 2016), developmental supportive care (Rheeder et al. 2017), and exclusive breastfeeding across South Africa (Nieuwoudt et al. 2019), with a renewed emphasis on involvement of the family, bonding, and attachment (Maree and Downes 2016). The success of implementation of the various strategies though varies.

The latest changes that are taking place are related to dealing with neonates amidst the Covid-19 pandemic. The pandemic forced the hospitals to change many policies, including policies affecting maternal and neonatal care to comply with the Covid-19 maternal and newborn care guidelines as published by the National Department of Health of South Africa (2020).

Reflective Practice of Betina, A Neonatal Nurse:

"I found my passion and the area in which I wanted to specialize during my training and since I graduated, I've been working with the little miracles in the Neonatal Unit. I can't describe the immense amount of belonging I feel when nursing these small and innocent beings. They are so vulnerable and completely powerless, yet such strong and determined fighters. I learn something new from them on a daily basis. We spend most of our lives at work, therefore finding a career where you want to get up in the mornings is of the utmost importance and I am truly blessed when I say that I am convinced I have found that, not only in being a nurse, but being a nurse in the NICU.

I experienced first-hand the effect of skin-to-skin contact to settle a very stressed preemie and how those small little ones' pain levels visibly decrease after a drop of sucrose. There is a feeling of achievement to observe the appreciation of a mother and a father touching their little one for the first time and knowing that I might have witnessed some building of bonding and attachment that should endure."

9.5   Conclusion

Neonatal care in South Africa is provided on different levels in the public and private sectors by a team of professionals. An important part of the team is the nursing staff who are trained on different levels, with a limited number being specialized in neonatal care. The system in nursing education and training is in a phase of transition, but neonatal specialization will not be included in the range of specializations. In spite of this, evidence-based practice is a high priority and is driven by a number of professional organizations and associations with the common aim of reducing neonatal mortality and morbidity.

References

Cuttini M, Forcella E, Rodrigues C, Draper ES, Martins AF, Lainé A, Willars J, Hasselager A, Maier RF, Croci I, Bonet M, Zeitlin J (2020) What drives change in neonatal intensive care units? A qualitative study with physicians and nurses in six European countries. Pediatr Res 88:257–264. https://doi.org/10.1038/s41390-019-0733-9

Department of Health, RSA (2015) South Africa's national strategic plan for a campaign on accelerated reduction of maternal and child mortality in Africa (CARMMA) http://www.health.gov.za/index.php/shortcodes/2015-03-29-10-42-47/2015-04-30-08-18-10/2015-04-30-08-24-27?download=584:south--africa-strategic-plan-on-accelerated-reduction-of-maternal-and-child-health-mortality-in-africa-carmma

Department of Health, RSA (2018) Road to Health Booklet. http://www.health.gov.za/index.php/shortcodes/2015-03-29-10-42-47/2015-04-30-08-29-27/2015-04-30-08-33-30/category/545-immunisation-survey?download=3388:road-to-health-booklet

Department of Statistics, RSA (STATSSA) (2019) Recorded live births: 2018. http://www.statssa.gov.za/?page_id=1854&PPN=P0305&SCH=7671

Feucht U, van Rooyen E, Skhosana R, Bergh A-M (2016) Taking kangaroo mother care forward in South Africa: the role of district clinical specialist teams. S Afr Med J 106(1):49–52. https://doi.org/10.7196/SAMJ.2016.V106I1.10149

Health Systems Trust (2012) National health care facilities baseline audit. https://www.health-e.org.za/wp-content/uploads/2013/09/National-Health-Facilities-Audit.pdf

Maree C, Downes F (2016) Trends of family-centered care in NICU. J Perinat Neonatal Nurs 30(3):265–269. https://doi.org/10.1097/JPN.0000000000000202

Maree C, Lubbe W, Barlow H, Davidge R, Prullage GS, Scheepers M, van Heerden C (2021) South African neonatal nurse specialization—is professional licensing justifiable? Neonatal Nurs 27:69–7

Minister of Higher Education and Training, RSA (2013) The Higher Education Qualifications Sub-Framework, Notice 1040 of 2012; Government Gazette No. 36003 of 14 December 2012 in terms of the National Qualifications Act, 2008 (Act No. 67 of 2008) and as contemplated in the Higher Education Act, 1997 (Act No. 101 of 1997). Government Printing Works, Pretoria

National Department of Health, RSA (2020) COVID-19 Maternal and newborn care guidelines. https://www.hst.org.za/Covid19/Documents/COVID-19%20Maternal%20%20newborn%20care%20guidelines%202020-04-30%20-%20revised.pdf

Nieuwoudt SJ, Ngandu CB, Manderson L, Norris SA (2019) Exclusive breastfeeding policy, practice and influences in South Africa, 1980 to 2018: a mixed-methods systematic review. PLoS One 14(10):e0224029. https://doi.org/10.1371/journal.pone.0224029

Nordic and Quebec Working Group (2015) Neo-BFHI: the baby-friendly hospital initiative for neonatal wards—Core document with recommended standards and criteria. http://portal.ilca.org/files/resources/Neo-BFHI%20Core%20document%202015%20Edition.pdf

Rheeder A, Lubbe W, van der Walt CSJ, Pretorius R (2017) Compliance with best practice guidelines for neurodevelopmental supportive care in South Africa: a situational analysis. J Perinat Neonatal Nurs 35(4):E83–E96. https://doi.org/10.1097/JPN.0000000000000275

Rhoda NR, Velaphi S, Gebhardt GS, Kauchali S, Barron P (2018) Reducing neonatal deaths in South Africa: progress and challenges. S Afr Med J 108(3 Suppl 1):S9–S16. https://doi.org/10.7196/SAMJ.2018.v108i3.12804

Scheepers M, Maree C, Janse van Rensburg ES (2020) Competencies for structured professional development of neonatal nurses in South Africa. Afr J Health Prof Educ 12(3):154–160

South African Nursing Council (SANC) (2015) Postgraduate Diploma: Nurse/Midwife/Accoucheur Specialist Qualification Framework. http://www.sanc.co.za/pdf/Post%20graduate%20diploma%20Nurse%20Midwife%20specialist%20qualification%20framework.pdf

South African Nursing Council (SANC) (2016) Registration of additional qualifications. https://www.sanc.co.za/education_and_training.htm

South African Nursing Council (SANC) (2020a) Education and training guidelines for postgraduate diploma programmes. https://www.sanc.co.za/education_and_training.htm

South African Nursing Council (SANC) (2020b) Registrations and listed qualifications—calendar year 2019. https://www.sanc.co.za/stats/stat2019/Stats%202019%20-%202%20Registrations%20and%20Listed%20Qualifications.pdf

Young M (2016) Private vs. public healthcare in South Africa. Honors Theses 2741. https://scholarworks.wmich.edu/honors_theses/2741

Websites

https://bettercare.co.za/
https://www.sanc.co.za/
https://nnasa.org.za/
http://www.lincare.co.za

Eastern Africa

10

Andre Ndayambaje, Fauste Uwingabire, Pacifique Umubyeyi, Ruth Davidge, Bartholomew Kamiewe, Geralyn Sue Prullage, Carole Kenner, and Noreen Sugrue

10.1 Introduction

The Sub-Saharan Africa neonatal mortality rate in 2019 was 27/1000 live births (WHO 2019, 2020). The Sustainable Development Goals call for a reduction in this rate to 12/1000 live births by 2030 (UNICEF 2020). To reach this milestone, many changes in care and education of health professionals, especially nurses, will have to occur. The challenges as well as the opportunities for improvement will be presented. COINN is actively involved in working with African neonatal nurses, governmental, and nongovernmental organizations to address the challenges and leverage the opportunities. Examples of this work are illustrated.

10.2 Neonatal Nursing

Many African countries have a general nursing workforce shortage which leads to substandard nurse to patient ratios. Day or night shifts may have only one nurse regardless of the number of patients or the clinical conditions. Similar shortages are also experienced in critical care areas including the neonatal intensive care unit (NICU). Throughout most of Africa, neonatal nursing is not recognized as a specialty, and there is little incentive for nurses to seek specialty training as it may not lead to career advancement or a higher salary. With severe budgetary shortages, health departments justifiably focus on primary preventative health care, often at the expense of high

A. Ndayambaje
University of Global Health Equity (UGHE), Kigali, Rwanda

Council of International Neonatal Nurses, Inc. (COINN), Yardley, PA, USA

F. Uwingabire
College of Medicine and Health Sciences, School of Nursing and Midwifery, University of Rwanda, Kigali, Rwanda

P. Umubyeyi
Rwanda Military Hospital, Kigali, Rwanda

R. Davidge
Kwa-Zulu Natal Department of Health, Neonatal Nurses Association of Southern Africa (NNASA), Johannesburg, South Africa

B. Kamiewe
YML, Lusaka, Zambia

G. S. Prullage
Council of International Neonatal Nurses, Inc. (COINN), NNP SIU School of Medicine, Alton, IL, USA

C. Kenner (✉)
School of Nursing, Health, and Exercise Science, The College of New Jersey, Ewing, NJ, USA

Council of International Neonatal Nurses, Inc. (COINN), Yardley, PA, USA

Alliance of Global Neonatal Nursing (ALIGNN), Honolulu, HI, USA

N. Sugrue
Latino Policy Forum, Chicago, IL, USA

J. Petty et al. (eds.), *Neonatal Nursing: A Global Perspective*, https://doi.org/10.1007/978-3-030-91339-7_10

cost curative care. Training therefore is focused on meeting these needs.

Following completion of a general nursing diploma or degree, a nurse may be assigned by a health department to any unit requiring staff—including a neonatal unit. This basic training generally only includes care of the well-mother–baby dyad with little included in the care of the small and sick newborn. When the nurse commences work in a neonatal intensive care unit, they may or may not receive orientation for this type of care. Due to staff shortages and the focus on generalized training, there is frequent rotation of staff out of neonatal units. This results in poor retention of skills, little experience, and lack of buy in or passion for developing neonatal competencies. This, in turn, leads to poor continuity of care and loss of institutional memory.

Formal education for the neonatal nursing specialty is nonexistent in most African countries or only offered through self-study courses while there may be some courses offered at the postgraduate level. Health departments may avoid high cost postgraduate training for highly specialized nurses believing that these nurses may seek overseas appointments or academic posts and, therefore, not provide benefit for the clinical needs of patients within the health system.

For any meaningful change to occur, standardized curriculum and formal orientation for neonatal nurses are needed. To accomplish that goal, ministries of health, nursing councils, and other governmental agencies must work with nongovernmental agencies such as UNICEF, USAID, WHO, Save the Children, Project Hope, COINN, and many others to set the standards for education and practice.

In Rwanda, one university has developed a postgraduate course; however, not many nurses can take advantage of that level of education and to date those who have undertaken this specialization are employed as general nurses. Zambia too is starting to explore a graduate level neonatal nursing curriculum. Nigeria and Ghana are also interested in elevating neonatal nursing expertise. One challenge for any of these programs is the lack of in-country faculty with neonatal expertise. To address this challenge in Sierra Leone and Malawi, Project Hope is partnering with the Council of International Neonatal Nurses, Inc. (COINN), international schools of nursing, and neonatal nursing expert volunteers, in order to support these countries' governments to raise the standards of neonatal nursing education. This is being achieved by upskilling and development of neonatal faculty and the preparation of a neonatal/pediatric nursing bachelor degree (https://www.projecthope.org/maternal-neonatal-child-health/).

Key "Think Points" for Learning

- Neonatal nursing is not recognized as a specialty in many African countries.
- No scope of practice or regulations exist for neonatal nursing.
- Neonatal nursing education/training may consist of unit orientation, self-study or in-service training but rarely includes formal standardized course work.
- Marked rotation of staff results in few experienced or skilled staff.
- Few experienced neonatal nurses are available to mentor nurses and faculty.
- Nurses assigned to neonatal units should not be shifted to other units. Only when there is a stable, well-qualified neonatal nursing workforce, will neonates and their families thrive.

10.3 Structure of Neonatal Care Provision

Globally neonatal care is organized using the World Health Organization (WHO) three levels of care as outlined in Survive and Thrive: *Transforming Care for Every Small And Sick Newborn* (2020). Level I: Primary or Essential Newborn Care; Level II: Secondary or Special Newborn Care; and Level III: Tertiary or Intensive Newborn Care. Providing care at any of these levels can be quite challenging as the following reflections illustrate.

Reflective Practice: Bartholomew Kamiewe, Zambia

I was caring for a 23-week-old baby that lived for only about 12 h. We did what we could to save it at our hospital. I also used support/advice from other neonatal nurses on an online platform because I work in a rural health facility which is quite far, about 280 km from the nearest referral hospital in Lusaka. From the time I was exposed to neonatal care from the S.T.A.B.L.E. Course and the Rwanda conference in 2018, there has been a difference in the way I care for neonates. That online support system is always there on hand, if I have questions here they always respond, they give me guidance, they sort of encourage me on what I should do. That support system is quite strong, and it has been there for the last 2 years. A challenge we have is the lack of equipment. We have basic equipment like IV bags, masks, but when we have a complex case that may need special equipment like CPAP, we lack the necessary equipment. A CPAP machine is quite expensive, and it is found at only high-level hospitals. We have, however, been taught to make a modified version of it using a bottle and a tubing placed in a bottle, and you connect it to an oxygen machine. That one also helps to function as a continuous positive airway pressure (CPAP) machine by giving oxygen with pressure, but of course the ideal one would have CPAP available. Other barriers would include few staff trained in neonatal care, lack of adequate space in facilities where neonates can be cared for and long distance to the nearest referral hospital. At one time, one of the medical officers at our institution said to me that "we need to have someone who is specifically looking at the neonates at this institution." That was very true as it would lead to continuity of care even when I am not around. So, we need to grow the team to combat the lack of adequately trained staff in neonatal care.

Reflective Practice: Andre Ndayambaje, Rwanda

When asked what I need to provide quality care I reflected on my years of practice as a midwife and neonatal nurse. The first thing I need is passion, passion to provide quality care. Compassion is needed too. I also need knowledge and skills. Being trained and equipped for care. I need a good space to conduct my skills and apply knowledge. I need a team; you know working in the unit. The team includes families. I need support from leadership. Finally, I need a system that has policies, guidelines, protocols, which are validated and that assess the quality of care that I am delivering. We must stop the "conflict of power" between and among the doctors and nurses as we all want to provide the best care possible. We must also ensure that once a baby is discharged that the community can provide the follow-up care. In Rwanda, many babies still die after discharge. The community-based care is a gap that must be addressed by healthcare policies and financing.

Reflective Practice: Pacifique Umubyeyi, Rwanda

What do you need to provide high-quality care? For the moment, I work as a unit manager in the neonatal intensive care unit here in my country. So, what I need are three things. The first thing I need is trained nurses to work in the unit with me. I need more skills and knowledge. But, at least me…I had the fortunate opportunity…to go to a master's program for neonatal nurses, but all of the team I work with, they did not have that opportunity. They receive some on the job training. Currently, in my country, there is no dedicated program for neonatal nurses in an undergraduate program. At least we started to have the master's program or postgraduate in neonatal nurs-

ing even though there is no clear scope of practice for neonatal nurses. But before there was no dedicated teaching for neonatal care. It was just general nursing. So, most of the nurses working together, they did general nursing, some were midwives, they did not receive a special course for caring for neonates. If we could basically have a little neonatal care knowledge there for the unit, if it was possible to train all nurses and midwives and if we had instruments for the care, all these things would help. In the city where I work, for example, we have only two CPAP machines, which are working perfectly. Yesterday, I saw, we have little babies need CPAP machines we do not have enough instruments but I said, It is good to be well equipped with functioning medical equipment including CPAP machines in order to care for these sick babies, but sometimes we do not have what we need and it is very challenging to provide care. What I want people to understand or to put into consideration, is that the neonates need special care. They need attention from the government, nongovernmental organizations, the authorities, the hospital authorities, so that they take it as a special service, they really need special nurses.

Fauste Uwingabire, Rwanda

Most people providing care, they are not having a chance to have a background exposure to neonatal science, so they just apply general principles of nursing care, they bring them to newborns. Even though we have a shortage of personnel, at least when we have, if they knew what the best option was, or the best way to care for the newborn and their family. It is not just for nurses, even for midwives, even for doctors, they do not really have the basics, even the

basics, for managing newborns. This is a systems problem that needs a consistent voice to remind institutions that just increasing the number of nurses and doctors is not enough to provide quality care but rather we need skillful, competent people who have had at least the basic knowledge of how to care for babies and families. Doctors have some protected time, but nurses do not. There is not even a good opportunity to mentor each other. Our district hospital is like the second level of care. Currently all district hospitals have at least a unit dedicated to neonatology and separate staff dedicated for neonatal care. Those nurses are over rotated from various hospital departments, due to the general assumption that "a nurse is a nurse" which is not true. When it comes to specialized/complex care like those needed by the small and sick newborns and their families. Monthly indicators related to neonatal morbidity and mortality are shared from healthcare facilities to the national level; the latter compiles, analyses the data so they can do like and give feedback to hospitals to see their level of performance. So, your hospital may struggle to maintain or try to improve their neonatal indicators. There is a performance-based financing system linked to this. There is one national neonatal group that is called National Technical Working Group, which is a group that links the nurses, midwives, physicians, mostly pediatricians from the central level, local associations, and nongovernmental organizations (NGOs) whose scope of work includes neonatal care. This is where most official issues of neonatal are discussed such as how the hospital performs on specific indicators—different equipment needed, neonatal standards, neonatal protocol development, and/or review. There is a kind of national commitment really to make it change, in terms of newborn care, and newborn indicators, but it is a journey.

Ruth Davidge, South Africa

I started caring for neonates in 1994. Those were in the days before developmentally supportive care, before we really understood pain in neonates, before kangaroo mother care (KMC) and family-centered care. The nurse was the sole care provider, and the parents generally were only considered as visitors. Supporting and empowering parents as the primary caregivers is still a huge challenge in Africa. With the steep increase in litigation many healthcare providers are fearful of family involvement in care and their presence in the unit. Unit visiting policies are often restrictive (particularly for fathers) and most frequently mothers are only seen as providers of breastmilk and often berated when they provide inadequate volumes.

However, this is slowly changing. Hospitals now are required to provide lodging facilities for mothers. Guidelines and systems are now in place to support family-centered care. Through the development and provision of parental educational brochures and the "Road to Health" booklet, families are being empowered to play a more central role in their child's care and ongoing health and development. This however is a slow process. In one hospital, where I was trying to increase the levels of parental involvement and had stated that parents should be present with their babies during the medical round, the consultant was most indignant stating that this would be disruptive and inconvenient as there is insufficient space. COVID-19 has also had a very negative impact on parental presence as all visiting for the small and sick babies has been banned resulting in decreased breastfeeding, bonding, and the provision of KMC. Currently, a South African parental support group is actively lobbying against this policy.

Kangaroo mother care (KMC) is now a standard of care, and South Africa is a

leading country supporting research and implementation of KMC. This has been such a change during my career. I always say I am the best advert for how evidence can change practice. When KMC was first introduced in our unit, it was part of a national research project. We sent one nurse for training, and when she returned stating, we must remove babies from their incubators and nurse them on their mothers' chests, I stated as the unit manager, "Over my dead body. We have good standards here and I am not taking a baby out of a perfectly good incubator and putting it on its mother's chest. We do not practice bush medicine here!" I was totally resistant to the idea as it came as instruction without any evidence or training to its benefits. Now 20 years later (and having read all the evidence and attended many conferences), I am passionately advocating for its universal implementation. Sadly, critical thinking, reflective practice, the need to look for data or evidence, or the latest research to support your practice, is still not a reality for the majority of our nurses.

Specialized postgraduate training of neonatal nurses stopped in 2003, and many of the neonatal nurses that were trained have emigrated or pursued academic roles due to the lack of specialized career pathing. Advanced pediatric and midwifery courses do not adequately cover care for the small and sick newborn. We consequently lack leadership and mentorship for nurses currently working in neonatal units. The average nurse in my province has not had the advantages I had: Specialized training, access to neonatal journals, international conferences, networking with national and international colleagues, and years of dedicated experience. They are dependent on the historical practices in their unit and the orders of the usually very junior and inexperienced and frightened community service doctors. Nurses lack the independence, confidence, and empowerment to question orders or reflect on their practice. I am therefore now responsible for trying to standardize and improve the delivery of neonatal care in 52 hospitals training from Level I through Level III. We have rolled out a standardized package of neonatal care including norms and standards, guidelines, skills assessments, standardized records, clinical management checklists, clinical governance audit tools, and a reporting and mentoring framework. I try to access the best available evidence, translate it into user-friendly clinical tools, and then support the healthcare workers to understand and implement the best possible care. In this way, the nurse on the frontline who knows nothing, who does not really care, who has just been allocated because they need a body, and has no mentor or leader to show her, has a piece of paper that can at least tell her what she needs to know and empowers her to implement this care even if the doctor's orders are contradictory. Changing attitudes and practices is a slow process but perseverance wins the race and slowly we are seeing progress.

10.4   Conclusion

This chapter highlights neonatal nursing care and education in Africa. It offers insights into the challenges and opportunities for neonatal nurses on that continent.

References

UNICEF (2020) Child survival and the SDGs. https://data. unicef.org/topic/child-survival/child-survival-sdgs/

World Health Organization (WHO) (2019) Newborns: improving survival and well-being. https:// www.who.int/news-room/fact-sheets/detail/ newborns-reducing-mortality

World Health Organization (WHO) (2020) Survive and thrive: transforming care for the small and sick newborn. https://www.healthynewbornnetwork.org/ resource/survive-and-thrive-transforming-care-for-every-small-and-sick-newborn/

Asia (Japan)

11

Wakako Eklund, Miki Konishi, Aya Nakai,
Aya Shimizu, Kazuyo Uehara,
and Noriko Nakamura

11.1 Introduction

In the history of the development of neonatology as a focused specialty, Japan has made critical contributions, both technological and scientific, toward supporting neonatal care and improving neonatal outcomes. A non-invasive continuous monitoring device to measure arterial blood oxygen saturation,

the Pulse Oximeter was first developed in Japan by Dr. Aoyagi, an engineer at Nihon Kohden Corporation in the mid-1970s (Aoyagi 2003; Aoyagi and Miyasaka 2002). Dr. Aoyagi devoted his research with the dream of detecting oxygen saturation without requiring actual blood specimens (Bhattacharya 2020). Use of pulse-oximetry is an essential tool for neonatal care in resuscitation, managing respiratory conditions, assessing the severity of apnea and bradycardia events, or to conduct pre-discharge screening for critical congenital heart disease (CDC 2018; Eklund and Mooneyham 2022). Pulse oximetry's presence extends to the entire healthcare system from infants to the patients in the operating room settings, to the geriatric population, making Dr. Aoyagi's contribution globally historic. Dr. Aoyagi passed in April 2020 when pulseoximetry may have become more important than any other period during his lifetime.

Artificial surfactant, with its unique biochemical composition, was found by Dr. Fujiwara of Japan in late 1970s after many years of trial and error research (Fujiwara et al. 1980). The news of his findings spread globally, and the story even made the Time Magazine (1980). This discovery accelerated the global efforts to bring this miracle substance to the bedside, and likely also contributed to propelling neonatal nursing as a specialty over time.

Improved survival of extremely low birth weight infants, made possible by the arrival of

W. Eklund (✉)
Pediatrix Medical Group of Tennessee,
Nashville, TN, USA

Bouvé College of Health Sciences, School of
Nursing, Northeastern University, Boston, MA, USA

Council of International Neonatal Nurses, Inc.
(COINN), Yardley, PA, USA
e-mail: wakako.eklund@pediatrix.com

M. Konishi
School of Nursing, Dokkyo Medical University,
Tochigi, Japan

A. Nakai
Graduate School of Nursing, Chiba University,
Chiba-City, Chiba, Japan

A. Shimizu
Graduate School of Nursing, Kyoto Tachibana
University, Kyoto-City, Kyoto, Japan

K. Uehara
Child Health Nursing, Okinawa Prefectural College
of Nursing, Naha, Okinawa, Japan

N. Nakamura
Seirei Hamamatsu General Hospital,
Naka-ku, Hamamatsu, Shizuoka, Japan

J. Petty et al. (eds.), *Neonatal Nursing: A Global Perspective*,
https://doi.org/10.1007/978-3-030-91339-7_11

surfactant or other technological advances led to an increase in chronic lung disease (Keller et al. 2017; Higgins et al. 2018; Steinhorn et al. 2017), neurodevelopmental/psychosocial challenges (Wilson-Costello et al. 2005; Laptook et al. 2005; Johnson and Marlow 2017), or other long-term problems resulting from complications such as necrotizing enterocolitis (Fullterton et al. 2017). This was observed globally.

Japan has since consistently maintained low infant mortality rates with a rigorous approach to the care of premature or sick infants. Efforts to care for infants who were once thought to be impossible to save still continue today. A remarkable survival of an infant born at 24 weeks gestation weighing 268 gm in Tokyo was recently reported (Arimitsu et al. 2021). This unique case was shared widely in Japan and abroad after the infant was discharged in 2019. A report of detailed care that included not only meticulous considerations to minimize pain but also other negative stimulations, while promoting what is known to be neuroprotective; all the while emphasizing the power of family presence which is incredibly heart-warming. Neonatal nurses work in multidisciplinary teams with physicians and other partners with passion and desire to improve the neonatal outcomes for every neonatal patient and their families.

Japan, however, faces a unique challenge, not seen in other parts of the world, of having an increasingly aging population curve and decline in annual births generating national attention and prioritization of resources to the aged. In 2015, the proportion of people 65 and older was 26.5%; however, the proportion of the older population in entire Japan is expected to reach 40% by 2060. The under-15-year population, however, was 12.7% in 2015 and it is expected to decline to 9% of the population by 2060 (JNA 2016a). These phenomena drive national policies and even impact the overall standards for nursing education. The current national direction emphasizes the fortification of the healthcare workforce to address those who live longer with complex health conditions. Despite the focus shifting to the older adult, perinatal and neonatal nursing is still important to the viability of Japanese society. Japanese perinatal care organization is an impor-

tant concept to highlight nursing's role as an essential member of a multidisciplinary team not only in NICUs, but also in academic and community settings. Attainment of strong neonatal outcomes is not possible by scientific or technological advances alone. Advocacy to promote quality perinatal/neonatal care is needed to ensure high-quality care in this population. Japanese neonatal nurses are central to support NICU infants and families and their transition to home. Continued nursing contributions support neonates in Japan in the past, today, and in the future.

> **Key "Think Points" for Learning**
>
> - Japanese perinatal healthcare delivery is a regionalized system.
> - Japanese Academy of Neonatal Nursing (JANN) is the neonatal-specific professional nursing organization to support neonatal nurses and neonatal/family care. JANN leads in research, education, and advocacy.
> - There are multiple educational pathways to enter Japanese nursing; however, neonatal-specific education is limited.
> - Japanese neonatal nurses contribute to various aspects of neonatal care, both in academic, healthcare delivery, and community settings.
> - Japanese neonatal nurses have opportunities to contribute to furthering evidence-based nurse-led research and projects.

11.2 Organization of Neonatal Care

11.2.1 Regionally Organized Perinatal Care System (Nakai and Konishi)

The Ministry of Health, Labour and Welfare of Japan (MHLWJ), in 2010, issued guidance to fortify regionalized perinatal care at prefectural level (similar to state or provincial) in response to highly publicized unfortunate outcomes related to high-risk perinatal cases, also in accordance with the national effort to counter the trend of dwindling annual births (Ministry of Health 2010a, b; Eklund 2010). The MHLWJ continued to update the guidance over subsequent years (Ministry of Health 2017b; Eklund 2010). The Japanese Regional Perinatal Referral Centers offer the highest level of perinatal care today. Multiple non-referral perinatal centers support each Regional Referral Center in every prefecture (a total of 47 prefectures exist in Japan).

According to the most recent 2017 guidance (Ministry of Health 2017b), each Regional Perinatal Referral Center must be equipped with, but is not limited to, the following: 6 and greater maternal-fetal ICU beds, 9 and greater (preferably 12 or more) neonatal intensive care unit (NICU) beds (not including the stepdown beds), 24 hour in-house coverage by obstetrician and a neonatologist (physicians), 24 hour transport response capability, and laboratory availability to conduct relevant studies, along with availability of mental health support for families and staff. Each prefectural perinatal committee is recommended to design and implement systems of communication to coordinate emergency transport, or disaster response. This guidance also encourages continued education for physicians, nurses, midwives, and mental health specialists. Non-referral regional perinatal centers are under less strict guidelines; however, MHLWJ recommends a workforce be provided that is similar to the regional perinatal referral centers. MHLWJ reports a total of 110 regional and 298 non-referral regional perinatal centers as of May first, 2020 (Ministry of Health 2020).

Additionally, there are numerous birthing clinics as well as many additional hospitals with obstetric services that are not designated as regional centers. Those deliveries deemed non-high risk are managed in these settings. These small birthing hospitals and clinics request the services from the regional centers in emergencies or when high-risk situations arise. In 2015 nearly half the births (45.5%) occurred at clinics while 53.7% of births occurred in hospitals. Midwife-supported birthing centers were used in 0.7% of cases (Ministry of Health 2017b).

Japan has experienced a notable decrease in annual births in the last several decades. The number of births in 1973 was over 2 million, but by 2019, births decreased to 864,000 (Cabinet Office, Government of Japan). In spite of this decrease and the overall population decrease, birth rates for preterm infants (<37 weeks), low birth weight infants, or extremely low birth weight infants have all increased in the last few decades. Infant mortality rate, however, has decreased from 2.6/1000 births in 1990 to 0.9/1000 births in 2015 (Ministry of Health 2017b). These changes underscore the value of a sophisticated perinatal system and well-trained multidisciplinary team members including neonatal nurses.

11.3 Multidisciplinary Team in NICU (Shimizu and Uehara)

Each Japanese NICU requires a high functioning multidisciplinary team. Team members include obstetrics, pediatrics (neonatology is a part of pediatrics), pharmacy, biomedical engineering, nutrition, rehabilitation, mental health, informatics, social service/case management, purchasing/central supply, in addition to the department of nursing and medicine. As a multidisciplinary team, members ensure the following; necessary devices are maintained and updated; accurate doses of correct medications/intravenous solutions are available for the infants; breast milk is stored and dispensed in safe manner; nutritional status and growth and development of each infant is followed, physical/occupational therapies are available and utilized for developmental support; psychosocial needs of parents are assessed and supported; nurses and physicians are trained and educated to align with the patient needs; provision of necessary supplies to care for the patients are available; and systems security is maintained for safe keeping of all patient data. The extent of the support available does differ based on the level of care provided by every institution.

The primary workforce to care for the day-to-day needs of NICU patients consists of neonatal nurses and physicians. By far nurses as a collective workforce is the largest group of professionals who support NICU patients. Staff neonatal nurses directly care for their assigned patients in coordination with nursing leadership, physician colleagues, and other members. In the Japanese system, the current recommendation for nurse patient ratio is 1:3 in high-risk neonatal care, and 1:6 in convalescent or stepdown care (Ministry of Health 2017b). This is a minimum staffing guidance given by MHLWJ and dependency level is adjusted based on the infants' acuity.

Some NICU nurses have globally recognized added qualifications such as Newborn Individualized Developmental Care and Assessment Program (NIDCAP 2020) or the International Board of Certified Lactation Consultant (IBCLE 2020). However, there is a unique program in Japan to qualify nurses as "Certified Nurse in Neonatal Intensive Care" (CN-NIC) (please see more detailed discussion regarding CN-NIC under education). These CN-NICs are an essential part of the multidisciplinary team in many NICUs. Preliminary analysis of distribution of CNs among the institutions revealed that, where gestationally smaller infants are admitted, a greater number of CNs were available per unit (Shimizu et al. 2019).

Nurses also serve in the role of a discharge planner or post-discharge coordinator, working closely with members of primary care, public health nurses, or home health nursing services in the community. Many medically dependent NICU graduates benefit from neonatally trained nurses as their understanding and experience is a necessary support to transition the infant and family to home (Ministry of Health 2017a). There are also neonatal nurses who are actively engaged with parent groups nationwide to advocate for the voices of parents and their neonates who have ongoing health concerns common among NICU graduates.

11.4 Role of Professional Associations (Shimizu and Uehara)

Neonatal nursing addresses both newborns and their families. The Japanese Nursing Association (JNA) (JNA 2016a), Japan Academy of Neonatal Nursing (JANN), and Japan Academy of Midwifery (JAM 2020) are the primary professional organizations that are important resources for the nurses who work with newborns and their families. Each organization supports national policies aimed at maternal and child health and promotion of healthy society for families (Ministry of Health 2001, 2010a; Cabinet Office, Government of Japan 2020), while being cognizant of the global trends in policy and practice recommendations.

JNA, a member of the International Council of Nursing, was founded in 1946, and it is the largest professional nursing association for all three distinct areas of nursing including public health nurses, midwives, and nurses (JNA 2016a). JNA offers specialty added recognitions for Certified Nurse Specialists (CNSs) which is conferred upon completion of specialized master's level education. Additionally, JNA offers the Certified Nurses (CN) designation in various specialties. CN programs are not graduate programs, and the program is 6–12 months long based on the specialty. The NICU-specific CN program will be discussed under the education section.

JANN is the national organization that advocates for neonatal nurses and neonates (JANN). JANN, founded in 1991, has contributed to the advancement of neonatal-specific nursing education and research. JANN voted to join the Council of International Neonatal Nurses, Inc. (COINN) in 2017 and has strengthened neonatal nursing as a specialty, joining hands with global colleagues. JANN published, "Standardized Care for NICU Neonates and their Families," and recently published the clinical ladder system. These will be discussed in the education section. JANN's efforts are important in maximizing the utilization of the currently available neonatal nursing workforce. In addition, JANN published "Neonatal Pain Management Guideline" in collaboration with neonatologists. The updated 2020 version is available in Japanese (JANN 2020a, b). JANN also set up an international committee to closely link JANN members with COINN and to disseminate global information to the Japanese members while informing the global colleagues with Japanese nurses' accomplishments. The international committee assisted with abstract/posters for JANN delegates preparing to attend COINN meetings or collaborated with global partners to translate English materials into Japanese when relevant. Four of the co-authors of this chapter served on the JANN's international committee at the time of the manuscript preparation.

JAM, founded in 1987, is a member of the International Confederation of Midwives (ICM 2018). JAM is an academic organization that contributes to the improvement of maternal and child health and welfare (JAM). Aligned with the ICM statement on the essential competencies of midwives, JAM plays the role in education for newborns, and supporting families. Breastfeeding and mental health support of families in crisis are two important areas for neonatal nurses and midwives.

11.5 Practice Regulation (Konishi)

The current nurse's scope of practice in Japan is primarily governed by the "The Act on Public Health Nurses, Midwives and Nurses," which was adopted in 1948 (JNA 2016a; Konishi 2016). Nursing was recognized as an essential partner to promote public health after World War II while Japan was under the occupied force. The nursing department was placed within the Health Ministry of Japan during this time. Extensive efforts were made by all the nursing stakeholders to organize and modernize the three separate existing nursing regulations into one Act. This Act has served as the legal basis to regulate the scope of nursing practice. The Act contains language that describes the nurse's role as more supportive or assistive to the medical role, likely contributing to Japan's traditionally limited scope of practice for nurses in all settings, but especially in neonatal settings compared to their global counterparts. Some of the interventions that are viewed as nursing globally may not be considered part of the nurse's role in Japan. Examples include administering medications via intravenous push (IVP), starting peripheral intravenous lines, or performing a venepuncture or heel stick. An additional legisla-

tive amendment was made to allow nurses to administer intravenous push medications in 2002; however, it is still rare to find NICU nurses who regularly perform IVPs for neonates (Konishi 2016). The Japanese NICU nurses, however, are experts in providing meticulous and detailed care for infants, including those extremely low birthweight (ELBW) infants during the most critical period. NICU nurses, for many years, have contributed to upholding high-quality care such as skin care, developmental care, parental support, and environmental care (management of lights, sound, humidity, temperature).

In recent years, the Japanese pioneers in nurse practitioner (NP) education advocated for the expansion of the scope of practice, thus challenging the current Act. Adult NP programs at graduate level have been in existence for the last 14 years. Those who are trained to perform the advanced practice role, do so under their original nursing license, regulated by the amended Act. This amendment allows them to perform certain interventions and decision-making under the direction of physician colleagues. Considerable discussions took place regarding neonatal NP needs in response to the perinatal care delivery crisis which identified shortages of neonatologists and NICU beds (Eklund 2010). To date, Japan has not passed legislation to recognize NP as a licensed independent profession.

11.6 Education and Training (Nakai and Konishi)

11.6.1 Nursing Education and Licenses

Three distinct nursing roles organized under JNA are the public health nurses, nurse midwives, and nurses. Nursing education leading to licensure may be from a 4-year university, 3-year junior college, or 3–5-year specialty training. A license is attained after successfully passing the basic national nursing examination. Public health and Midwifery education are both offered at both university level or at a graduate level in addition to the basic nursing education. Both pathways lead to the same midwifery or public health licensing exam eligibility (JNA 2016a). JNA submitted an official petition to the Ministry of Education in 2018 to permanently affirm the 4-year university education as the foundation for nursing education, and to support the graduate level education as the standard education for public health and midwifery specialties. This action supports the increasing nursing demands and changing role (JNA 2018).

11.6.2 Neonatal Content in University Nursing Education

Neonatal content is scant in basic nursing education. The full-term healthy newborn care comprises the majority of didactic and clinical hours. Nursing care for vulnerable neonates is included in the pediatric nursing textbook used at many universities. However, in-depth discussions of high-risk neonatal assessment, pathophysiology, or developmental care are not possible. Neonatal content comprises 1.5 to 4.5 lecture hours and there are also only a few neonatal licensure questions. An analysis of examination questions from 2013 to 2018 revealed one question concerning a case of a low birth weight infant in 2014. Published content standards for the nursing examination have moved away from using expressions such as "perinatal" or "low birth weight infants" (Konishi 2018a). This trend is driven by national efforts to address the aging population trend in Japan.

Midwifery educational content and examinations contain more neonatal content (Ministry of Health 2018b). The revised 2019 educational standards for public health nurses and midwives suggested adding didactic and clinical hours across the board, while specifically adding more neonatal/perinatal content to midwifery education, such as perinatal mental health, care of high-risk pregnant mothers, and advanced skill and knowledge to respond to certain high-risk perinatal/neonatal events (Ministry of Health 2019). Most midwifery graduates seek employment in the obstetrical department serving in the labor and delivery or postpartum care and not in NICUs. Current trends driving the policy are

potentially overlooking the vulnerable infants' needs, although the responses are logical in view of rapidly aging Japanese society.

11.6.3 Challenges Against Education for Nurses in NICUs

The Japanese government directed perinatal care regionalization in 2010 in response to highly publicized maternal/neonatal case that exposed the vulnerability of the perinatal health system (Eklund 2010; Ministry of Health 2010b). Efforts were made to increase NICU beds. By 2014, the national average had reached 30.4 beds per 10,000 births meeting the national perinatal goal. Thus, workforce demands increased for all involved including nursing and challenged the nursing organization and healthcare settings regarding the methods and quality of training/education to equip nurses to align with the increased NICU beds and patient needs.

It is common for new nursing graduates to arrive in NICU without any neonatal-specific preparation. It is also very common to not be trained in Neonatal Cardiopulmonary Resuscitation (NCPR, equivalent to the Neonatal Resuscitation Program or NRP) (NCPR 2020) until they have worked for several months in the NICU. Methods of bedside training and the gradual exposure to neonatal-specific content vary widely according to the employing institution. Traditionally, when hired, nurses belong to the larger nursing body under the director of nursing, rather than to a specific department such as the NICU. It is common practice to conduct frequent inter-departmental transfers of nurses from one division to another without the individual nurse's specific desire (Furukawa 2012). This practice has negative implications. Primarily, the investment and efforts to train nurses to become experts in a certain field is defeated. The nursing administration may simply move a very capable nurse who has excelled in high-risk neonatal care to an adult intensive care unit (ICU) with a very good reason, such as exposure to wider areas, thus grooming the nurse to be a leader in the organization. Infants and families, however, lose dedicated nursing staff who have the hands, eyes, ears, and mind to care, assess, hear, and critically think about the high-risk neonates and their families.

11.6.4 NICU-Specific Clinical Competencies

JNA recognizes the strengths of expert nurses and advocates for training from novice to expert, by issuing a competency guideline containing five progressive levels (JNA 2016b). In response, a JANN committee launched an effort to develop a neonatal-specific competency ladder document. The initial version was published in January of 2019 (JANN 2019). This competency document will serve as a guide for future designing of any NICU-specific training or continuing education (CE) programs. Any educational content must be tailored to meet the specific patient population, for example, at an institution where a large number of ELBW babies are admitted, or surgical cases are seen, specific content must be reinforced. The competency document will also serve as a tool for neonatal leadership to evaluate and nurture the NICU nurses. Education program types, both orientation and CE, however, rely largely on the institutional policies, budget, and the direction of leadership; therefore, nurses' access to educational opportunities varies widely. JNA does not require renewal of nursing licenses or CE credits for license maintenance. This factor may impact institutions or even individuals from placing a high priority to increase access to CE offerings.

JANN annually holds an educational conference and additional seminars; however, not every nurse is able to attend annually due to the cost constraints of travelling, paying for the tuition, and staffing logistics. Other private entities, industry partners, healthcare facilities, or academic institutions often collaborate with JANN to design additional educational opportunities. The recent COVID-19 pandemic may have uncovered an area of continuing education that Japanese nursing organizations or healthcare facilities have yet to fulfil. On demand access to view educational programming recorded earlier or participating in virtual webinars from home may increase the nurses' access to cost-effective

education. Japanese nurses are enthusiastic about learning opportunities and JANN's annual neonatal conference draws approximately 1000 participants. In addition to the CE offerings, more formal education for added qualification is discussed in the following section.

11.6.5 Certified Nurses in Neonatal Intensive Care (CN-NIC)

JNA launched an added qualification system in various specialties for a nurse to become a certified nurse (CN) in 1995. The CN education in neonatal intensive care (CN-NIC) began in 2003 to encourage nurses with strong knowledge and skills to lead the neonatal team at the bedside (JNA 2016a). Eligibility to enrol in this six-month course includes having 5 years of clinical experience as a licensed nurse with three of those years in NICU. As of the end of the year 2020, a total of 441 have attained the CN-NIC designation (JNA 2020a). All components are completed on-site, without a virtual component. The program was once offered at two locations, however, recently, it was offered at only one university campus near Tokyo. CN-NIC curriculum consists of six competencies: optimize the outcome of neonates, promote developmental/family-centered care, advocate for the rights of newborns and their families, promote multidisciplinary collaboration, coach others, and serve as consultants. The CN-NIC program has seen a decline in enrolment. As of 2020, this program is on hold; however, while the CN program in Pediatric Primary Care will carry on including certain neonatal content, it does not include an in-depth neonatal intensive care content. Currently, emphasis is placed on addressing the needs of medically dependent children in the community, and added efforts are being made to prepare specialized nurses for this population, rather than increasing the number of nurses with NICU-specific training (Saiseikai Yokohamashi Tobu Hospital 2016). This trend, again, is logical due to the decreasing annual births; however, it can lead to a challenge for neonatal nurses to gain specialty education. At the time of the final review in early 2022, there is a move among the neonatal passionate educators to revive neonatal specific added training through a different pathway, incorporating expanded content starting in 2023. (Personal Communication with M. Konishi, January, 2022).

Leadership is evident in NICUs where CN-NICs are serving. CN-NICs are critical to train new nurses and to develop protocols. Some CNs advance into administrative positions instead of remaining in clinical roles. Other CNs seek further studies to gain research skill by advancing to graduate school, since the CN program does not include the scholarly component in the training. The CN-NIC program has made a difference in NICUs.

11.6.6 Nurse Specialists (CNS) in Child and Women's Health Nursing

JNA in collaboration with the Japanese Association of Nursing Programs in Universities (JAMPU) also developed graduate level specialized programs to confer the Certified Nurse Specialist (CNS) credential. Since the neonatal-specific CNS program was never developed, some neonatal nurses who seek higher levels of education have enrolled in child health or women's health CNS programs. At the end of 2020, there were 279 CNSs in child health and 87 CNSs in the women's health specialty in Japan (JNA 2020b) A handful of CNSs are serving in roles dedicated to NICU across Japan; however, it is not common. Certification for CN and CNS status do require renewal every 5 years, unlike the basic nursing license which does not require renewal, with a range of requirements that candidates must complete to maintain the designation.

The current CNS curriculum underwent a critical transition during the last decade, partially impacted by the emergence of master's level education, which began to train nurse practitioners. In 2019, the JANPU made official adjustments to the CNS curriculum requirement and increased the total credit hours from 26 to 38 credits (JANPU 2019). The new curriculum fortifies the skills and knowledge in physical assessment, pathophysiology, and clinical pharmacology. CNSs do not have prescriptive authority and do not perform independent clinical practice making medical diagnosis or initiate treatment without the direct physician supervision. It is evident, however, that a high level of clinical understanding strengthens the overall ability of CNSs to serve in any role.

A new trend which may change the landscape of nurse workforce and challenges NICU education and training further, is emerging. Nurse candidates from southern Asian countries with whom Japan has an Economic Partnership Agreement with since 2008, have increased the foreign/migrant nurses who work in Japan. These candidates are primarily from Indonesia, the Philippines, and Vietnam, but this program is expected to expand (JICWELS 2020). As the project with foreign countries expands, the Japanese NICU workforce becomes more diverse both educationally and culturally. Additionally, NICU patients are also becoming more diverse with increased migrant workers living in Japan. These observed changes along with current trends underscore the urgent need to fortify neonatal-specific curriculum to educate future nursing graduates or foreign nurses who seek NICU employment, if a quality neonatal workforce is to be sustained.

A neonatal-specific graduate level program for advanced practice is not being considered at this time; however, expansion of the nurse's scope of practice has been attempted at the institutional level in a few organizations. To increase the overall nursing impact, more collaboration of nurse specialists in clinical settings and nurse scholars in educational institutions who understand research is desired. NICU nursing specialists who are also prepared at a doctoral level such as a Doctor of Nursing Practice (DNP) are also desired to lead quality improvement projects and research to increase nurse-led evidence generation and NICU practice changes. Japan is early in the DNP offering, and its impact on neonatal settings is not fully understood.

Task shifting and task-sharing are becoming increasingly common topics of discussion in healthcare settings. The next 10 years may bring more changes to the landscape of neonatal nursing from an educational perspective. Improvements in the quality of neonatal care may be achieved by enabling nurses to maximize their abilities to not only perform clinical skills and render effective judgements, but also to have tools to impact the organizational or national policies to improve the future care of the vulnerable neonates. Advanced education is definitely the backbone to fortify the neonatal nursing collective workforce.

11.7 Evidence-Based Practice (Nakai and Konishi)

Many barriers impede neonatal nurses' abilities to fully promote and guide evidence-based practice (EBP). Presence of EBP in NICUs reduces practice variations from place to place, or from one nurse to another, and it aims to continuously improve patient outcomes. Japan has, for example, begun adopting EBP related to neonatal pain in the last decade, now making neonatal pain a topic that is addressed in every NICU in Japan. The superb infant outcomes related to extremely premature infants in Japan has been a source of inquiry by neonatal nurses from other Asian countries. Japanese nurses are increasingly invited to share their expertise with international colleagues (Eklund & Konishi 2013). However, there are still opportunities for change. One challenge that nurses face concerns Kangaroo Mother Care (KMC) or simply the practice of parents engaging with, and holding their infants on the night shift. Due to decreased night shift staffing, involving parents in caregiving is often discouraged or prohibited. This is observed, even in facilities where KMC is promoted. One reason for this challenge may lie in the lack of adequate educational provision for neonatal nurses. Justification for investment in neonatal/pediatric-specific education is often a challenge at any organizational level as previously stated. However, inadequate education has negative practice implications since it prevents the full realization of nurse empowerment. The Nursing Now Campaign (2018–2020) jointly promoted by WHO and the International Council of Nurses (ICN) and endorsed by COINN, addresses exactly this point and encourages the need to fortify nurses' voices to lead in healthcare settings, as well as promote a greater investment in nursing workforce (WHO 2020). When nurses are not able to confidently stand by and promote EBP, such as KMC, which is well-established globally, non-evidence-based safety concerns that

are raised by the administration or physician team can easily overrule nursing, and new policies or rules are enforced against sound evidence.

EBP in neonatal intensive care is also challenged by the limited number of neonatal nurses trained to conduct systematic reviews to develop evidence-based guidelines. Only a handful of neonatal nurses have attained doctoral education, primarily PhD. Once doctoral education is achieved; however, very few clinical career options are available in Japan, thus forcing them to enter academic careers without leaving the opportunity to make an impact in clinical settings. The gap between research and practice that exists must be addressed before neonatal nursing practice can align with the recommendations by the Nursing Now Campaign.

11.7.1 Neonatal Resuscitation in Japan

Most deliveries occur at settings where trained professionals are present; however, only half of the annual deliveries occur in hospitals where multidisciplinary specialists are present. When high-risk deliveries are anticipated in settings outside hospitals, pediatricians or neonatologists are not readily available (Ministry of Health 2017b). Japan has a representative to the International Liaison Committee on Resuscitation (ILCOR), and evidence-based training sessions have been provided to meet the specific needs in Japan since 2007 under the direction of the Japanese Society of Perinatal and Neonatal Medicine (Hosono et al. 2019). Although the Japanese version of neonatal resuscitation (NCPR) began as a physician-led evidence-based project, nurse experts such as neonatal nurses and midwifery professionals gradually began to engage in the NCPR as not only providers but also as instructors. Awareness of skilled nurses' presence at birth has led to an increase in NCPR certified nurses. By the end of 2020, 52,418 professionals had completed the advanced NCPR (nurses 30.2% and midwives 49.6%). This training included clinical knowledge/skills of the full scope of resuscitation including intubation and drug administration (nurses would not perform these functions without the physician's direction unless with additional training designated by the amended law). A total of 10,459 professionals (nurses 34.0% and midwives 43.1%) completed the basic NCPR provider course by the end of the year 2020 (NCPR 2020a). One NCPR certified nurse was available per 15.8 newborns per year nationwide in 2020 (MDs, 1:90.8) providing additional coverage for deliveries where physicians were not always available (NCPR 2020b, c). An increase in the number of nurses trained in NCPR would ensure that no infant would be born without NCPR certified nurses in the delivery room even at birthing clinics in any community.

Out of the 5033 NCPR instructors in Japan at the end of 2019, a total of 3203 taught the advanced course (nurses 14.6%, midwives 22.2%). A total of 1820 were basic course instructors with nursing engagement more significantly noted among this group (nurses 22.7%, midwives 59.5%) (NCPR 2020a). It is encouraging to observe quality improvement in delivery room settings, such as prevention of hypothermia, which is increasingly nurse-led.

11.7.2 Nurses' Contribution in Prenatal Diagnosis and Assisted Reproductive Medicine

Although ethical discussions continue regarding use of non-invasive prenatal genetic testing (NIPT) using maternal blood, NIPT is becoming widely available ahead of sufficient regulatory and policy provision or recommended standards, such as to only offer NIPT at tertiary centers to ensure availability of support and ethical transparency. It is known that mothers who are informed of undesirable fetal diagnosis experience significant shock regardless of the type of diagnosis (Awazu et al. 2015). Evidence-based standards must become available for ethical, safe, and effective use of NIPT or to set standards on how best to counsel those who undergo NIPTs. What methods of genetic counselling, post-testing emotional, or decision-making support are effective have not been well studied or understood, and current support is not adequate.

Today, nearly one in 60 births is the result of in-vitro fertilization in Japan. This phenomenon is multifactorial. Many Japanese couples are delaying childbearing, and increasingly, younger cancer patients are electing to receive fertility-preservation treatment. Increasingly, oncology and reproductive collaboration to refine the care for both parents and their newborns is being considered (Takai 2018). The nursing profession has an opportunity to build evidence to bridge the current gap in care so that parents who face complex experiences through NIPT, or have infants born after complicated fertility experiences, will receive adequate psychosocial support to achieve optimal family outcomes.

Opportunities to address maternal psychosocial challenges placing infants at risk.

Annually, 40,000 pregnant women suffer from mental health conditions requiring treatment. Maternal psychosocial challenges are often the contributing factors (Nakai et al. 2017). Child abuse among women suffering from postpartum depression is a public health crisis. When the medical fee schedule was revised in 2018, care of "High-Risk Mothers with Mental Health Conditions" received an additional credit (1000 points per month to the primary point of care) to allow reimbursement for the evaluation and implementation of multidisciplinary support during the prenatal visits. The care is coordinated among the team members of obstetrics, psychiatry, nursing, community health, and local health authorities to seamlessly support the mother from pregnancy to post-discharge after the birth of the child (Ministry of Health 2018c). There is paucity of data regarding the care of mother/infants when mothers suffer mental health conditions. Mothers with previous or existing diagnoses are known to experience difficulties in managing both self-care and parenting, often due to both the condition itself and drowsiness/fatigue as result of pharmacologic treatment (Kanamaru et al. 2017). New evidence is urgently needed with a strong nursing perspective to maximize the utilization of nurse-led resources (KMC, breastfeeding, Childcare Support, discussions, counselling, peer support, collaboration with community support) for "at risk mother/infant dyads" toward successful adaptation to life with the new child.

11.7.3 Disaster Preparedness

Past experiences with major disasters such as the Great Hanshin-Awaji Earthquake, the Great East Japan Earthquake and Tsunami, or the Kumamoto Earthquake led Japan to design highly coordinated and sophisticated systems to address disaster preparedness. Every prefecture has a designated point of contact which coordinates the regional perinatal needs in time of disaster (Ministry of Health 2017b). A total of 155 disaster health coordinators have been appointed as of 2018 to address perinatal/pediatric health, with 98% physicians (44% OBGYN, 52% Peds), and 1% midwives (Ministry of Health 2018a). It is recognized that an increase of nurses and midwives to serve in this role is needed. Additionally, significant challenges exist during a disaster to maintain and coordinate support for medically dependent infants at home who may have disruption in power, availability of clean water, or simply a safe place to live. A 2016 report estimated that nearly 17,000 medically dependent infants live in Japan (Ministry of Health 2017a). Rigorous nursing research as a part of a multidisciplinary team within the context of disaster management is needed.

Reflective Practice

Promoting developmental care (DC) at one institution in the greater Tokyo area. (Nakai)

Much progress has occurred in Japanese NICUs during the last 20 years in terms of understanding how best to provide developmentally sensitive care. Bright lights used to be common in NICUs, and repositioning and feedings were offered mechanically every 2 to 3 hours for very low birth weight infants without an in-depth understanding of infants' state transition. Crying infants were offered pacifiers, but little was done to truly soothe them. Families were often outside the NICU. The author was in NICU as a young third year staff nurse in 2004 when a developmental care (DC) training opportunity was offered. Along with the author's superior, efforts were made to disseminate the DC knowledge. The goals were set, and practice changes were implemented with unit wide education and training in spite of staff pushback. Recruiting the entire NICU team members including physicians was essential to avoid exposing infants to excess stimulations/procedures without concerns for the state transition. After the successful adoption of the new care approach, it was visibly noticeable that infants appeared calm, slept, and fed better with the lights and sounds controlled and state-sensitive care consistently provided. Nurses gained understanding of infants' responses to care and contributed to parental understanding of their infants. It was the author's perception that even the parental disposition improved when the DC concept was fully adopted. Saving critically ill or very premature lives do not always offer better long-term prognosis. Observing changes recognized in the infants and their families inspired the team to continue to progress and refine the NICU caregiving.

IBCLC-CNS collaboration to conduct Quality Improvement Project (Nakai)

A pediatric CNS at one tertiary center near Tokyo conducted a quality improvement project to increase the time infants can spend with parents, regardless of the mode of feeding or time of the day. The NICU considered unsafe on night shift for parents to breastfeed or hold infants who are tube-fed. The CNS proposed to the institution's Breastfeeding Support Working Group to relax these restrictions. The WG members conducted a hearing with the NICU and stepdown nursing and medical staff to evaluate the benefits and gain consensus. As a result, the WG approved pilot work in the stepdown unit. Nurses drafted parental educational materials to maintain safety. One physician who holds IBCLC status, consulted with the medical safety division at the institution to obtain clearance to launch parental engagement even on night shifts. The pediatric CNS and the lead stepdown unit nurse collaborated to ensure that the protocol was evidence-based. Three-months post-launch, a survey assessed the perceptions of stepdown unit nursing staff regarding the new practice. Results revealed favorable support for the practice change. The high-level care unit still has obstacles preventing the launch of this practice, thus, additional evidence-based strategies for NICU culture change are needed.

11.8 Future Challenges

The more critical the infants' conditions are, the stricter the institutional policies governing nursing practice can become. All in the name of safety, both nursing and parental care contributions may become restricted. The 2020–2022 ongoing global Pandemic with COVID19 and its impact may be a good example. Without evidence, many institutions eliminated the presence of families from bedside or highly restricted their presence to care for and to get to know their hospitalized vulnerable child. Concerns remain as to what long-term impact this restricted parent-child contact will have on both infants and families, and nurse-led research is greatly desired to minimize the negative impact. (Please refer to Chap. 18 for further discussion on the indirect impact of pandemic-led practice modifications).

Safety concerns have traditionally prevented nurses from performing many invasive procedures, although global neonatal nursing colleagues have long viewed peripheral intravenous line placements, heel sticks, or changing central line infusion tubing as nursing interventions. Recent findings revealed that many nursing administrators (30%) consider nurses' involvement in invasive care unnecessary, while 18% perceived it necessary and 50% of the respondents selected neutral (Konishi 2018b). To realize

high-quality family integrated care and maximize nursing contributions in all aspects of neonatal care, barriers must be overcome using a strategic evidence-based approach to promote the value of NICU nursing.

Case Studies

Case: Unique cultural challenges in Okinawa islands: An NCU Nurses' passion makes a difference (Uehara)
The Okinawa prefecture consists of 160 remote islands (47 inhabited), with Okinawa island, the largest, extending over 1000 km east to west, and 400 km north to south. Okinawa has 1.43 million population as of 2019. Nine percent of 1.43 million reside on remote islands away from Okinawa's main island. Okinawa's population has increased since 2000 with 40% coming from abroad. The top three countries contributing to the increase include China, the United States, and the Philippines (Okinawa Times 2019). Currently 1% of the Okinawan population is non-Japanese.

Due to the mismatch of female verses male population, the arrival of foreign brides from Southeast Asia also increased especially in remote areas (Nishihara 2019) as evidenced by 0.8% of maternal/child health handbooks being issued to foreign mothers. These handbooks which keep records of immunizations or records from check-ups are issued to every mother who delivers an infant in Japan. Okinawa has a higher childbirth rate per woman (the number of children every woman delivers in life between 15 and 49 years of age) compared to the national average (1.89 and 1.42, respectively). There are also higher under-19 age pregnancies than nationally (2.41% and 0.96% respectively). The low birth weight rate is also higher (12.4% and 10.5%, respectively) (e-Stat 2018). The main Okinawa island has two tertiary

NICUs (total 30 beds) and three secondary NICUs. Two other small NICUs are located on 2 of the remote islands. When there is a risk of premature birth in areas without NICUs, mothers are transported by the prefectural operated helicopter or by a fixed wing operated by a not-for-profit organization. During the evening hours, helicopters by the Self-Defense Force are often deployed. When premature infants are born on remote islands, physicians are sent via helicopter for infant retrieval. Thus, perinatal services are available throughout Okinawa.

A Filipino mother who was 28 weeks pregnant was transported from one of the remote islands to Okinawa Prefectural Nanbu Medical Center located on the main island. She delivered a 1112-g male infant with respiratory distress requiring ventilator support; however, he progressed without significant complications. The Filipino mother and the Japanese husband remained at the hospitality house nearby and visited their son regularly during the first several days. This Filipino mother had just recently arrived in Okinawa as a new bride not speaking either Japanese or English sufficiently. One of the NICU nurses informed the mother with a Tagalog-Japanese dictionary aided by gestures how her son was doing, or how to perform care including breast milk expression. The father was obligated to return home to tend to the family farm several days after the birth. Soon afterwards, the frequency of mother's visits declined due to anxiety in spite of her husband's daily phone call. Worried that his wife was depressed, the father took the initiative to call the NICU nurse to ask to reach out to his wife.

Nurse Noriko, when she visited the mother, found the mother in tears, distraught, and defeated. Noriko gently embraced her and asked, "How do you take care of babies in the Philippines? You can do the Filipino way for your baby."

Gradually, the mother warmed up to Noriko. With a smile returning, she resumed visiting NICU daily. With the continued progress over months, the infant was ready to be discharged on home-oxygen. Home-oxygen, however, had never been used for infants on the island where the family lived. This presented a major challenge.

Noriko, committed to a successful transition for this family to home, coordinated care to ensure that oxygen delivery devices could be maintained, and necessary supplies regularly delivered to the island. With the support from the clinic nurse, the only nurse residing on the island, meticulous and detailed follow-up plans were made, and the family began their new life at home. Noriko was delighted to see the mother and her thriving son at the follow-up clinic months later. She was also proud to find that mother's Japanese communication abilities were improving. A successful family adjustment to island life was visible.

This case demonstrates the contribution of a neonatal nurse and her team to strategically coordinate the care of infants and families with multiculture/communication, to resource challenges during the NICU stay and to follow through beyond the NICU graduation. Assessment of the needs of the family and the resources available in the community allowed the successful follow through. Increasing number of multicultural families will be seen in hospitals, not only in Okinawa, but throughout Japan. Psychosocial assessment and providing culturally sensitive support while also exploring the resource needs was made possible when nursing members are able to strategize with the passion to nurture families as Noriko did. The author hopes that this example inspires our nurse colleagues globally.

Case: Culturally Sensitive Grief/ Bereavement Care. (Nakamura)
When a family loses a child in NICU, the memory of the child is often left behind in the NICU. Once the family leaves the NICU,

the process of accepting the child's death, or absence of the child, while struggling through complex emotions of grief continues. The quality of the NICU family grief/bereavement support that is made available while in NICU greatly impacts the bereavement experience for parents after leaving the NICU empty handed, without their baby.

Traditionally Japanese culture viewed a child's death as a socially unacceptable topic for discussion among family members or friends; however, this trend is changing. With an increased number of publications on the topic of death and grief by bereaved parents, followed by recent national recommendations, open discussions have been promoted. The number of NICUs with private rooms has increased globally; however, private room NICU is not common in Japan. The family-centered care concept guided Seirei Hamamatsu General Hospital in Hamamatsu City to design the first Japanese NICU with private-room-like pods (only 4 beds/ pod) and additional full private rooms, which can be used for highly personalized palliative/bereavement care.

Interventions Aimed at Supporting Families Who Are Grieving

Once palliative care is elected by the family, the NICU team explores and discusses how the parents wish to spend their last days or hours with their child. The nurses propose possible interventions; however, every effort is made to hear the family's wishes and desires. The following is a list of care interventions often utilized at this institution for grieving parents.

- Allowing a stroll in the NICU as well as the hospital grounds when the weather and infant's condition permit.
- Making hand and footprints with family members.
- Making monthly birthday cards for the infant during the NICU stay.

- Having family room-in using the private room space (equipped with traditional Japanese home-like setup with futon mattress, Japanese style deep bath and other limited, but soothing decor) as often as possible, including encouraging the Japanese style "family bathing" experience (this is symbolic of family happiness and togetherness).
- Inviting the family to join the infant during any NICU events, such as Holiday celebrations.
- Setting up a special environment where a discharged twin can return to spend time with the dying sibling.
- Sending families a bereavement journal with nursing entries (it describes the family's experience of anticipatory grieving and observation of the infant's life from nursing perspective).
- Sending families annual holiday greetings to express that the NICU team remembers the child.

Feedback from the Bereaved Family Members

After a private space was constructed, frequencies of family visits as a part of their grieving increased. Letters received from families after the deaths of children often expressed satisfaction with the care they received using the private room. The following are actual words from families, either expressed in letters or in conversation during actual visits families had with the hospital staff afterwards.

> "It really felt like we were at home when we spent time with our dying child in the private family room. I did the 'routine' care for my baby in the middle of the night or any time without the worry of bothering other NICU babies."
> "The hours and days we were given to spend time as a family unit in the private family room was precious. We are able to live on with smiles on our faces today because of the precious opportunities we were given."

"The journal entries by the nurses were simply precious and receiving the journal encouraged us to move forward"

"When we received the holiday card, it reminded us fondly of the previous year when we celebrated the holiday together with our child at the hospital!"

"Receiving the holiday greeting from the hospital made us say, 'Thank you for remembering us!"

"The sibling (of the baby who passed away) loved seeing the greeting card that came from the hospital because she too has special memories of spending time with her baby sibling."

"Yes, we miss our baby boy who passed away,,,,, but it is not devastating us every day. We have no regrets in terms of what we were able to do for our baby, Ao-chan. We miss the physical presence, but we know Ao-chan is not too far away from us."

"I was so PROUD of the coffin we made of cypress tree ourselves (father stated proudly) for Ao-chan, and we were able to use a brand-new car to carry his precious tiny coffin! It could not have been more perfect to honour my precious "BOY" who lived so bravely than to have such a cool car for him! Having had the moments with Ao-chan in the private room before he left us allowed us to find more ways to honour our child with a positive attitude." (With family's request, Ao-chan's real name is included in these father's words to honour his son).

Reflection

The private room offered a home-like experience for the families, creating meaningful memories aligned with the home-like routines, such as a family bath in Japanese traditional style. The private room maximized the quality of the family experience during the last days and hours and encouraged them to engage in caregiving as well as just being together. Liberal use of the family room may be highly useful for families to cope with their grief. Some of the families' experiences appeared to have a lasting impact after the loss, enhancing the quality of bereavement experience. The sense of control to maintain a degree of normalcy

was important to many families, and parents having the freedom to be "family" in a home-like setting proved highly effective while making meaningful memories for not only parents, but also for siblings. Ao-chan's case was particularly special to the author who was the NICU manager at the time of Ao-chan's entire stay. Ao-chan remains alive in the hearts of the family members as well as in the author's (Nakamura).

11.9 Conclusion

This chapter highlights Japanese neonatal nursing education, practice, and healthcare delivery system. It presents the challenges and opportunities for the future changes. Global challenges in addressing increasingly complex needs of the neonates and their families both in NICU and in the community post-discharge call for the neonatal nurses to act locally with cultural sensitivity, act nationally to impact the policies, and act globally joining hands with global colleagues.

References

Aoyagi T (2003) Pulse oximetry: its invention, theory, and future. J Anesth 17:259–266

Aoyagi T, Miyasaka K (2002) Pulse oximetry: its invention, contribution to medicine, and future tasks. Anesth Analg 94:S1–S3

Arimitsu T, Wakabayashi D, Tamaoka S, Takahashi M, Hida M, Takahashi T (2021) Case report: intact survival of a marginally viable male infant born weighing 268 grams at 24 weeks gestation. Front Pediatr 8:628362

Awazu F, Yoneda M, Soyama S (2015) 出生前診断において胎児異常を告げられ た女性の心理に関する文献的考察 [Japanese]. Review of maternal psychological experiences upon being informed of abnormal fetal diagnosis. Ishikawa J Nurs 12:105–114

Bhattacharya K (2020) Takuo Aoyagi—a tribute to the brain behind pulse oximetry. Indian J Surg 20:1–2. https://doi.org/10.1007/s12262-020-02365-x

Cabinet Office, Government of Japan (2020) 少子化社会対策大綱 概要 [Japanese]. National Strategies to improve Japanese annual birth rates. [Online]. https://www8.cao.go.jp/shoushi/shoushika/law/pdf/r020529/shoushika_taikou_g.pdf

Cabinet Office, Government of Japan. Current Situation of Dwindling Births. https://www8.cao.go.jp/shoushi/shoushika/whitepaper/measures/w-2021/r03webhonpen/html/b1_s1-1-2.html

Center for Disease Control and Prevention DC (2018) Congenital heart defects. Information for the Healthcare Providers [Online]. https://www.cdc.gov/ncbddd/heartdefects/hcp.html

Eklund W (2010) Japan and its healthcare challenges and potential contribution of neonatal nurse practitioners. J Perinat Neonatal Nurs 24:155–166

Eklund W, Konishi M (2013) Evidence based practice, and the spirit of inquiry: the Asian example. J Neonatal Nurs 19:233–237

Eklund W, Mooneyham S (2022) Chapter 17: Critical congenital heart disease screening: History and concept. In C. Kenner & M. Boykova (Eds.). Neonatal nursing care handbook. An evidence-based approach to conditions and procedures. (3rd ed., pp. 586–595). Springer Publishing.

E-STAT (2018) Portal site for official statistics of Japan. e-Stat

Fujiwara T, Maeta H, Chida S, Morita T, Watabe Y, Abe T (1980) Artificial surfactant therapy in hyaline-membrane disease. Lancet 1:55–59

Fullterton BS, Hong CR, Velazco CS, Mercier CE, Morrow KA, Edwards EM, Ferrelli KR, Soll RF, Modi BP, Horbar JD, Jaksic T (2017) Severe neurodevelopmental disability and healthcare needs among survivors of medical and surgical necrotizing enterocolitis: a prospective cohort study. J Pediatr Surg

Furukawa H (2012) NICUに配置転換となった看護師の教育を考える ハイリスク新 生児ケアを担う配置転換となった看護師教育の課題を考える.[Japanese]. Considering the educational needs of nurses who are transferred to NICU without prior experience. J Jpn Acad Neonat Nurs 18:26–27

Higgins RD, Jobe AH, Koso-Thomas M, Bancalari E, Viscardi RM, Harters TV, Ryan RM, Kallapur SG, Steinhorn RH, Konduri GG, Davis SD, Thebaud B, Clyman RI, Collaco JM, Martin CR, Woods JC, Finer NN, Raju TNK (2018) Bronchopulmonary dysplasia: executive summary of a workshop. J Pediatr 197:300–308

Hosono S, Tamura M, Isayama T, Sugiura T, Kusakawa I, Ibara S, Neonatal Resuscitation Committee Japan Society of Perinatal Neonatal, M (2019) Neonatal cardiopulmonary resuscitation project in Japan. Pediatr Int 61(7):634–640. https://doi.org/10.1111/ped.13897

International Board of Certified Lactation Consultant (2020) IBCLC Certification [Online]. https://iblce.org/step-1-prepare-for-ibclc-certification/#

International Confederation of Midwives (2018) https://www.internationalmidwives.org

Japan Academy of Midwifery (2020) https://www.jyosan.jp/modules/english/index.php?content_id=1

Japan Academy of Neonatal Nursing (2019) 看護師のクリニカルラダー(日本看護協会 版)をもとにしたNICU看護師のクリニカルラダー案 [Japanese]. NICU-specific clinical ladder for nurses based on the JNA version [Online]. http://www.jann.gr.jp/wp-content/uploads/2019/01/be755be9716a-b13050ee5300011567191.pdf

Japan Academy of Neonatal Nursing (2020a) http://www.jann.gr.jp

Japan Academy of Neonatal Nursing (2020b) NICU に入院している新生児の痛みのケア ガイドライン 2020 年(改訂)版 [Neonatal pain management guidelines for NICU infants. Updated in 2020]

Japan Association of Nursing Programs in Universities (2019) 高度実践看護師教育課程 基準 [Japanese]. Advance Practice Nursing Educational Standard [Online]. https://www.janpu.or.jp/download/pdf/cns.pdf

Japan International Corporation of Welfare Services (2020) EPA 看護・介護受け入れ事業 [Japanese] Economic Partnership Agreement for Migrant Nurses and Assistive Care professionals. [Online]. https://jic-wels.or.jp/?page_id=14

Japan Nursing Association (2016a) Nursing in Japan. https://www.nurse.or.jp/jna/english/pdf/nursing-in-japan2016.pdf

Japan Nursing Association (2016b) 看護師のクリニカルラダー [Japanese]. Clinical Ladder for Nurses [Online]. https://www.nurse.or.jp/home/publication/pdf/fukyukeihatsu/ladder.pdf

Japan Nursing Association (2018) 文科省に要望書を提出 [Japanese]. Request submitted to the government. strengthen policies that guide nursing education and training. [Online]. JNA. https://www.nurse.or.jp/up_pdf/20180427105839_f.pdf

Japan Nursing Association (2020a) 認定看護師 [Japanese]. Certified Nurses [Online]. https://nintei.nurse.or.jp/nursing/wp-content/uploads/2020/12/CN_map_202012.pdf

Japan Nursing Association (2020b) 専門看護師 [Japanese]. Certified Nurse Specialist [Online]. https://nintei.nurse.or.jp/nursing/qualification/bunyatodofukentizu_cns

Johnson S, Marlow N (2017) Early and long-term outcome of infants born extremely preterm. Arch Dis Child 102:97–102

Kanamaru T, Mochizuki M, Nakamura N, Sato N, Nakai A (2017) Support provided by, and needed for, family members of mothers with mental health conditions who are raising young children. In: Paper presented at the 20th East Asian Forum of Nursing Scholars, p 85

Keller RL, Feng R, DeMauro SB, Ferkol T, Hardie W, Rogers EE, Respiratory Outcomes P et al (2017) Bronchopulmonary dysplasia and perinatal characteristics predict 1-year respiratory outcomes in newborns born at extremely low gestational age: a prospective cohort study. J Pediatr 187:89–97e83. https://doi.org/10.1016/j.jpeds.2017.04.026

Konishi M (2016) Japanese neonatal nursing with a historic perspective. J Neonatal Nurs 22(5):218–222. https://doi.org/10.1016/j.jnn.2016.04.004

Konishi M (2018a) Evaluation of national licensure examination content from 2013–2018. Any questions about neonates? In: Poster presentation. Paper presented at the 18th National Neonatal Nurses Conference, September 5–8. New Orleans, USA

Konishi M (2018b) NICU看護師の注射、採血実践の躊躇 看護師長の視点から [Japanese]. Perceptions among NICU managers toward neonatal nurses' involvement in invasive procedures, such as injections, venous puncture, or heel sticks. In: Paper presented at the 28th Japan Academy of Neonatal Nursing Annual Conference, Tokyo, Japan

Laptook AR, O'Shea TM, Shankaran S, Bhaskar B, Network NN (2005) Adverse neurodevelopmental outcomes among extremely low birth weight infants with a normal head ultrasound: prevalence and antecedents. Pediatrics 115(3):673–680. https://doi.org/10.1542/peds.2004-0667

Ministry of Health Labor and Welfare of Japan (2001) Healthy Parents and Children 21 [Online]. http://sukoyaka21.jp/healthy-parents-and-children-21

Ministry of Health Labor and Welfare of Japan (2010a) 子供・子育てビジョン [Japanese]. Vision for the future to raise and nurture children. [Online]. https://www.mhlw.go.jp/bunya/kodomo/pdf/vision-zenbun_0001.pdf

Ministry of Health Labor and Welfare of Japan (2010b) 周産期医療体制整備指針 [Japanese]. Guidelines for perinatal regionalization. [Online]. https://www.jnanet.gr.jp/document/kan/shishin2010.pdf

Ministry of Health Labor and Welfare of Japan (2017a) 医療的ケアが必要な障害児への 支援の充実に向けて [Japanese]. Medically dependent pediatric/neonatal population in the communities: strategies to reinforce support. [Online]. https://www.mhlw.go.jp/file/06-Seisakujouhou-12200000-Shakaiengokyokushougaihokenfukushibu/0000180993.pdf

Ministry of Health Labor and Welfare of Japan (2017b) 周産期医療の体制構築に関わる 指針 [Japanese]. An updated standard for regionalized organization of perinatal services [Online]. https://www.mhlw.go.jp/file/06-Seisakujouhou-10800000-Iseikyoku/4_2.pdf

Ministry of Health Labor and Welfare of Japan (2018a) 災害医療コーディネート体制 [Japanese]. National Disaster Preparedness [Online]. https://www.mhlw.go.jp/content/10802000/000377340.pdf

Ministry of Health Labor and Welfare of Japan (2018b) 助産師国家試験出題基準 [Japanese]. The national midwifery examination standards in Japan [Online]. https://www.mhlw.go.jp/file/04-Houdouhappyou-10803000-Iseikyoku-Ijika/0000158946.pdf

Ministry of Health Labor and Welfare of Japan (2018c) 平成30年度診療報酬改定の概要 個別改定項目 [Japanese]. Updates to healthcare reimbursement for services, 2018. [Online]. https://www.mhlw.go.jp/file/05-Shingikai-12404000-Hokenkyoku-Iryouka/0000193708.pdf

Ministry of Health Labor and Welfare of Japan (2019) 看護基礎教育検討会報告書 [Japanese]. A report from the Investigative Commission for Nursing Basic Education] [Online]. https://www.mhlw.go.jp/content/10805000/000557411.pdf

Ministry of Health Labor and Welfare of Japan (2020) 周産期母子両センター施設リスト [Japanese] A complete list of perinatal centers in Japan, May 1, 2020 [Online]. https://www.mhlw.go.jp/content/10800000/000637424.pdf

Nakai A, Mitsuda N, Kinoshita K (2017) メンタルヘルスに問題がある妊産婦の頻 度と社会的背景に関する研究 [Japanese]. Pregnant mothers with mental health conditions and their psychosocial issues. J Jpn Soc Perinat Neonat Med 53:43–49

NCPR (2020a) 新生児蘇生法講習会 インストラクター累計(職種別)[Japanese]. The number of NCPR instructors by profession and the types of courses. [online]. https://www.ncpr.jp/pdf/202012/202012-14.pdf

NCPR (2020b) 新生児蘇生法修了認定者数(医師) 1人当たりで担当する1年間の新生 児数(都道府県別対比) [Japanese]. The number of patients per NCPR certified physician per year. [online]. https://www.ncpr.jp/pdf/202012/202012-8.pdf

NCPR (2020c) 新生児蘇生法修了認定者数(助産師あるいは看護師)一人当たりで担当する一年間の新生児数 [Japanese]. The number patients per NCPR qualified nurse professional per year. [online]. https://www.ncpr.jp/pdf/202012/202012-9.pdf

Neonatal Cardio-Pulmonary Resuscitation (NCPR) (2020) http://www.ncpr.jp/index.html

NIDCAP Federation International (2020) NIDCAP Training [Online]. https://nidcap.org/en/programs-and-certifications/nidcap-training/overview-2/

Nishihara T (2019) 沖縄県の離島における在日フィリピン人母親の子育て [dissertation, Filipino mothers' efforts to raise children in Japan]. PhD, Okinawa Prefectural College of Nursing

Okinawa Times (2019) 沖縄の在留外国人、中国が2600人で最多に 米国人を抜 き初 [Japanese]. Foreign residents in Okinawa: 2600 Chinese nationals ahead of the US natives. https://www.okinawatimes.co.jp/articles/-/454843

Saiseikai Yokohamashi Tobu Hospital (2016) 小児プライマリケア認定看護師教育課程 2,021年 4月開講 [Japanese]. Certified Nurse Program in Pediatric Primary Care opening in April in 2021. [Online]. Saiseikai Yokohamashi Tobu Hospital. https://www.tobu.saiseikai.or.jp/pediatric-primary-care/

Shimizu A, Muraki Y, Fujimori M, Konishi M, Uchida M, KInoshita C, Utoh H et al (2019) Neonatal nursing practice survey: data from Japanese Perinatal Medical Centers. In: Poster presentation. Paper presented at the Council of International Neonatal Nurses Conference 2019, May 5–8, 2019. Auckland, NZ

Steinhorn R, Davis JM, Gopel W, Jobe A, Abman S, Laughon M (2017) Chronic pulmonary insufficiency of prematurity: developing optimal endpoints for drug development. J Pediatr 191:15–21e11. https://doi.org/10.1016/j.jpeds.2017.08.006

Takai Y (2018) Recent advances in oncofertility care worldwide and in Japan. Reprod Med Biol 17(4):356–368

TIME Magazine (1980) The Cow-Lung concoction may save "preemies" from early death. TIME Mag 115(8):59. direct=true&db=a9h&AN=54217671&site=ehost-live&scope=site

Wilson-Costello D, Friedman H, Minich N, Fanaroff AA, Hack M (2005) Improved survival rates with increased neurodevelopmental disability for extremely low birth weight infants in the 1990s. Pediatrics 115:997–1003

World Health Organization (2020) Nursing Now Campaign [Online]. https://www.who.int/hrh/news/2018/nursing_now_campaign/en/

Middle East (Lebanon)

12

Lina Kordahl Badr, Lama Charafeddine, and Saadieh Sidani

12.1 Introduction

Lebanon, like most countries, has some variation in neonatal nursing care. This chapter is based on personal observations of 12 Neonatal Intensive Care Units (NICUs) as well as face to face reports from 26 head nurses in 26 NICUs from all districts of Lebanon. Although this may not capture 100% of the NICUs, it represents the majority.

> **Key "Think Points" for Learning**
> - Levels of care do exist in Lebanon but some NICUs claiming Level III (tertiary) status do not have sufficient equipment.
> - NICU developmental care such as noise control, positioning, and parental visit is often not present.
> - Transport guidelines do not exist.
> - No consistent standards exist for neonatal nursing training.
> - Neonatal care standards and policies must be updated on a regular schedule.

L. K. Badr (✉)
Azusa Pacific University, Azusa, CA, USA

The American University of Beirut, Beirut, Lebanon

L. Charafeddine · S. Sidani
The American University of Beirut, Beirut, Lebanon

> - There is a critical need to increase NICU beds.
> - There is also a critical need to increase specialty neonatal nurses' training/education.

12.2 Background

Lebanon is a small country located on the eastern shore of the Mediterranean Sea; it consists of a narrow strip of territory and is one of the world's smaller sovereign states. Its rugged, mountainous terrain has served throughout history as an asylum for diverse religious and ethnic groups and for political dissidents. Lebanon is one of the most densely populated countries in the Mediterranean area and has a high rate of literacy. It is approximately 100 miles (160 km) long and varies in width from 6 to 35 miles (10–56 km). Despite its small size, the country has developed a well-known culture and has been highly influential in the Arab world, powered by its large diaspora. Before the Lebanese Civil War (1975–1990), the country experienced a period of relative calm and renowned prosperity, driven by tourism, agriculture, commerce, and banking. Because of its financial power and diversity in its heyday, Lebanon was referred to as the "Switzerland of the East" during the 1960s, and

J. Petty et al. (eds.), *Neonatal Nursing: A Global Perspective*,
https://doi.org/10.1007/978-3-030-91339-7_12

its capital, Beirut, attracted so many tourists that it was known as "the Paris of the Middle East." At the end of the war, there were extensive efforts to revive the economy and rebuild national infrastructure with little success especially with the influx of over one million Syrian refugees since 2011. The population of Lebanon was estimated to be 6,859,408 in 2018; however, no official census has been conducted since 1932 due to the sensitive confessional political balance between Lebanon's various religious groups.

In terms of health, a recent study noted that almost 80% of the estimated 168 hospitals in Lebanon are privately owned and are more expensive than public hospitals. In comparison with other developing countries where 4–6% of the GDP is spent on health, Lebanon's health expenditures were approximately 12% of its GDP. Europe spends 10% of its GDP on health with far more superior provision of health services, compared with Lebanon where many indigent individuals and families often do not receive appropriate care (Kronfol 2006; Tabbarah 2000). In addition, many people in rural areas are not able to access a functioning health facility either because this facility has been seriously damaged in the war or because it does not have the basic supplies or manpower required to provide health services. Lebanon has 2.88 beds per 1000 population—one of the highest ratios in the Middle East; however, the occupancy rate is as low as 60% in most hospitals. In 2009, there were 31.29 physicians and 19.71 nurses per 10,000 inhabitants, which is opposite to most countries where the ratio of nurses to physicians is much higher and the ratio of nurses to inhabitants is higher. The life expectancy at birth was 72.59 years in 2011. Many, if not all, health professionals speak English and/or French in addition to Arabic. The fertility rate was 1.75 in 2004 (no new data were available at the time of writing this chapter).

The rate of prematurity in Lebanon is between 9% and 12%, and low birth weight (LBW) is between 6% and 8%, with both showing an upward trend in the past decade (Sather et al. 2010). There are higher rates in the Syrian refugee camps. Around 18,000 preterm babies are born each year in Lebanon, half of them are Syrian babies which reflects the higher rates of premature birth among refugees than in the local population. The mortality rate in Lebanon is 20/1000 live births. There are 156 NICU beds in Lebanon in both private and public hospitals. Almost 50% of the private and public hospitals claim to have a neonatal intensive care unit (NICU), although it is not clear which level of care is provided. Furthermore, because the provision of NICUs is not regulated by the Lebanese government, there is a lack of standardized care (Firth and Ttendo 2012). The etiology of preterm birth (PTB) in Lebanon and, indeed, worldwide, remains unclear. Consanguinity, which is still common in the Middle East, may be a potential risk factor for PTB. The incidence rate of major birth defects in Lebanon was 16.5 per 1000 live births in 2009. The neonatal mortality rate for Lebanese children is 4.4% per 1000 births, and for non-Lebanese it is 6.3% with the largest incidence in infants weighing between 1000 and 2000 g. The next section deals with the care of preterm infants in the NICUs in Lebanon.

12.3 Care and Design

Although there is a growing number of NICUs in Lebanon, only a couple qualify as level III units. Even NICUs that claim to have level III units do not have the equipment to stabilize or provide neonatal resuscitation. Although essential equipment for safe maternal and newborn health care such as infusion pumps and fetal monitoring equipment are available in most public and private hospitals, some NICUs lack the basic equipment for a level III unit. For example, in some NICUs, oxygen saturation monitors are not available to all infants; neither are portable X-rays nor blood gas analysis available on the unit. In terms of bedside monitoring of infants, most NICUs have monitors for heart rate and respiratory rate assessments. Monitoring of oxygen saturation and delivery in preterm infants is also available in most facilities. Mercury and digital thermometers are readily available and in many NICUs, rectal temperature taking is still being used. A micro-laboratory is not present in any of the hospitals visited and observed by the authors. Most hospitals observed have the NICU as a distinct area within the health care facility, with controlled access and a controlled environment (Fernández and Antolín-Rodríguez 2018). However, not all NICUs exclude passage to other services. All the hospitals have the NICU in close and controlled proximity to the area of the hospital where births occur. Often, seriously ill infants are not separated from healthy infants and are not near the nurses' station for close observation. Free hand-washing stations for hand hygiene and areas for gowning and storage of clean and soiled materials are noted in the majority of the hospitals. In some NICUs, the sinks are within the patient care area and are often too small to control splashing. On observation of hospitals, only one hospital had a family-infant room to encourage overnight stays by parents and the infant in the NICU. Despite the awareness of most nurses that high noise levels in the NICU may negatively impact infants, literature supports the fact that only a few NICUs have a written policy related to noise reduction and a machine to measure noise levels (Almadhoob and Ohlsson 2020; Casavant et al. 2017; Shogan and Schumann 1993; Walsh-Sukys et al. 2001; Zahr and de Traversay 1995). Moreover, close to only 50% of NICUs appear to have guidelines regarding ambient light and practiced covering the isolettes with blankets to reduce light (Lasky and Williams 2009).

12.4 Transport

It was not clear from the units observed whether there are clear guidelines regarding the safe transport of infants to other facilities that provide more advanced care. Often, a red cross ambulance may be called for transportation; however, these ambulances are usually not equipped for the safe transfer of sick or ventilator-dependent infants. It is worth noting that traffic in Beirut is extremely congested and drivers do not give way to ambulances so that even the best equipped ambulances do not reach their destination in time to save lives.

12.5 Neonatal Staff

Nurses To date, Lebanon lacks an official reporting mechanism to survey nurses or to monitor continuing education credits. However, most nurses are required to take a neonatal resuscitation course offered in conjunction with the Ministry of Health. The American and European standards for providing trained neonatal nurses are non-existent in Lebanon. Thus, the skills required for nurses to provide safe and high-quality neonatal intensive nursing care are not present. There are also no regulations related to the ratio of nurses to babies, although most NICUs indicated that for high-dependency infants, one nurse is responsible for one or two babies, and for less acute infants, the ratio is one nurse to three or four babies. The majority of nurses are not certified in certain skills such as intravenous (IV) peripheral cannula insertion or venepuncture, although many receive on-site training.

Physicians In university hospitals, there is a designated neonatologist, pediatrician, or pediatric resident on call who is responsible for the care of high-risk infants. However, this may not be the case in several hospitals. In fact, on observation, in one hospital with a level II NICU, neither a pediatrician nor a neonatologist on call was available. There is no NICU intensivist at night anywhere in Lebanon which is understandable due to poor resources to finance a full-time neonatologist 24/7. There are 16 certified neonatologists with 6 pediatricians experienced in neonatology. The indefinite presence of Syrian refugees in Lebanon has put additional pressure in NICUs for neonatologists (Blanchet et al. 2016). To be registered at the Lebanese order of physicians, one only needs proof of 2 years of experience in neonatology; there is no board requirement or subspecialty colloquium. There are only a handful of neonatologists who have formal neonatology training. Many of those trained in Europe have a combined pediatric intensive care unit (PICU) and NICU training (Kassak et al. 2006). Many NICUs in the country are attended by pediatricians with "experience" in neonatology.

12.6 Policies

Although most NICUs visited by the authors had some written policies and standards of care, some of these policies had not been updated for years. There were limited and often non-existent protocols for several essential procedures such as for transportation, for evaluation and treatment of retinopathy of prematurity, for resuscitation, and for the recognition of seizures or necrotizing enterocolitis among others (Charafeddine et al. 2016).

12.7 Parents

While there is a trend in some NICUs to engage parents in the care of their babies, 70% of NICUs do not have flexible parental visiting hours. Parental involvement is restricted to holding the baby with few NICUs practicing kangaroo care (Nyqvist et al. 2010; Pineda et al. 2018; Roque et al. 2017). Many physicians express skepticism about the benefits of kangaroo mother care (KMC) based on their apprehension for increasing the risk of infection. Breastfeeding is encouraged in all the NICUs and in the majority, there is a special room for expressing and for storing breast milk. In some NICUs, formula is offered to infants, because mothers do not want to express their milk or nurses were concerned about breast milk being contaminated. None of the NICUs have any program for lending breast pumps.

12.8 Monitoring of Outcomes and Physical Parameters

Lebanon lacks a national system for the organization and distribution of the quality of maternal health services. The ministry of health began collecting data a decade ago on maternal and newborn health outcomes, but the data remain inconsistent. In terms of bedside monitoring of infants, most NICUs have monitors for heart rate and respiratory rate assessments. Monitoring of oxygen saturation and delivery in preterm infants

is also available in most facilities. Mercury and digital thermometers are readily available. However, in many NICUs, rectal temperature is still being used. No guidelines have been noted in relation to the frequency of recording vital signs for seriously ill infants compared with less sick infants. Daily weights are recorded in all NICUs; however, premature infant charts are not being used in most NICUs, and the assessment of head circumference and abdominal girth does not appear to be routinely done.

12.9 Infection Control, Sepsis

All hospitals have a designated area for an isolation room. However, it is not clear if these rooms had appropriate ventilation systems for negative air pressure or tight seals to prohibit potentially harmful air infiltrating the NICU environment from the outside or from other airspaces. All the NICUs previously observed have had protocols for infection control such as using sterile techniques for the change of tubing and stopcocks and for flushing syringes on a regular basis. Furthermore, some NICUs did not have a system for reporting infections in the NICUs as required by Western standards (Vergnano et al. 2011). Again, this finding reflects the lack of governmental monitoring of data on neonatal outcomes. Nurses, doctors, and visitors are required to use a long gown upon entry to the NICU. Hand hygiene includes scrubbing hands after removing any jewelry or using hand-sanitizing gels, although this is not often observed when moving from one baby to another. Individual stethoscopes, thermometers, and wash basins are available at each bedside. Other equipment such as scales and probes are washed with a chlorhexidine alcohol solution, and incubators are wiped clean daily by the bedside nurse. There is no noted hand hygiene monitoring via volunteers, staff, or infection control task forces in place. Infants with suspected sepsis receive sepsis workup and antibiotics. However, what is required for workup and the choice of antibiotics is at the discretion of physicians because no standard policy has been observed. The most commonly prescribed antibiotics are a penicillin/gentamicin combination, followed by cefotaxime and vancomycin.

12.10 Feeding

The initiation of breastfeeding is encouraged in most facilities, although many are placed on formula milk as soon as they are stable. Most NICUs do not have the adequate equipment to collect and store breast milk. Daily fluid intake is routinely commonly recorded by nurses, but energy intake is done by residents or physicians. Feeding protocols vary between facilities, but in general, feeds consists of formula provided at 90–100 cal/kg/day slowly via a feeding tube (sizes between 3FG and 8FG or French-FR in many countries) inserted via the nasogastric route. Use of the oral route for the gastric tube and facilitating sucking with a pacifier is not commonly practiced. Residuals are checked before each feed, and the feeding tube remains in place and is changed every 8–24 h. No evidence-based guidelines or algorithms based on Western standards for the safe placement and assessment of feeding tubes by pH testing or radiographs (the gold standard) are observed in most NICUs. Total parenteral nutrition (TPN) is given to infants who cannot tolerate formulas or who are seriously ill according to the physician's written orders. In some NICUs, the nurses prepare the TPN solution. It is unclear if there are any standards for TPN orders or for sterile preparation of TPN under laminar flow hoods. The provision of intralipids or standard order sets is noted in few NICUs.

12.11 Intravenous Lines

Peripheral arterial lines and central lines are inserted by neonatologists, pediatricians, or pediatric residents, whereas peripheral IV lines are inserted by nurses. Umbilical lines are also used in some NICUs. All the hospitals visited had a policy to change IV lines every 72 hours. Umbilical lines are kept for a maximum of 7–10 days. Nurses draw blood from umbilical lines as requested by physicians. Although catheter-associated bloodstream infections are a serious threat to NICU patients, only a few NICUs had protocols for assessing the incidence of catheter-associated bloodstream infections in umbilical or peripheral lines, for monitoring the occurrence.

12.12 Thermoregulation

Protocols for thermoregulation are not noted in most NICUs, and the prevention of heat loss in low birthweight (LBW) infants by the use of kangaroo care, head caps, or polyethylene occlusive skin wrapping is not observed in the majority of the NICUs. Most NICUs do not have clear policies to monitor hyperthermia or hypothermia during delivery or transport to the NICU (Dauger and Jones 2017).

12.13 Developmental Care

Developmental care is becoming trendier, especially in university hospitals. One neonatologist and a developmental care nurse have acknowledged the benefits of developmental and have implemented a developmental care follow-up clinic in one university hospital including Newborn Individualized Developmental Care and Assessment Program® (Boston, MA) (NIDCAP) training for nurses. The majority of NICU graduates are followed up by a pediatrician who refers a developmentally delayed infant to a neurologist. It is hoped that many more NICUs around the country will recognize the benefits of follow-up developmental care. Several NICUs are implementing cluster care to allow the infant to sleep. Nesting devices and positional aids are used in some NICUs, although the most common position of infants in most NICUs is supine with no support.

12.14 Pain Management

Repetitive painful stimuli may persistently alter pain processing in humans. Several studies have found an association between excessive painful stimuli and later developmental and behavioral problems (Badr et al. 2007; Cong et al. 2017). However, most NICUs have not taken serious measures to alleviate pain in premature infants. Two NICUs were found to have standardized tools for pain assessment (e.g., Neonatal Pain, Agitation and Sedation Scale—NPASS, Neonatal Infant Pain Scale—NIPS, or *C*rying, *R*equires Oxygen for arterial oxygen saturation greater than 95, *I*ncreased Vital Signs, *E*xpression, *S*leepless—CRIES) and three NICUs use sucrose during painful procedures. No written protocols for pain assessment or the management of pain nonpharmacologically or pharmacologically have been observed in most NICUs.

12.15 Discharge Planning

Few NICUs have written discharge planning protocols. While discharge planning is coordinated between the charge nurse and the neonatologist/pediatrician, most NICUs discharge infants based on weight and not on the individual readiness of the mother and baby (van Kampen et al. 2019). Discharge teaching and the need for follow-up appointments are performed as needed by nurses or physicians on a one-to-one basis. Discharge booklets for parents have been noted in two NICUs, and teaching parents about cardiopulmonary resuscitation or the use of car seats is noted in two university hospitals. However, there is no law that fines parents for not placing their infants in car seats.

12.16 Long-Term Follow-Up

Unfortunately, none of the NICUs have a defined protocol for neurodevelopmental follow-up or a close liaison with local child development teams. Most infants are followed up by their pediatrician. This can be explained by the fact that most physicians are reluctant to send their babies to another provider for care. The result is that babies at risk for neurodevelopmental and learning disabilities especially in the very LBW infants are often missed or not diagnosed until it is too late for any beneficial intervention. One university hospital has recently begun a premature follow-up clinic with developmental assessment which was funded by private donations. Although this clinic provides free care, most families who attend are of low income while most middle- and high-income families revert to follow-up with their private pediatricians.

12.17 Conclusion

Overall, the limitations in premature infant care may be related to a lack of national standards and limited collaboration between public and private sectors, between obstetric and neonatal providers, and between public health professionals and business groups, who ideally should be working toward a common goal to encourage quality care to all premature infants. Lebanon's NICUs are facing tremendous challenges as there is an economic crisis and the government is not able to pay hospitals. Rural hospitals are more at jeopardy as they lack qualified health professionals and a there is a dearth of technology for advanced support and equipment. Overall, there is an urgent need to increase the number of NICU beds and to introduce new medical monitoring and treatment therapies. There is also a serious and pressing need to increase the number of qualified, trained neonatologists and to train more nurses in the care of sick, small and premature infants to help enhance future outcomes for them and their families.

Personal Reflection
I graduated from my bachelor's in nursing (BSN) program in Lebanon in 1973 at the age of 20 years and came to Houston to study for my master's in nursing (MSN) degree. With no money to support me,

I sought a night shift position in several hospitals at the medical center with no avail. After a month of trying to find a position, I landed one at a public hospital working night shifts. With no experience except for my clinical rotations during my university years, I was assigned the charge nurse of a 60-bed pediatric ward where 10 isolettes were assigned to premature infants. With one LVN and one nurse helping me, needless to say that many of these premature infants did not survive a day or two after birth. We have come a long way in the past 48 years thanks to dedicated neonatal physicians and nurses.

References

Almadhoob A, Ohlsson A (2020) Sound reduction management in the neonatal intensive care unit for preterm or very low birth weight infants. Cochrane Database Syst Rev 1:CD010333. https://doi.org/10.1002/14651858.CD010333.pub3

Badr LK, Abdallah B, Balian S, Tamim H, Hawari M (2007) The chasm in neonatal outcomes in relation to time of birth in Lebanon. Neonatal Netw 26(2):97–102. https://doi.org/10.1891/0730-0832.26.2.97

Blanchet K, Fouad FM, Pherali T (2016) Syrian refugees in Lebanon: the search for universal health coverage. Confl Heal 10:1–5

Casavant SG, Bernier K, Andrews S, Bourgoin A (2017) Noise in the neonatal intensive care unit: what does the evidence tell us? Adv Neonatal Care 17(4):265–273. https://doi.org/10.1097/ANC.0000000000000402

Charafeddine L, Badran M, Nakad P, Ammar W, Yunis K (2016) Strategic assessment of implementation of neonatal resuscitation training at a national level. Pediatr Int 58(7):595–600. https://doi.org/10.1111/ped.12868

Cong X, Wu J, Vittner D et al (2017) The impact of cumulative pain/stress on neurobehavioral development of preterm infants in the NICU. Early Hum Dev 108:9–16. https://doi.org/10.1016/j.earlhumdev.2017.03.003

Dauger S, Jones P (2017) Passive hypothermia (≥35 - <36°C) during transport of newborns with hypoxic-ischaemic encephalopathy. PLoS One 12(3):e0170100. https://doi.org/10.1371/journal.pone.0170100

Fernández D, Antolín-Rodríguez R (2018) Bathing a premature infant in the intensive care unit: a systematic review. J Pediatr Nurs 42:e52–e57. https://doi.org/10.1016/j.pedn.2018.05.002

Firth P, Ttendo S (2012) Intensive care in low-income countries – a critical need. N Engl J Med 367(21):1974–1976. https://doi.org/10.1056/NEJMp1204957

Kassak KM, Ghomrawi HM, Osseiran AM, Kobeissi H (2006) The providers of health services in Lebanon: a survey of physicians. Hum Resour Health 17:4–9

Kronfol NM (2006) Rebuilding of the Lebanese health care system: health sector reforms. East Mediterr Health J 12:32–39

Lasky RE, Williams AL (2009) Noise and light exposures for extremely low birth weight newborns during their stay in the neonatal intensive care unit. Pediatrics 123:540–546

Nyqvist KH, Anderson GC, Bergman N et al (2010) State of the art and recommendations. Kangaroo mother care: application in a high-tech environment. Breastfeed Rev 18:21–28

Pineda R, Bender J, Hall B, Shabosky L, Annecca A, Smith J (2018) Parent participation in the neonatal intensive care unit: predictors and relationships to neurobehavior and developmental outcomes. Early Hum Dev 117:32–38. https://doi.org/10.1016/j.earlhumdev.2017.12.008

Roque ATF, Lasiuk GC, Radünz V, Hegadoren K (2017) Scoping review of the mental health of parents of infants in the NICU. J Obstet Gynecol Neonatal Nurs 46(4):576–587. https://doi.org/10.1016/j.jogn.2017.02.005

Sather M, Fajon AV, Zaentz R, Rubens CE (2010) Global report on preterm birth and stillbirth (5 of 7): advocacy barriers and opportunities. BMC Pregnancy Childbirth 10(1):5

Shogan MG, Schumann LL (1993) The effect of environmental lighting on the oxygen saturation of preterm infants in the NICU. Neonatal Netw 12(7–13):468

Tabbarah R (2000) The health care system of Lebanon. http://www.who.int/entity/chp/knowledge/publications/case_study_lebanon.pdf

van Kampen F, de Mol A, Korstanje J et al (2019) Early discharge of premature infants < 37 weeks gestational age with nasogastric tube feeding: the new standard of care? Eur J Pediatr 178(4):497–503. https://doi.org/10.1007/s00431-018-03313-4

Vergnano S, Menson E, Kennea N et al (2011) Neonatal infections in England: the Neon IN surveillance network. Arch Dis Child Fetal Neonat 96:F9–F14

Walsh-Sukys M, Reitenbach A, Hudson-Barr D, De Pompei P (2001) Reducing light and sound in the neonatal intensive care unit: an evaluation of patient safety, staff satisfaction and costs. Perinatology 21:230–235

Zahr LK, de Traversay J (1995) Premature infant responses to noise reduction by earmuffs: effects on behavioral and physiologic measures. J Perinatol 15:448–455

Part II

Key Topics for Neonatal Nursing Across the Globe

Continuity of Neonatal Care in the Community: Post-discharge Care for Preterm, Small, and Sick Babies

13

Andre Ndayambaje

Key "Think Points" for Learning

- The majority of neonatal deaths are preventable.
- Neonatal deaths occur after discharge to home so community-based approaches to care must be strengthened to improve these outcomes.
- Community-based interventions should include family empowerment through health education.

The United Nations for Children and Families (UNICEF) (2020) reported that the global neonatal mortality rate was 17 deaths per 1000 live births in 2019 with around 6700 neonatal deaths occurring daily. UNICEF (2020) stated that, although there has been a reduction of infant and child mortality, neonatal mortality continues to decrease more slowly. From 1990 to 2019 neonatal mortality declined by 2.5% compared to 3.6% decrease among children aged 1–59 months during the same time period. Around 75% of neonatal deaths occur during the first week of life and

the majority of these deaths are due to preventable intrapartum-related complications such as lack of assistance to breath at birth, infections, and poor or lack of thermocare at birth (World Health Organization (WHO) 2020). Besides the remaining avoidable facility-based deaths, many other neonates continue to die in the community/at home after being discharged or among those born at home. A study on post-discharge infant mortality prediction in Sub-Saharan Africa reported that up to 13% of discharged infants deteriorate in the communities and many of them die (Madrid et al. 2019). The same study concluded that "No predictive models of post-discharge mortality among all cause admissions in resource-constrained hospitals or among infants have been developed to date" (Madrid et al. 2019). The evidence indicated that home-based group counselling of mothers and family members has moderate effects on the reduction of neonatal morbidity and mortality in limited and low-income settings. Hanson et al. (2017) conducted a meta-analysis of community-based health education models that focused on newborn care, breastfeeding, and how to care for a sick newborn. They found that when these strategies were employed there was a 25% reduction in neonatal mortality (Hanson et al. 2017). However, these interventions had more effect in south Asia than sub-Saharan Africa and were less effective if the neonate was facility born (Hanson et al.

A. Ndayambaje (✉)
University of Global Health Equity (UGHE), Kigali, Rwanda

Council of International Neonatal Nurses, Inc. (COINN), Yardley, PA, USA

J. Petty et al. (eds.), *Neonatal Nursing: A Global Perspective*,
https://doi.org/10.1007/978-3-030-91339-7_13

2017). In 2013, another systematic review of seven trials of women's groups based on participatory learning and action cycles published found a 20% decrease in neonates' deaths (Prost et al. 2013). In 2014, the WHO launched a call entitled "Evidence and recommendation on community mobilization through facilitated participatory learning and action cycles with women's groups for maternal and newborn health" as one of key strategies to improve health outcomes of vulnerable neonates in communities. This chapter describes the importance of the continuum of newborn care at community and home level and its impact on neonatal morbidity and mortality in remote and low-income settings.

According to the 2017 WHO bulletin on neonatal survival trends, community-based neonatal approach composes one of key strategies to achieve the Sustainable Development Goal (SDG 3) which is to decrease neonatal mortality to 12 deaths per 1000 live births by 2035 (Hanson et al. 2017). The neonatal community-based approach includes the decentralization and provision of high quality of care at community and home level by skilled health professionals, community health workers (CHW), and parents (Guta et al. 2018). The package should include neonatal health promotion, prevention, curative and rehabilitation approaches with active community participation and mobilization (Guta et al. 2018). Post-discharge follow-up and care includes home-based counselling and behavior-change education to enable the parents to detect, respond, and report the danger signs of health issues to the health professionals and/or community health workers (CHWs). Mothers and other family members are trained on what to look for and to seek medical assistance when a neonate presents with one of the danger signs such as difficulties with breastfeeding, losing weight, seizures, difficulty breathing, hyperthermia ($>37.5°C$) or hypothermia ($<36.4°C$) and jaundice. In home-based counselling sessions are aimed to promote exclusive breastfeeding, skin-to-skin contact for small and preterm neonates; kangaroo mother care (KMC) for term babies, timely seeking care for sick newborns, immunization and weight gain monitoring. Mothers and other family members

when given this information are empowered and able to mobilize the community resources. These actions will help mitigate factors associated with neonatal morbidity and mortality.

All neonates whether term, preterm, low birth weight (LBW) and those discharged from newborn care units should have continuity of essential newborn care until six weeks of life. Exclusive breastfeeding is recommended to continue until six months of life (World Health Organization (WHO) 2021). Before discharge mothers receive counselling and education on how to provide adequate and effective essential newborn care at home.

13.1 Continuity of Neonatal Care at Community and Home Level

Continuum care promotes exclusive breastfeeding which means to feed a baby only human milk until 6 months of life except some medications, oral rehydration salts, vitamins, and fortifiers under medical indications and prescriptions. When exclusive breastfeeding is combined with the practice of Kangaroo mother care (KMC) or skin-to- skin contact (SCS), this creates a strong relationship between a mother and her baby and increases breastfeeding rates (Sharma 2016).

A well breastfed baby gains enough weight and acquires safe nutrients in the breastmilk needed for the baby to grow and build his/her immune system against childhood sickness. Although exclusive breastfeeding is one of the most effective strategies for increasing survival of infants, unfortunately the practice of exclusive breastfeeding is still low especially in African countries with the average 37% among the infants under six months (Bhattacharjee et al. 2019). In some rural communities, babies are fed cow's milk, while in urban settings where the mothers return to work a few weeks after giving birth, they prefer to use a different formula. Unfortunately, the types of formula are poorly prepared which leads to food intolerance, gastrointestinal tract infections, sepsis, and other conditions related to unbalanced diet intake.

13.2 Role of Community Health Workers in Promotion of Continuum Newborn Care

The evidence indicates that well trained, supplied, supported and supervised community health workers (CHWs) can play a great role in the reduction of neonatal morbidity and mortality by identifying, reporting and where possible treating most neonatal danger signs (Bhutta et al. 2005). During pregnancy, the CHW promotes antenatal care, helps prepare for birth, and prepares the mothers for optimal newborn care practices. After birth and when a neonate is discharged from a facility, a CHW conducts three home visits to assess the newborn for any danger sign, help with breastfeeding and thermal care, weigh the baby, and advise on care for mother and baby.

Studies conducted in Bangladesh, India, and Pakistan reported that the community health workers, through home visits can contribute up to 61% reduction in newborn deaths in settings with high neonatal mortality (Aboubaker et al. 2014). The same studies showed that "among infants who survived the first day of life, neonatal mortality was 67% lower in those who received a CHW visit on day one than in those who received no visit and that for those who survived the first two days of life, receiving the first visit day two was associated with 64% lower neonatal mortality than those who did not receive a visit" (Aboubaker et al. 2014).

The remaining questions need to be explored around community-based neonatal approaches. There is an urgent need to scale up the community and home-based neonatal approaches to ensure the continuum of newborn care until 6 weeks of life. However, there are still many barriers regarding implementation of neonatal healthcare programs that demand additional operational research. Several areas in need of strengthening through research are: availability and implementation of policies and protocols, evidence-based guidelines for care, metrics and how the data are collected to measure success, workforce shortage including the specialized education and knowledge of the present healthcare workforce and their impact on neonatal outcomes (Khurmi et al. 2017).

Which cadre of health workers can most effectively provide the needed services at the community level? How will these cadres be trained, supervised, and supported to ensure they can provide the evidence based and high quality of newborn care? What is a scope of community-based neonatal care delivery (e.g., health promotion, prevention, curative or rehabilitation)? Is there a need to deploy a professional team down to community level to work closely with the CWHs and mothers, particularly for the preterm, small, and sick neonates? Can effective implementation of a behavior-change communications package at the domiciliary level, without active case management of newborn illness by health workers, improve neonatal outcomes? What is the added benefit and cost-effectiveness of active identification and management of neonatal illness, particularly serious bacterial infections and intrapartum hypoxia/birth asphyxia? What are the most feasible and effective ways to deliver lifesaving newborn resuscitation and antibiotic therapy in the community? How can barriers to care seeking for newborn illness be overcome most effectively so that home-based care and care seeking can be effectively linked with referral-level care at facilities? What is the impact and cost-effectiveness of postnatal visitation for promotion of healthful behaviors and recognition of neonatal illness? Can the same worker address the postnatal needs of both mothers and newborns? What is the optimal timing and number of routine visits with a health-care provider? What special skills/training do personnel need if they are caring for the small and sick newborn?

Reflective Practice

In 2018 I was a mentor in a remote District Hospital of Rwanda in a Low Dose High Frequency Mentorship program called Helping Mothers and babies survive. This hospital is located in one of the coldest regions of Rwanda where the population survives from agriculture and elevage or upbringing. It is a rural and mountainous region with poor geographical accessibil-

ity to the health facilities especially in the rainy season. Due to the fact that pregnant mothers were involved in heavy work with poor and unsafe living conditions, many pregnancies ended with premature rupture of membranes and preterm births. Many of those preterm babies died in communities before reaching the health facilities and many others died a few days or weeks after being discharged from the hospital. The major causes of neonatal deaths in that cold region are hypothermia and neonatal infections. The main concern was that the discharged preterm and small babies accompanied their mothers to work in the fields very early in the morning returning later in the evening. With this exposure, many of those babies deteriorated in the community and died. In order to mitigate those neonatal deaths, we initiated community outreach and educated mothers about kangaroo mother care (KMC) and skin-to-skin contact (SSC), the identification and reporting the danger signs to the community health workers (CHWs) and behavior-change counselling sessions on seeking health assistance when the baby was sick. Clothes were donated to the mothers to keep the babies warm as well as feeding cups to keep adequate intake at home. We conducted a mentorship program among the community health workers on home-based essential care for every baby and small/sick babies. The outcome was impressive; there was increasing neonatal survival in the community especially among the preterm and low birth weight babies. We learned that the continuum of neonatal care at community and home levels could contribute to the elimination of the remaining preventable and available neonatal deaths in low-income countries. However, there still is a need to link the facility-based neonatal approaches to the community

interventions. The neonatal community-based intervention should comprehensively be adapted on socio-cultural, economic, and geographical health determinants among the members of the society.

13.3   Conclusion

This chapter has presented the use of community-based approaches to improve neonatal survival. My personal experiences have been shared.

References

Aboubaker S, Qazi S, Wolfheim C, Oyegoke A, Bahl R (2014) Community health workers: a crucial role in newborn health care and survival. J Glob Health 4(2):020302. https://doi.org/10.7189/jogh.04.020302

Bhattacharjee NV, Schaeffer LE, Marczak LB et al (2019) Mapping exclusive breastfeeding in Africa between 2000 and 2017. Nat Med 25:1205–1212

Bhutta ZA, Darmstadt GL, Hasan BS, Haws RA (2005) Community-based interventions for improving perinatal and neonatal health outcomes in developing countries: a review of the evidence. Pediatrics 115(2):519–617. https://doi.org/10.1542/peds.2004-1441

Guta YR, Risenga PR, Moleki MM, Alemu MT (2018) Community-based maternal and newborn care: a concept analysis. Curationis 41(1):e1–e6. https://doi.org/10.4102/curationis.v41i1.1922

Hanson C, Kujala S, Waiswa P, Marchant T, Schellenberg J (2017) Community-based approaches for neonatal survival: meta-analyses of randomized trial data. Bull World Health Organ 95:453–464. https://doi.org/10.2471/BLT.16175844

Khurmi MS, Sayinzoga F, Berhe A, Bucyana T, Mwali AK, Manzi E, Muthu M (2017) Newborn survival case study in Rwanda-Bottleneck analysis and projections in key maternal and child mortality rates using the lives save tool (LiST). Int J MCH AIDS 6(2):93–108

Madrid L, Casellas A, Sacoor C, Quinto L, Sitoe A, Varo R, Acacio S, Nhampossa T, Massora S, Sigauque B, Mandomando I, Cousen S, Menendez C, Alonso P, Macete E, Bassat Q (2019) Post discharge mortality prediction in sub-Saharan Africa. Pediatrics 143(1):320180606

Prost A, Colbourn T, Seward N, Azad K, Coomarasamy A, Copas A, Houweling TAJ, Fottrell E, Kuddus A, Lewycka S, MacArthur C, Manandhar D, Morrison J, Mwansambo C, Nair N, Nambiar B, Osrin D, Pagel C, Phiri T, Pulkki-Brannstrom A-M, Rosato M, Skordis-Worrall J, Saville N, More NS, Shrestha B, Tripathy P, Wilson A, Costello A (2013) Women's groups practising participatory learning and action to improve maternal and newborn health in low-resource settings: a systematic review and meta-analysis. Lancet 381(9879):1436–1446

Sharma A (2016) Efficacy of early skin-to-skin contact on the rate of exclusive breastfeeding in term neo-nates: A randomized controlled trial. Afr Health Sci 16(3):790–797

UNICEF (2020) Levels & trends in child mortality. UNICEF, New York

World Health Organization (WHO) (2020) Newborns: improving survival and well-being. https://www.who.int/news-room/fact-sheets/detail/newborns-reducing-mortality

World Health Organization (WHO) (2021) Exclusive breastfeeding for optimal growth, development and health of infants. https://www.who.int/elena/titles/exclusive_breastfeeding/en/

Patient and Family Centered Care in Neonatal Settings

14

Andréia Cascaes Cruz, Luciano Marques dos Santos, and Flavia Simphronio Balbino

14.1 Introduction

The arrival of a newborn baby is an event permeated by changes in roles and family dynamics. When birth is accompanied by illness and hospitalization of the newborn in a neonatal intensive care unit (NICU), the family is challenged by the short-, medium- and sometimes long-term implications imposed by the baby's health condition, especially in prematurity situations. To reduce the impact on family life and improve indicators related to newborn health, it is recommended to implement patient and family centered care (PFCC), a concept synonymous with that of 'Family-Integrated Care' (FiCare) in other countries. Implementation of PFCC requires a relational practice based on partnership and the principles of dignity and respect, sharing of information, collaboration and participation that guide institutional policies and professional practice.

At the end of reading this chapter, the reader will be able to: recognize the impact of newborn (NB) hospitalization in the Neonatal Intensive Care Unit (NICU) on the family, define Patient and Family Centered Care (PFCC), describe the principles of the PFCC, describe actions that characterize the implementation of PFCC at institutional level and in clinical practice of nurses in NICU and list benefits resulting from the implementation of PFCC as a care model in the NICU.

Key "Think Points" for Learning

- Recognizing the impact of newborn (NB) hospitalization in the neonatal intensive care unit (NICU) on the family is essential. The reader should also be able to;
- define patient and family centered care (PFCC);
- describe the principles of the PFCC;
- describe actions that characterize the implementation of PFCC at institutional level and in clinical practice of nurses in NICU and;
- list benefits resulting from the implementation of PFCC as a care model in NICU.

A. C. Cruz (✉)
School of Nursing, Federal University of Sao Paulo, Sao Paulo, Brazil

Council of International Neonatal Nurses, Inc. (COINN), Yardley, PA, USA

L. M. dos Santos
Estadual University of Feira de Santana, Feira de Santana, Bahia, Brazil

F. S. Balbino
School of Nursing, Federal University of Sao Paulo, Sao Paulo, Brazil

14.2 Newborn Hospitalization in the NICU and Impact on the Family

NICUs have advanced technology and therapies to ensure the survival of newborns with complex clinical conditions resulting from prematurity, congenital malformations, perinatal asphyxia, congenital infections, or other causes. Among the numerous consequences related to neonatal hospitalization, a number of changes, challenges, and obstacles faced by families stand out. The impact on the family system is present in the short, medium, and long term. The fear of losing the child is part of the parents' experience, especially in the first visit to the NICU, considered the worst and the most difficult situation. The NICU environment and the technological equipment connected to the baby is perceived by both mothers and fathers and/or partners as enigmatic and threatening, contributing to negative feelings, stress, increasing fear, and prolonging uncertainty (Fernández Medina et al. 2018; Roque et al. 2017).

Throughout the experience, there is a mixture of feelings, such as joy, love and tenderness, anxiety, fear, distress, sadness, pain, frustration, shame, worry, and helplessness. Guilt is the strongest maternal feeling during neonatal hospitalization in the NICU and after hospital discharge (Fernández Medina et al. 2018).

With regard to the creation of parent–child bonds and parenting, it is known that a baby needs early contact with parents for optimal physiological and psycho-emotional development. Parents also need meaningful relationships with their babies to establish their identities as mothers and fathers. The hospitalization of a baby can disrupt these processes (Roque et al. 2017).

In the context of the NICU, parents' physical and psychological proximity to their babies (Ainsworth et al. 2015) can be compromised when they are unable to provide direct care to the baby. This distance may occur because of the baby's fragile health status, limitations imposed by NICU interventions and routines, distance between the family home and the hospital, and the balance of domestic duties with the time that the

parents remain within the NICU. The incubator, machines, lighting, noises, design of the NICU, restriction of hours, and lack of information constitute serious barriers to the development of a relationship between parents and their children and the bonding process (Heydarpour et al. 2017).

Parental negative feelings and stress are described as the main reasons for delaying the normal transition to parenthood and the performance of parental roles (Al Maghaireh et al. 2016). In addition to stress, there is evidence that parents of babies at the NICU have higher levels of depressive symptoms than parents whose babies were not in the NICU. Risk factors for the development of significant depression in parents included the lack of support from the nursing staff, newborns with younger gestational ages, longer periods of hospitalization, and preterm newborns with more serious clinical problems (Roque et al. 2017).

It is also necessary to consider the impact of birth and hospitalization on the lives of the newborn siblings. The mother ends up moving away from the children who are at home due to the need to stay in the NICU with the newborn, who becomes a priority in her life (Carvalho et al. 2019). In general, the presence of hospitalized newborn siblings in NICUs is prohibited or restricted, justified by the increased risk of infection. However, there is already evidence proving that the entry of siblings in the NICU does not increase viral infections (Horikoshi et al. 2018). In order to minimize the impact of this experience on the newborn and family lives, and to generate better results in the short, medium, and long term, it is recommended to implement the PFCC model in NICUs (Davidson et al. 2017; Mann 2016).

14.3 Definition of Patient and Family Centered Care (PFCC)

Patient and Family Centered Care is a care approach that respects and responds to the individual needs and values of families. All family members are recognized as recipients of care (Davidson et al. 2017). In the context of the

NICU, PFCC is defined as an "interdisciplinary, comprehensive, and holistic care of neonates and families maintaining their respect and dignity. Family, as a constant member in a neonate's life and one of the main participants in healthcare, collaborate mutually with healthcare workers. Complete information exchange without any bias leads to promotion of quality of care provided for neonates and their families" (Ramezani et al. 2014).

14.4 Principles of the PFCC approach and its Interface with the NICU

The central concepts of the PFCC are: dignity and respect, participation, information sharing, and collaboration, based on a partnership relationship between the healthcare team and families (Institute for Patient- and Family-Centered Care 2012).

- Dignity and respect: Healthcare professionals must listen to and honor the perspectives and choices of patients and families, and should incorporate their knowledge, values, beliefs, and cultural contexts into the planning and provision of care.
- Information sharing: Healthcare professionals must communicate and share complete and impartial information with patients and family members, so that they are affirmative and useful. To participate effectively in care and decision-making, patients and families must receive timely, complete and truthful information.
- Participation: Patients and families should be supported and encouraged to participate in the care and decision-making processes at the level they choose.
- Collaboration: Patients and families must work together with institutional leadership in the development, implementation, and evaluation of policies and programs, in the planning of care facilities, in professional education and together with healthcare professionals, in the planning and provision of direct care to the patient.

In NICUs, the PFCC concepts are applied as: (Ramezani et al. 2014)

- Family care: assessment of family and evaluation and provision of its needs.
- Equal family participation: family participation in care planning, decision-making, and providing routine and special care.
- Collaboration: interprofessional collaboration with the family and its involvement in regulating and implementing care plans.
- Maintaining family's respect and dignity: includes two specifications—the importance of families' differences and recognizing their tendencies.

Partnership is the central attribute of the PFCC approach; sharing, reciprocity, and common goals are fundamental values of the partnership. Specifically, in regard to the value of reciprocity, it is important to consider that this implies the consideration of the needs of both parties, and that both the healthcare team and the family assume responsibility for a positive outcome (Institute for Patient- and Family-Centered Care 2017).

The incorporation of the PFCC principles in clinical practice favors the effective relationship between staff and family members, and can positively influence the well-being of families and, consequently, the health of newborns.

14.5 Implementation of PFCC in the Clinical Practice of Nurses in the NICU

The first issue to consider for the implementation of the PFCC is its description in institutional policies. The lack of this description in the official documents is one of the main barriers to the implementation of this model of care in clinical practice (Abraham and Moretz 2012).

Other important issues for the implementation of the PFCC are to abolish restrictions on visits to families and to encourage the presence of the family (Gasparini et al. 2015). In this approach to care, family is not a visiter; the family is should be considered an essential member of the healthcare team. Institutional policies must guarantee the presence of families 24 h a day, 7 days a week (Dokken et al. 2015).

There should be no restriction on access to the NICU due to the age of the family member or degree of kinship, since PFCC family is defined as "two or more people who are related in some way, biologically, legally or emotionally." Thus, it is the individuals/patients and family members who define who is part of the family and the level of involvement that each family member will have in aspects related to the care of the newborn (Davidson et al. 2017). Limiting visiting hours, the number of visitors or the age of visitors can put patients at greater risk of errors, contribute to the emotional distress of the patient and family, create distrust between staff and families, and can decrease patient and family satisfaction in relation to their hospitalization experience (Dokken et al. 2015).

The design of care environments can also be a facilitator or a barrier to the inclusion of families in care practice. The literature shows that, in some situations, restrictions on visiting family members were due to space limitations and lack of facilities, rather than an institutional objection for families to be present (Shields et al. 2012). In order to implement PFCC, good communication is still needed between the nurse and other members of the healthcare team with the family. Therefore, among other strategies, active listening, expressions of empathy and affirmative statements should be included in conversations with families. It is also recommended to hold routine interdisciplinary meetings with the family to improve their satisfaction with communication, trust in the team, and reduce conflict between family members and the team (Davidson et al. 2017).

Participation in a collaborative way with the family requires that they participate in the care of the baby and in decision-making as they wish, through a negotiation process. This includes considering and respecting families who do not want to participate in care or decision-making related to the baby. Nurses responsible for the care provided must teach/train the parents to provide care

to their newborn. In this case, there is sharing of knowledge, valuing the family's capacities and strengths to take care of the child (Brødsgaard et al. 2019).

Another strategy for integrating PFCC concepts in the NICU is the so-called family-centered developmental care, which involves the family as an essential collaborator for the provision of individualized care and support for the baby's development (Craig et al. 2015). Providing families with hospitalization care in the NICU in Single Family Room Units is also a way to provide greater involvement of parents in the care of the newborn, with the privacy they need (Toivonen et al. 2017).

Chart 14.1 Actions to Implement the PFCC in the Clinical Practice of Nurses (Bastani 2015; Carvalho et al. 2019; Yu et al. 2017)

- Consider the family as an essential member of the healthcare team.
- Encourage and support the family to interact with the baby and participate in the baby's care.
- Offer parents of critically ill newborns the option of being taught how to help care for their critically ill children, in order to increase parental confidence and competence in their role as caregiver and improve parents' psychological health during and after NICU hospitalization.
- Establish with the family how they want to be included in care.
- Ask the family about their questions and concerns.
- Provide families with leaflets with information about the NICU environment to reduce family members' anxiety and stress.
- Include the newborn's siblings in the care plans.
- Provide information on an ongoing basis to families.
- Create a relationship of trust with families.
- Communicate with families using language they understand.
- Welcome the families' doubts and feelings.

- Respect families' choices and beliefs.
- Offer, as appropriate, the family the option of being present during cardiopulmonary resuscitation (CPR) efforts if the situation arises, with a team member assigned to support them.
- Let the family decide when they will be present at the bedside, providing support and positive reinforcement to the healthcare team, so they can work in partnership with families in all decision-making processes.
- Offer families the option to participate in interdisciplinary team visits to improve communication satisfaction and increase family involvement.
- Include family education programs as part of clinical care.
- Implement peer support groups (parents-parents) to improve family satisfaction, reduce parents' stress and reduce depression.
- Implement the NICU diaries, in which families write about the day-to-day lives in the NICU, helping to reduce the anxiety, depression, and post-traumatic stress of family members.

Source: Created by the authors

14.6   Benefits from the Implementation of the PFCC as a Care Model in the NICU

The implementation of interventions guided by the PFCC is linked to the reduction of parental stress, improves the competence of parents in the care of their baby, increases breastfeeding rates, offers more opportunities for families to solve communication problems with the healthcare team and obtain information about the care of their baby, as well increases the receptivity of the members of the healthcare team to the presence of the parents (Balbino et al. 2016).

There is also a reduction in hospitalization rates to the NICU (Bastani 2015; Segers et al. 2019; Yu et al. 2017), a reduction in readmission after discharge (Bastani 2015), and a reduction in long-term morbidity, with better neurobehavioral performance and in the indicators of feeding and growth verified up to 24 months after discharge (Yu et al. 2017). Parental involvement in the care of their baby can result in increased family satisfaction (Bastani 2015). Evidence indicates that parents are more satisfied when collaboration with healthcare professionals improves. Therefore, collaboration between parents and professionals, including decision-making situations, should be incorporated into care in the NICU (Segers et al. 2019). The implementation of Family Single Rooms can improve maternal safety and confidence, strengthening the relationship between mother and/or partner/father and baby (Twohig et al. 2016).

NICUs in Brazil that implemented the Patient and Family Centered Care Model concluded that there was a contribution to the reduction of parental stress (Balbino et al. 2016). In India, there was an improvement in pre-discharge breastfeeding rates when the PFCC was implemented (Verma et al. 2017). In China, groups of parents included in an intervention that promoted their participation in the care of the newborn for at least 4 hours a day resulted in an increase in the breastfeeding rate and greater weight of the babies at discharge, when compared to the group of parents who followed the routine hospital care model, which did not allow parents to participate in baby care (Lv et al. 2019).

Parental education programs have shown beneficial effects, such as reducing anxiety, depression, post-traumatic stress, and generalized stress. This has improved family satisfaction with the care provided by the team (Carvalho et al. 2019). The success of the PFCC model in NICUs is directly related to the participation of parents in the care of their baby during hospitalization, as their involvement ensures that they are the primary caregivers of their children. Therefore, parents feel empowered by the experience, with greater competence and security in their roles.

Reflective Practice

Joseph was born at 24 weeks of gestational age, weighing 680 g. He was intubated in the delivery room and transferred to the NICU shortly after birth. Joseph's mother was only able to meet him at the NICU two days after delivery. Doctors from the NICU team went twice a day during those 48 hours to talk to her in the obstetric inpatient unit, bringing information about Joseph. Joseph's father stayed with his son for the first 24 hours since his admission to the NICU. On the second day of hospitalization to the NICU, the team explained to the father about the NICU environment and delivered an information leaflet with the main rules and routines of the unit. On the parents' first visit to the NICU, members of the medical and nursing staff went to talk to the couple, trying to understand their fears, anxieties, and expectations. Beginning at the mother's first meeting with the child, the nurses encouraged her to touch him and asked if she wanted to help with changing diapers. The mother felt useful for being able to perform this task. On the twentieth day of hospitalization, Joseph was diagnosed with necrotizing enterocolitis and the parents were called by the team to talk about the need for surgery and possible ileostomy. After more than an hour of conversation, the parents and the team decided that it was best to submit the baby to surgery, and the parents opted to leave the decision about performing the ileostomy at the discretion of the surgical team. The day after the surgery, the team informed the family that Joseph needed to receive a blood transfusion and asked if they had any opposition to this procedure. On the thirtieth day of hospitalization, Joseph had a cardiopulmonary arrest, the parents were next to the incubator and were asked if they wanted to leave or remain close to their son during the cardiopulmonary resuscitation proce-

dure. They decided to stay. A nurse was assigned to stay with the family during the maneuvers, explaining everything that was going on. Joseph survived and after 5 months of hospitalization, he was discharged home.

14.7 Conclusion

The implementation of the PFCC in clinical practice firstly requires its incorporation into the philosophy and institutional policies. Its applicability by the team working in the NICU implies the incorporation of its principles—dignity and respect, information sharing, participation, and collaboration—to the actions taken individually and collectively. To this end, training aimed at improving the skills necessary for a relationship based on partnership must be continuously developed. Scientific evidence has demonstrated the benefits resulting from the implementation of the PFCC, mainly due to the participation of families in the care of their baby in the NICU, such as greater satisfaction of the healthcare team and families, reduction of parental stress, reduction of both length of stay and hospital readmissions. Although this model of care is beneficial for newborns, families, institutions, and health professionals, its implementation is still a challenge.

References

Abraham M, Moretz JG (2012) Implementing patient- and family-centered care: part I - understanding the challenges. Pediatr Nurs 38(1):44–47

Ainsworth MDS, Blehar MC, Waters E, Wall SN (2015) Patterns of attachment: a psychological study of the strange situation. Patterns Attach 2015:1–417

Al Maghaireh DF, Abdullah KL, Chan CM, Piaw CY, Al Kawafha MM (2016) Systematic review of qualitative studies exploring parental experiences in the Neonatal Intensive Care Unit. J Clin Nurs 25:2745–2756

Balbino FS, Balieiro MMFG, Mandetta MA (2016) Measurement of family-centered care perception and parental stress in a neonatal unit. Rev Lat Am Enfermagem 24:104

Bastani F (2015) Effect of family-centered care on improving parental satisfaction and reducing readmission among premature infants: a randomized controlled trial. J Clin Diagn Res 9:4–8

Brødsgaard A, Pedersen JT, Larsen P, Weis J (2019) Parents' and nurses' experiences of partnership in neonatal intensive care units: a qualitative review and meta-synthesis. J Clin Nurs 28(17–18):3117–3139

Carvalho SC, Facio BC, de Souza BF, Abreu-D'Agostini FCP, Leite AM, Wernet M (2019) Maternal care in the preterm child's family context: a comprehensive look towards the sibling. Rev Bras Enferm 72(3):50–57

Craig JW, Glick C, Phillips R, Hall SL, Smith J, Browne J (2015) Recommendations for involving the family in developmental care of the NICU baby. J Perinatol 35(1):5–8

Davidson JE, Aslakson RA, Long AC, Puntillo KA, Kross EK, Hart J et al (2017) Guidelines for family-centered care in the neonatal, pediatric, and adult ICU. Crit Care Med 45(1):103–128

Dokken DL, Kaufman J, Johnson BH, Perkins SB, Benepal J, Roth A et al (2015) Changing hospital visiting policies: from families as "visitors" to families as partners. J Clin Outcomes Manag 22(1):29–36

Fernández Medina IM, Granero-Molina J, Fernández-Sola C, Hernández-Padilla JM, Camacho Ávila M, López Rodríguez M (2018) Bonding in neonatal intensive care units: experiences of extremely preterm infants' mothers. Women Birth 31(4):325–330

Gasparini R, Champagne M, Stephany A, Hudson J, Fuchs MA (2015) Policy to practice. JONA J Nurs Adm 45(1):28–34

Heydarpour S, Keshavarz Z, Bakhtiari M (2017) Factors affecting adaptation to the role of motherhood in mothers of preterm infants admitted to the neonatal intensive care unit: a qualitative study. J Adv Nurs 73(1):138–148

Horikoshi Y, Okazaki K, Miyokawa S, Kinoshita K, Higuchi H, Suwa J et al (2018) Sibling visits and viral infection in the neonatal intensive care unit. Pediatr Int 60(2):153–156

Institute for Patient- and Family-Centered Care (2012) http://www.ipfcc.org/about/pfcc.html

Institute for Patient- and Family-Centered Care (2017) Advancing the practice of patient-and family-centered care in primary care and other ambulatory settings: how to get started. Inst Patient Family Care 20814(301):1–22

Lv B, Gao X, Sun J, Li T, Liu Z, Zhu L et al (2019) Family-centered care improves clinical outcomes of very-low-birth-weight infants: a quasi-experimental study. Front Pediatr 12:7

Mann D (2016) Design, implementation, and early outcome indicators of a new family-integrated neonatal unit. Nurs Womens Health 20(2):158–166

Ramezani T, Hadian Shirazi Z, Sabet Sarvestani R, Moattari M (2014) Family-centered care in neonatal intensive care unit: a concept analysis. Int J Commun Based Nurs Midwif 2(4):268–278

Roque ATF, Lasiuk GC, Radünz V, Hegadoren K (2017) Scoping review of the mental health of parents of infants in the NICU. J Obstet Gynecol Neonatal Nurs 46(4):576–587

Segers E, Ockhuijsen H, Baarendse P, van Eerden I, van den Hoogen A (2019) The impact of family centred care interventions in a neonatal or paediatric intensive care unit on parents' satisfaction and length of stay: a systematic review. Intensive Crit Care Nurs 50:63–70

Shields L, Zhou H, Taylor M, Hunter J, Munns A, Watts R (2012) Family-centred care for hospitalised children aged 0-12 years: a systematic review of quasi-experimental studies. JBI Database Syst Rev Implement Rep 10(39):2559–2592

Toivonen M, Lehtonen L, Löyttyniemi E, Axelin A (2017) Effects of single-family rooms on nurse-parent and nurse-infant interaction in neonatal intensive care units. Early Hum Dev 106:59–62

Twohig A, Reulbach U, Figuerdo R, McCarthy A, McNicholas F, Molloy EJ (2016) Supporting preterm infant attachment and socioemotional development in the neonatal intensive care unit: staff perceptions. Infant Ment Health J 37(2):160–171

Verma A, Maria A, Pandey RM, Hans C, Verma A, Sherwani F (2017) Family-centered care to complement care of sick newborns: a randomized controlled trial. Indian Pediatr 54(6):455–459

Yu Y-T, Hsieh W-S, Hsu C-H, Lin Y-J, Lin C-H, Hsieh S et al (2017) Family-centered care improved neonatal medical and neurobehavioral outcomes in preterm infants: randomized controlled trial. Phys Ther 97(12):1158–1168

Brain Development, Promoting Sleep and Well-Being in the Context of Neonatal Developmental Care

15

Julia Petty and Agnes van den Hoogen

15.1 Introduction

Newborns of earlier gestations and lower birth weights than ever before are now surviving (Santhakumaran et al. 2018). More sophisticated technology and advances in medicine have increased the ability of neonatal healthcare teams to treat even the most premature babies. This means that it is ever more essential to pay particular attention to the long-term outcomes and associated quality of life of these babies and their families. Premature birth can bring with it a number of potentially negative effects, ranging from mild developmental delay to severe disability. Babies born very premature at less than 32 weeks of gestational age (GA) have poorer neurobehavioral outcomes than those born at term (>37 weeks of GA), including poorer school performance and higher rates of attention deficit disorder (Glass et al. 2015). To add, the neonatal intensive care environment causes additional stress to the baby, compromising neurodevelopmental stability. There is growing evidence of how critically important, yet stressful, medical and nursing care interventions may negatively impact on the baby's neuromotor, behavioral, growth milestones as well as sleep patterns (Sanders and Hall 2018; Beltrán et al. 2021). To address these challenges requires an approach that will minimize any long-term adverse effects. Developmental care is such an approach that should be employed as early as possible in the neonatal unit using individualized strategies in partnership with parents (Spittle et al. 2015). In this chapter, the terms 'baby' and 'neonate' will be used interchangeably.

> **Key "Think Points" for Learning**
>
> - Considering the importance of understanding brain development and sleep as an essential component of normal functioning, to promote well-being in the neonate is vital.
> - Considering the nature of neonatal sleep and what influences its development is also vitally important.
> - An important question is: What can we do to improve sleep? We must consider the strategies to promote and protect sleep in our vulnerable babies with vital components of an integrated developmental care model.

J. Petty (✉)
Department of Nursing, Health and Wellbeing, School of Health and Social Work, University of Hertfordshire, Hatfield, Hertfordshire, UK

Council of International Neonatal Nurses, Inc. (COINN), Yardley, PA, USA
e-mail: j.petty@herts.ac.uk

A. van den Hoogen
University Medical Centre of Utrecht (UMCU), Wilhelmina Children's Hospital, Utrecht, The Netherlands

Council of International Neonatal Nurses, Inc. (COINN), Yardley, PA, USA

© The Editor(s) (if applicable) and The Author(s), under exclusive license to Springer Nature Switzerland AG 2022
J. Petty et al. (eds.), *Neonatal Nursing: A Global Perspective*, https://doi.org/10.1007/978-3-030-91339-7_15

15.2   Model and Definitions

Developmental care is an approach that uses a range of nursing and medical interventions to reduce the stress of preterm/sick neonates in the neonatal intensive care unit (NICU) (Als and McAnulty 2011). These interventions are designed to allow optimal neurobehavioral development of the neonate in close and constant partnership with the family. This is a core feature of Family Integrated Care, known as "FiCare" (O'Brien et al. 2015). A key element of developmental care is not only the recognition of the need for individualized care for each baby (Craig et al. 2015) but that of a commitment to using a range of strategies to ensure optimum well-being of the baby is promoted throughout the neonatal stay and beyond. A model that encompasses all of these essential elements including the promotion of sleep, is the excellent, comprehensive neonatal integrative developmental care model of Altimier and Phillips (2016) (Fig. 15.1).

The integrated model comprises seven core measures for neuroprotective developmental care

of premature/sick babies (1) Safeguarding sleep; (2) Healing environments; (3) Positioning and handling; (4) Minimizing stress and pain; (5) Protecting skin; (6) Optimizing nutrition; and (7) Partnering with families. Each one of these seven measures is a topic in its own right. This chapter focuses mainly on the topic of sleep but will discuss it within the context of all aspects of the model as a whole.

15.3   Brain Development

To fully understand the impact of the NICU environment on sleep and well-being, it is important to have underpinning knowledge of the developing brain in-utero and beyond. This includes the vulnerability of the brain and nervous system in the fetal and neonatal period and why it is at risk of external stressors/influences. In utero, the fetal period begins at the end of 10th week of gestation and the fetus is considered as full term between 37 and 40 weeks which means there is sufficient development for life outside the uterus.

Fig. 15.1 The integrated model. Source: Adapted from Altimier and Phillips (2016)

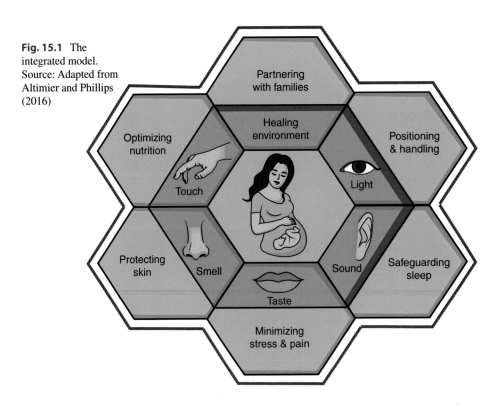

Bennet et al. (2018) summarizes clearly the development of brain and neural pathways in utero. By the end of the embryonic phase at the 12th week of gestational age (GA), the basic structures of the central and peripheral nervous systems are in place (Sanders and Hall 2018). In humans, neuron production starts around embryonic day 42 and this process is largely complete by mid-gestation, and neural migration effectively completed by 26–29 weeks GA (Thaise et al. 2017). The antenatal period of life is critical for white matter and subsequent cortical neuronal development, the latter itself requiring appropriate maturation of white matter (Back 2017; van Tilborg et al. 2018). It is also a critical time for establishing functional connectivity of the neural network which is important for sleep regulation. However, preterm birth disrupts the establishment of the neural connectivity framework, and this impacts on the development and efficiency of sleep.

15.4 Causes of Neonatal Stress and Sleep Disruption

Throughout pregnancy, the fetus develops within the uterine environment which is protective, warm, dark, providing boundaries and safety from external stressors. Noise is "muffled" by the abdominal wall and the amniotic fluid. The NICU environment is, by comparison, noisy, bright, and cooler compared to the intrauterine environment. There are no boundaries and the baby can be faced with a multitude of interventions resulting in a very stressful situation (Williams et al. 2018). The differences between term and preterm neonates must also be considered. Term babies have developed and organized behavioral states, the ability to regulate self-quiet/calm and they can remain in a deep sleep for up to 90 minutes with adequate muscle tone. However, the premature baby has reduced muscle tone, an extended posture and movement, poor flexion/extension balance and control of movements and limited ability to self-quiet/calm regulation. Their immature physiological systems lead to poor heat production and significant heat loss as well as an inability to self-regulate leading to sleep patterns that are disrupted. Known effects of a stressful environment are hypoxia, bradycardia/tachycardia, increase in intracranial pressure, apnea, malabsorption leading to poor weight gain, hearing problems, restlessness, and sleep disturbances.

15.5 Promoting and Protecting Sleep

Sleep is essential for brain development and brain maturation in babies (Allen 2012). They require extensive sleep for further development of the neurosensory systems, structural development of the hippocampus, pons, brainstem, and midbrain and optimizing physical growth. According to Barbeau and Weiss (2017), sleep is a necessary function of life. Studies consistently show the importance of sleep in its role for cognitive functioning and developing memories. Most importantly, sleep solidifies new information. Sleep deprivation in adults leads to ineffective attention, learning, emotional regulation, and decision-making. Neonates and children show a similar response. At about 6 months of age, REM sleep comprises about 30% of sleep. Babies spend 50% of their time in each of these states and the sleep cycle is about 50 minutes. By the time children reach preschool age, the sleep cycle is about every 90 minutes (Jawabri and Raja 2020).

Inadequate sleep in children has been associated with increased adiposity, poor emotional regulation, poor overall well-being, and decreased academic performance. Because fetuses and babies spend most of their day asleep, ensuring adequate sleep is important, especially so in neonates born preterm because brain development mainly takes place in the latter part of pregnancy. A busy, noisy and bright environment such as the NICU also affects the sleep of admitted neonates. Protecting infant sleep is a critical component of providing developmentally appropriate care for premature and full-term babies in the NICU because many of them are hospitalized during one of the most critical periods of brain development. Interventions to enhance comfort and sleep in the critically ill baby are outlined in Table 15.1.

Table 15.1 Types of interventions to enhance comfort and sleep in the NICU (adapted from Allen 2012; Kudchadkar et al. 2017; Pineda et al. 2017)

• Environmental interventions, including but not limited to earplugs, headphones, alarm modifications, white noise, music therapy or unit-based "quiet hours," lighting control/cycling, eye masks, and bright light therapy, or a combination (Beltrán et al. 2021)

• Behavioral interventions, including but not limited to kangaroo care (skin-to-skin contact), massage, music therapy, and guided imagery

• Physical therapy interventions such as mobility or exercise during the day

• Complementary and alternative therapies such as aromatherapy and acupressure or acupuncture. This summary below with examples may be particularly useful:

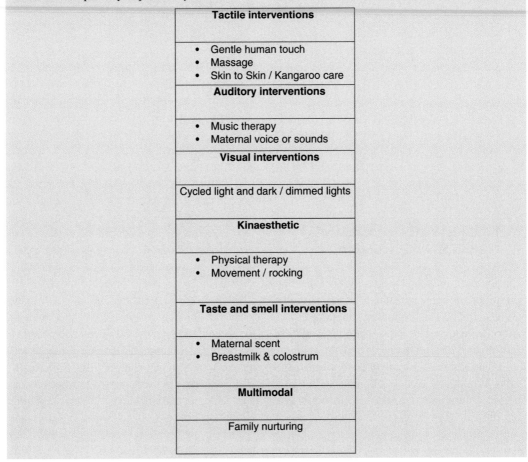

| **Tactile interventions** |
| • Gentle human touch
• Massage
• Skin to Skin / Kangaroo care |
| **Auditory interventions** |
| • Music therapy
• Maternal voice or sounds |
| **Visual interventions** |
| Cycled light and dark / dimmed lights |
| **Kinaesthetic** |
| • Physical therapy
• Movement / rocking |
| **Taste and smell interventions** |
| • Maternal scent
• Breastmilk & colostrum |
| **Multimodal** |
| Family nurturing |

To best provide developmentally appropriate care, close behavioral assessment including identification of sleep-wake states is necessary. So far, no instrument for measuring sleep has turned out to be valid and reliable in the neonatal period. The golden standard polysomnography cannot be applied in neonates because of adhesives or patches attached on a relatively small head and numerous cables that can disturb sleep. Sleep-wake states can be distinguished both through electroencephalography (EEG) and biobehavioral techniques. EEG can be useful in the detection of sleep-wake states and cycles in neonates, but most nurses are not trained to interpret EEGs.

However, in the NICU it is possible to determine sleep states by key observational assessment. This can lead to valuable insights and direct the performance of developmental care. Thereby, parents/caregivers can plan and coordinate their care and interventions according to wake and sleep patterns and maintain a clear and ongoing insight including an overview of changes and incidents (Werth et al. 2017). Therefore, it is a key nursing role to utilize observation of biobehavioral responses to determine changes in sleep-wake states. Sleep-wake states are observable behaviors regulated by neuronal-controlled physiologic mechanisms recurring longitudinally in babies. Sleeping and waking evolve into distinct states as the brain continues to develop the neural structures and connections necessary for cyclical synchronization with other physiologic mechanisms (e.g., heart rate variability, thermoregulation). If the neonate's brain has not reached the necessary stage of development to perform certain behaviors, they will be unable to display the overt behaviors associated with various sleep-wake states. Thus, as premature babies develop, so do their behaviors displayed through the range of sleep-wake states in their behavioral repertoire.

Scales to describe sleep-wake states have been used for decades to better understand how the neonate interacts with his environment. The underlying objective of the scales is to identify behaviors and their relationship to phases of development that are portrayed through their individual responses to their environment. The Brazelton Neonatal Behavioral Assessment Scale (BNBAS) was an early scale that was developed for term neonates and measured four dimensions: interactive capacities, motor capacities, response to increased stimulation, and physiological response to stress. The BNBAS was later adapted for use in premature neonates and is known as the Assessment of Preterm Infants' Behavior (APIB). Other researchers describe sleep-wake behaviors based on eye movement, respiratory pattern, gross motor movement, and muscle tone. Identification of the behaviors associated with specific sleep-wake states is important because endogenous stimulation occurs during the active sleep state and this aids in the development of neurosensory systems (touch, vestibular, auditory, and visual). Animal models suggest that

deprivation of sleep, both active and quiet sleep, can result in impaired development and loss of brain plasticity (Graven 2006).

Circadian rhythms gradually emerge between birth and the first several months of life (Logan and McClung 2019). The circadian rhythm is synchronized to the light-dark cycle promoting both wakeful and restful activities depending on the timing of the cycle. In infancy, premature babies engage in longer, lighter, and more active sleep than those born at term. As preterm babies develop, their sleep patterns gradually begin to resemble those at term, although their sleep tends to be more variable and less consistent across the first year of life when compared to term babies. During their NICU stay, sleep patterns of preterm babies appear to follow a distinctly different pattern than sleep at other stages of development and these differences may predict later developmental outcomes (Schwichtenberg et al. 2016).

In summary thus far, safeguarding sleep is a vital part of developmental care, for the following reasons: It is essential for normal neurodevelopment, gives adequate growth and healing, energy restoration and maintenance of body homeostasis. In addition, preservation of brain plasticity (the ability of the brain to constantly change its structure and function in response to environmental change) and longer-term, positive learning outcomes and continuing brain development.

Given the complexities of sleep-wake state development and the importance of sleep in relationship to long-term outcomes, neonatal nurses need to promote and protect sleep as much as possible, in vulnerable hospitalized infants. The importance of observing sleep-wake states in premature and critically ill term babies is to ensure that nursing care focuses on prevention of stress. Many interventions exist that have the potential to improve sleep and ongoing research continues to provide additional information about how to best deliver these interventions. Providing nursing care that promotes and protects sleep in the NICU is critical to ensuring vulnerable babies receive the best care possible.

In relation to strategies, conclusions of a review by van den Hoogen et al. (2017) are as follows:

- Many different interventions have been reported to promote sleep in babies who require intensive care.
- There is great variation across studies in methods of sleep assessment, the targeted sleep behaviors, and the study populations.
- While there seems to be insufficient evidence to recommend any new intervention to promote neonatal sleep in the NICU, the importance of sleep for the development of the neonatal brain remains strongly agreed.
- The review suggests some key guidelines based on moderate evidence, expert opinion, and parental values to improve sleep on the NICU and to direct future neonatal sleep studies.

Key recommendations from the review are:

- Recognize the significance of promoting sleep as a keystone of the treatment of neonates on the NICU via integrated teaching programs (e.g., e-learning, parent information, flyers) targeted to nurses, physicians, parents, and support personnel.
- Incorporating sleep measurements (e.g., observational scales (a) EEG, innovative non-obtrusive sleep measurements) into daily ward round assessments will increase awareness of sleep as a key factor in neonatal health and are necessary to improve sleep for NICU patients.
- Make regulations about elective care procedures, which can be postponed during sleep (e.g., routine lab, routine X-rays, routine cardiac assessments).

Finally, in this section, it is worth reminding the reader of other important conditions for growth and development; love and protection from parents/caregivers, healthy feeding for growth, prevention of stress and maintenance of enough sleep. With this in mind and in relation to specific interventions, the chapter now moves on

to address the remaining parts of Altimier et al.'s integrated developmental care module. These comprise the following important strategies: optimizing the NICU environment, safe and comfortable positioning, preventing pain and stress (to include clustering care, allocated quiet time, and cue-based caring), protecting skin integrity, and ensuring adequate nutritional status, in line with a family-integrated care philosophy.

15.6 Other Components of the Integrated Developmental Care Model

The chapter will now turn to further above mentioned vital elements of care that impact on sleep and well-being of the neonate in the NICU.

15.6.1 Optimizing the NICU Environment

Within the NICU, there should be enough spacing between cots/incubators to promote privacy and safety, including light and noise control. Light control is very important and dimmed lights during quiet time is recommended. The use of opaque curtains/blinds could be helpful as well as laying a padded cover on incubators. In addition, individual lighting should be used for procedures, being aware at all times to ensure adequate warmth and prevent any unnecessary heat loss. Preventing undue noise and stress can also be achieved by considerations often forgotten or done without intending to cause disruption, such as closing portholes gently, not placing anything on top of the incubator and removing water condensation from the tubing of ventilator circuits. The use of double walled incubators can help in reducing noise. Ward rounds and handover should be carried out away from the incubator. The neonatal team can plan for a designated quiet time and where noise is kept to a minimum without that from radios on the unit, not talking over the incubators with family or colleagues,

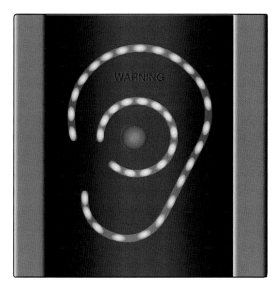

Fig. 15.2 Noise monitor

Table 15.2 Examples of noise levels within the NICU (source: Adapted from Joshi and Tada 2016)

Source of noise	Sound in decibels (dB)
Closure of doors	80–90
People talking	80–95
Ventilator alarms	80–90
Nebulizer	70–80
Telephones	75–85
Monitor alarms	60–85
Ventilator compressor	70–80
Intravenous pump alarms	65–75
Suctioning	70–85
Gas supply	80–90

being aware not to talk loudly in the room and turning down volume of alarms. Alarms and phone calls should be attended to and answered promptly. Attention should be paid in particular to when babies are being fed as the environment has been shown to have a potential negative impact on feeding (Pickler et al. 2013). Utilizing noise monitors within the NICU is a useful way to highlight and create awareness of noise levels (Fig. 15.2). The recommended noise level in NICU is no higher than 45 decibels (db) (Williams et al. 2018). Many common noises within the NICU however are much higher than this (Table 15.2).

15.6.2 Safe and Comfortable Positioning

One of the earliest interventions in NICU is therapeutic positioning. Premature infants miss their third trimester partly or all of it. The flexed position in the uterine environment is ideal. NICU staff should be aware of the importance of body posture and the principles of developmental care (Madlinger-Lewis et al. 2013).

Regardless of prone, supine or side lying, midline orientation should be pursued with the arms and legs in a flexed position close to each other and to the body, the head kept in a neutral position with respect to the torso which should be in a slightly flexed position (See Fig. 15.3a–e). Thermal regulation, bone density, sleep facilitation, calmness and comfort, skin integrity, optimal growth, and brain development will increase when babies are in the right position. Subsequently, for optimal musculoskeletal development and physiological function and stability, it is essential to create a position as closely as possible to the position the baby would have been in the womb. Supporting body containment with bendable positioning aids is helpful for a comfortable position and could help counteract any abnormal posture. Support of nurses in developing body awareness and movements in neonates is essential. Of course, positioning should not interfere with any nursing or medical interventions.

15.6.3 Preventing Stress and Pain

It is important in the harsh environment of the NICU to prevent stress and pain. Premature babies are subject to noxious sounds, bright lights, and painful procedures in the NICU along with repetitive, non-nurturing handling and usually, separation from parents. These altered sensory experiences can have negative effects on the baby's brain development, leading to poor cognitive and motor scores and impairment of growth

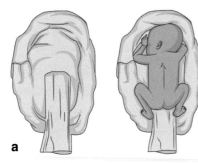
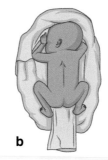

a   **b**

Prone 1:
Softly rolled sheet or blanket positioned in a complete circle. One smaller softly rolled sheet placed over the sheet circle and cover sheet, folded to support pelvic and thoracic lift. Arms and shoulders can be elevated to improve lung function, or fixed and tucked under the thorax, An additional cover may be needed to tuck under the nesting sheet. This serves to draw the nest closer into the infant, supporting flexed containment.

Prone 2:
Noppy roll length-wise under the body from head to hips. This may require additional rolls or blankets across the baby. The head can be supported at an oblique angle, if tolerated.

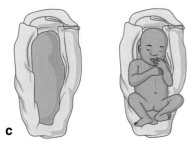
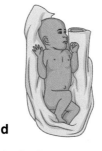
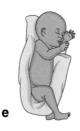

c   **d**   **e**

Supine 1:
Soft blanket or sheet rolled info a nest encourages flexion of lower limbs, brings shoulders forward and keeps the head in mid-line. If this continues round the contours of the head it may promote comfort. A small degree of neck flexion, if tolerated, can provide greater stability.

Supine 2:
Supine quarter turns can be utilised to vary position and reduce head flattening.

Side-lying:
One firmly rolled blanket in a 'U' shape. May need to be supported by tucked covers. Note the opportunity for tactile and visual stimulation in this position.

Fig. 15.3 (a–e) Correct positioning in the NICU

(Soleimani et al. 2020). In addition, there may be decreased white matter and subcortical gray matter maturation. Toxic stress has been linked to changes in the developing brain, negatively impacting the creation of neural connections, and this impact is likely to be more pronounced in preterm neonates (Weber and Harrison 2019).

Minimizing stress in preterm babies has many neurologic benefits such as reducing the likelihood of long-term abnormal stress responsiveness which will help preserve existing neu-

roplastic capacity (Altimier and Phillips 2016). Optimal caring is key. To avoid unnecessary pain periods, accurate monitoring and assessment using a validated pain tool is important as well as close and consistent clinical observation of both "time-out" signals and comfort signals (Table 15.3). Management of pain through pharmacologic and non-pharmacologic measures such as swaddling, positioning, and non-nutritive sucking is essential. Effective prevention and management of procedural and postopera-

Table 15.3 "Time-out" and "Comfort" signals

Time-out	Comfort
• Yawning	• Hand to mouth
• Facial grimacing	• Curled up/nested
• Finger splaying	position
• Tongue extending	• Eye contact
• Coughing	• Smiling/relaxed
• Hiccupping	posture
• Vomiting	• Stable vital signs
• Color changes	• Tolerance of
• Unstable vital signs (e.g.,	feeding
tachycardia)	• Easy to console

tive pain in neonates are required to minimize acute physiological and behavioral distress and may also improve acute and long-term outcomes. For common painful procedures, such as heel sticks, venepuncture, and orogastric tube (OG) insertions, non-pharmacological interventions should be the first choice in non-compromised babies. Non-pharmacological interventions that have demonstrated efficacy are maternal presence, breastfeeding, breastmilk, sucrose, non-nutritive sucking, facilitated tucking, swaddling, and developmentally supportive positioning. Maternal-related olfactory stimuli (mother's milk) have been associated with comfort and diminished pain responses in both term and preterm babies. These findings support the hypothesis that they remember, recognize, and prefer smell that is associated with their prenatal environment including maternal-related olfactory stimuli (mother's milk) and auditory recognition (mother's voice, heartbeat, and music).

15.6.4 Protecting Skin Integrity

Immature skin structures of premature neonates are very different from the skin of those born full-term. The premature baby has an under-developed skin barrier, which puts them at risk for high water loss, electrolyte imbalance, thermal instability, increased permeability, additional skin damage, delayed barrier maturation, and infection (Altimier and Phillips 2016; Kusari et al. 2019). Neonates in the NICU are at risk for skin compromise due to immature skin, compro-

mised perfusion, fluid retention, being immuno-compromised, medical diagnosis, as well as the presence of dressings, tapes, adhesives and various medical devices, such as intravenous lines or nasal prongs for example, that are essential to their care.

Skin protection is part of sound thermoregulation, fluid electrolyte balance, and barrier protection. Practices include bathing protocols, evidence-based skin care guidelines including a validated skin assessment tool, the use of emollient and adhesives, humidity practices, gentle and consistent handling and positioning. Such practices should be incorporated into unit practices and policies. Improved skin outcomes can be realized by utilizing the most evidence-based skin care guidelines available along with careful monitoring and gentle, consistent handling, positioning and care. The key to achieving optimum skin condition is through the utilization of validated skin assessment tools to assess the skin condition and evaluate attributes that indicate skin compromise.

15.6.5 Ensuring Adequate Nutritional Status

Adequate nutrition has well-documented effects on infant brain development. Because breast milk is the most well-tolerated substrate for enteral feeding in the premature, baby full enteral feedings are reached sooner when breast milk is used, thereby decreasing the total days of total parenteral nutrition (TPN) needed (Altimier and Phillips 2016). Evidence has consistently highlighted that breastfeeding is the optimal method of baby feeding and should be promoted and supported (Lau 2020). Because of the many documented benefits of human milk for the preterm baby, supporting mothers in the initiation and maintenance of adequate breast milk supply should be a major focus in the NICU. Immature feeding is a common reason for prolonged hospital stays and persistent poor feeding can result in hospital readmissions. Maturational and developmental issues affect oral feeding success because only 53% of brain cortical volume is present at

34-week gestation when a premature baby is just beginning oral feeds (Belfort and Ehrenkranz 2017).

Oral feeding is a complex task for premature babies and requires a skilled caregiver in assisting them infant in achieving a safe, effective, and pleasurable feeding experience. Infant-driven feeding scales that address feeding readiness, quality of feeding, as well as developmentally supportive caregiver interventions are beneficial when initiating oral feedings in the premature baby. Goals for successful baby-driven feedings are that they are safe, functional, nurturing, and individually and developmentally appropriate. State organization and ingestive functions are regulated by the same autonomic nervous system. The autonomic control of the stomach includes a cephalic phase that prepares the stomach for food, followed by a gastric phase. The cues for these phases are primarily olfactory, but also linked to state organization; therefore, consideration should be given to matching the neonate's feeding schedule to his own sleep cycle, rather than the clock.

Educating staff and parents about neonatal cues and specialized feeding techniques for breastfeeding and bottle feeding are essential as they are the foundation for continued success and prevention of future oral aversions. As with the previous core measures, a validated tool (feeding readiness, quality of feeding, and caregiver techniques) should be utilized to promote consistency in assessing readiness (Crowe et al. 2016), evaluating quality, as well as caregiver efforts and techniques.

Breastfeeding difficulties can impact the fragile mother–infant relationship; therefore, providing support for breastfeeding mothers in learning to feed their preterm babies at the breast, as well as learning to feed with a bottle (with expressed breast milk or preterm formula) is important. Daily skin-to-skin contact/holding can facilitate early "practice" breastfeeding sessions for mothers and babies. Key areas are essential for this component of the developmental care model: Cue-based feeding, assessment of readiness and milk tolerance, working closely with the families, and giving consistent support are essential.

15.6.6 Family Integrated Care

Premature babies have premature parents who are not prepared for the crisis in the NICU. Unexpected preterm delivery and admission of a baby to the NICU is a traumatic event associated with parental fear and is known to cause significant stress (Jubinville et al. 2012; Shaw et al. 2006; Vanderbilt et al. 2009; Wraight et al. 2015). Seeing the baby at the NICU connected to tubes and surrounded by technological equipment with unknown, various alarms, early separation after the delivery and not being able to touch their baby, are experienced as very stressful by parents (Caporali et al. 2020). Parental stress hampers the bonding process between baby and parents and is associated with a higher risk of acute stress disorder (Thaise et al. 2017). To a NICU parent, there is much uncertainty about their baby's future. Parents might experience financial stress because of not being able to work, extra cost, and travelling. It is the nurses' role to help families to achieve a positive outcome from their NICU experience. It is important that parents are not separated from their babies to ensure neurodevelopment. It is evident that early bonding makes a significant difference in brain development. Parents need support through education, coaching, and mentoring to become the primary caregiver of their baby. When practicing zero separation, families can ideally be present throughout the 24-hour period, within the NICU with their baby. Helping parents to achieve a positive outcome from the NICU should be the priority for staff. A prime example of a practice that facilitates parent partnering is skin-to-skin care which shall now be discussed to end the chapter, prior to the relevant case studies.

15.6.7 Skin-to-Skin Contact: Kangaroo Care

The foundation for neonatal care in the NICU is skin-to-skin contact, or Kangaroo Care, and is the ultimate nurturing environment for new borns. Skin-to-skin contact improves physiological regulation of function most optimally and is an essential component for neuroprotective family-centered care for preterm babies. It supports optimal brain development and facilitates attachment (Petty 2017) which promotes neonatal self-regulation over time. Skin-to-skin care increases oxytocin levels significantly for both parents and provides an opportunity to partner with families by providing them an active role. Skin-to-skin care facilitates supportive positioning and fosters optimal autonomic and physiologic stability to reduce pain and stress. In addition, skin-to-skin care provides proximity to maternal odors to contribute to sleep cycling and increases mothers' milk supply. In summary, nurses and other neonatal staff should strive to provide the opportunity to partner with families and facilitate skin to skin care (Pineda et al. 2016).

Skin-to-skin contact (Fig. 15.4) is also thought to be beneficial to premature sleep cycles and brain development. Research suggests skin-to-skin contact improves sleep-wake cycling, which

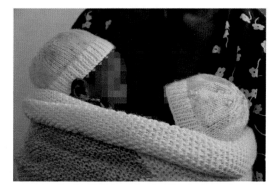

Fig. 15.4 Skin-to-skin contact. Source: Attribution: Lindsay Mgbor/Department for International Development (Creative commons licence for open access use)

may indicate accelerated brain maturation, in both preterm and term babies (Conde-Aguedelo and Díaz-Rossello 2016). The benefits of skin-to-skin contact may also be associated with improved arousal modulation, emotional regulation, and toy manipulation at 3 and 6 months of age for premature babies. Touch, massage, and music are emerging as possible interventions to improve sleep states with subsequent positive impact on early brain development. Further research about the effect of touch and/or massage on premature babies should elucidate the impact of touch and massage on premature brain development. When considering these interventions, it is important to refer back to the recommendations from the American Academy of Pediatrics (AAP), to limit sound to less than 45 decibels and that music within appropriate sound levels may be beneficial to premature neonatal development (Lasky and Williams 2009).

In an attempt to adjust nursing care to be more developmentally driven, the Newborn Individualized Developmental Care and Assessment Program (NIDCAP) has been recommended as a potentially useful way for nurses to provide care (Als and McAnulty 2011; Charafeddine et al. 2020). The program advocates for decreased light through covering the incubator, decreased noise, use of supportive bedding, and promotion of state transition to sleep by hand swaddling, non-nutritive sucking, or grasping. These studies found that premature babies who received the developmental care versus the standard care had increased sleep times in total sleep time, active sleep, and quiet sleep. However, other studies have failed to find any differences in quiet sleep of very low birth weight babies between developmental care (NIDCAP) versus standard care. The differences could be related to the study designs employed by each researcher and the differences between the sample characteristics. Additional research is necessary to understand the implications of an individualized, developmental care program on sleep-wake states.

Case Studies

Case study 1: Two-day-old premature baby

Arun is a 3-day-old baby boy born at 25 weeks gestation. Following a traumatic delivery requiring resuscitation, he is fully ventilated within a humidified incubator and is also having monitoring via a heart rate monitor, pulse oximetry, and arterial line blood gas analysis. He has an intravenous long-line in situ for nutrition and drugs. The postnatal surroundings pose a harsher and less protective environment to this baby compared to the in-utero environment. Being born too soon has led to him being more vulnerable to stressors such as loud noises, light, cold air, and other disturbances and he exhibits stress signs to this environment. High levels of sound in the neonatal unit lead to sleep disturbance and induce some physiological instability shown by fluctuations in heart rate, blood pressure, perfusion, and oxygen saturation.

Arun is currently in light sleep and upon handling, immediately becomes hyper-alert and agitated with extensor postures and "panicked" facial expression. There is difficulty in achieving a quiet, alert state with responsive and animated facial expression. He is showing a picture of infant stress.

Optimum environmental care is needed in this case which includes provision of a quiet, dimmed and calm room and the avoidance of stress. Individualized developmental care is also vital for Arun. This demonstrates how family-integrated, neuroprotective, developmentally supportive care includes creating a healing environment that manages stress and pain while offering a calming and soothing approach that keeps the whole family involved in his care. Interventions include one or more elements such as control of external stimuli (vestibular, auditory, visual, tactile), clustering of nursery care activities, and positioning or swaddling of the preterm baby. Literature supports this management of Arun's stress. Individual strategies have also been combined to form programs, such as the "Neonatal Individualized Developmental Care and Assessment Program" (NIDCAP). The effects of light and sound (noise) levels on preterm babies have been studied and it is generally accepted that a dimmer, quieter environment is important for the developing brain and modification of the environment could minimize the iatrogenic effects. Cue-based care is an important strategy for comfort and feeding. Minimal handling and responding to pain and stress signs is essential. Arun should also be positioned appropriately with head in the midline and cushioned/nested so that boundaries are maintained, and he can use his immature limbs to push against. This will also facilitate optimum ventilation.

Case Study 2: Three-week-old premature twin boys

Laila and Maya are 2-week-old twins who were born at 24 weeks gestation. Laila has suffered a grade 2 bleed (IVH) on her left side but regardless of this, she has progressed well and has been taken off all forms of ventilatory support just requiring some low flow oxygen in the special care unit. Maya, however, has not progressed so well, had become septic and was re-ventilated after being on high flow oxygen therapy, currently being nursed in the intensive care unit. She has been diagnosed with a grade 2 and 3 bleed on the right and left sides, respectively. Developmental care interventions should be individualized for each of the twins depending on their own cues and responses to stimulation/handling/interventions. Laila will be more able to tolerate stimulation than Maya who still requires ventilatory support and is more unstable; however, key principles of family-integrated developmental care must be provided for both. The parents can be supported to work with their babies' cues and can also be encouraged to provide positive touch and skin-to-skin contact if the conditions allow.

Managing the environment is essential to avoid unnecessary stressors and supportive strategies such as optimum positioning and providing certain positive sensory experiences have been linked to improved outcomes for both the baby and family. The neonatal multidisciplinary team should also be involved: Neonatal nurses, medical staff, developmental care specialist if available, physiotherapist, occupational therapist, speech and language therapist, feeding support specialist, counsellor/family support.

Case Study 3: Eight-week-old premature baby on a developmental care program

Baby Paulo was born at 23 weeks and is now 7 weeks old. After a very unstable few weeks, he is starting to show progress in all areas but remains oxygen dependent with difficulty tolerating his feeds. He has been reviewed by a developmental care specialist who is trained in "NIDCAP." Along with the parents, they explain to you about the importance of observing the reactions of Paulo in different environmental conditions. They also note the circumstance which supports his efforts to quieten and relax or reach alertness. They observe his behavior during periods of high activity and note the stress responses as well as comparing the state system stability in relation to the environment of care. These observations are important as part of NIDCAP interventions and are required to work towards discharge home, to minimize adverse outcomes; examples are Kangaroo care/skin-to-skin care, positive touch, optimum positioning, individualized cue-based care and feeding, appropriate sensory stimulation, minimal handling, and involvement of the multidisciplinary team—refer to the strategies highlighted in case studies 1 and 2.

Key Learning Points

- Protecting and supporting sleep is a core part of the neonatal integrative developmental care model and is vital in promoting positive outcomes and well-being in preterm, vulnerable neonates.
- Recognizing the causes and signs of neonatal stress within the NICU is an essential starting point in order for protective, developmentally supportive strategies to be put in place, in partnership with families.
- Developmentally supportive care principles that include, crucially, the protection of sleep may reduce the likelihood of long-term problems in preterm babies.
- It is strongly recommended that these principles are applied, working with parents, in any setting regardless of country of birth to optimize outcomes of our vulnerable babies.

15.7 Conclusion

The importance of preventing stress in premature and critically ill babies is an important part of neonatal nursing care particularly given the adverse outcomes that can ensue from the NICU; for example, leading to loss of caloric intake, physiologic alterations, and disruption to sleep with potential long-term consequences. Many interventions exist that have the potential to improve sleep in NICU babies. Providing nursing care that protects sleep in the NICU is critical to ensuring vulnerable babies receive the best care possible to prevent adverse outcomes. Promoting and protecting sleep in the neonatal intensive care unit is an integral component of individualized, developmentally appropriate, neuroprotective care. Learning the principles of neurodevelopment and understanding the meaning of preterm behavioral cues makes it possible for NICU nurses, caregivers, and parents to provide developmental care to each baby they care for, in any setting.

References

Allen KA (2012) Promoting and protecting infant sleep. Adv Neonatal Care 12(5):288–291. https://doi.org/10.1097/ANC.0b013e3182653899

Almgren M (2018) Benefits of skin-to-skin contact during the neonatal period: Governed by epigenetic mechanisms? Genes Dis 5(1):24–26. https://doi.org/10.1016/j.gendis.2018.01.004

Als H, McAnulty GB (2011) The newborn individualized developmental care and assessment program (NIDCAP) with kangaroo mother care (KMC): comprehensive care for preterm infants. Curr Women's Health Rev 7(3):288–301. https://doi.org/10.2174/157340411796355216

Altimier L, Phillips R (2016) The neonatal integrative developmental care model: advanced clinical applications of the seven core measures for neuroprotective family-centered developmental care. Newborn Infant Nurs Rev 16(4):230–244

Back DB, Kwon KJ, Choi DH, Shin CY, Lee J, Han SH, Kim HY (2017) Chronic cerebral hypoperfusion induces poststroke dementia following acute ischemic stroke in rats. J Neuroinflammation 14(1):216. https://doi.org/10.1186/s12974-017-0992-5. PMID: 29121965; PMCID: PMC5679180.

Barbeau DY, Weiss MD (2017) Sleep disturbances in newborns. Children 4(10):90

Belfort MB, Ehrenkranz RA (2017) Neurodevelopmental outcomes and nutritional strategies in very low birth weight infants. Semin Fetal Neonatal Med 22(1):42–48

Beltrán MI, Dudink J, de Jong TM, Benders MJ, van den Hoogen A (2021) Sensory-based interventions in the NICU: systematic review of effects on preterm brain development. Pediatr Res 2021:1–14

Bennet L, Walker DW, Horne RS (2018) Waking up too early–the consequences of preterm birth on sleep development. J Physiol 596(23):5687–5708

Caporali C, Pisoni C, Gasparini L, Ballante E, Zecca M, Orcesi S, Provenzi L (2020) A global perspective on parental stress in the neonatal intensive care unit: a meta-analytic study. J Perinatol 40(12):1739–1752

Charafeddine L, Masri S, Sharafeddin SF, Badr LK (2020) Implementing NIDCAP training in a low-middle-income country: Comparing nurses and physicians' attitudes. Early Hum Dev 147:105092

Conde-Aguedelo A, Díaz-rossello JL (2016) Kangaroo mother care to reduce morbidity and mortality in low birthweight infants. Cochrane Database Syst Rev 2016:149

Craig JW, Glick C, Phillips R, Hall SL, Smith J, Browne J (2015) Recommendations for involving the family in developmental care of the NICU baby. J Perinatol 35(1):5

Crowe L, Chang A, Wallace K (2016) Instruments for assessing readiness to commence suck feeds in preterm infants: effects on time to establish full oral feeding and duration of hospitalisation. The.

Cochrane Database Syst Rev 8:CD005586. https://doi.org/10.1002/14651858.CD005586.pub3

Glass HC, Costarino AT, Stayer SA, Brett CM, Cladis F, Davis PJ (2015) Outcomes for extremely premature infants. Anesth Analg 120(6):1337–1351. https://doi.org/10.1213/ANE.0000000000000705

Graven S (2006) Sleep and brain development. Clin Perinatol 33:693–706

Jawabri KH, Raja A (2020) Physiology, sleep patterns. In: StatPearls. StatPearls Publishing, Treasure Island

Joshi G, Tada N (2016) Analysis of noise level in neonatal intensive care unit and post-natal ward of a tertiary care hospital in an urban city. Int J Contemp Pediat 4(3):1358–1361

Jubinville J, Newburn-Cook C, Hegadoren K, Lacaze-Masmonteil T (2012) Symptoms of acute stress disorder in mothers of premature infants. Adv Neonatal Care 12(4):246–253. https://doi.org/10.1097/ANC.0b013e31826090ac. PMID: 22864005.

Kudchadkar SR, Barnes S, Anton B, Gergen DJ, Punjabi NM (2017) Non-pharmacological interventions for sleep promotion in hospitalized children. The. Cochrane Database Syst Rev 12:CD012908. https://doi.org/10.1002/14651858.CD012908

Kusari A, Han AM, Virgen CA, Matiz C, Rasmussen M, Friedlander SF, Eichenfield DZ (2019) Evidence-based skin care in preterm infants. Pediatr Dermatol 36(1):16–23

Lasky RE, Williams AL (2009) Noise and light exposures for extremely low birth weight newborns during their stay in the neonatal intensive care unit. Pediatrics 123(2):540–546

Lau C (2020) To individualize the management care of high-risk infants with oral feeding challenges: what do we know? What can we do? Front Pediatr 8:296. https://doi.org/10.3389/fped.2020.00296

Logan RW, McClung CA (2019) Rhythms of life: circadian disruption and brain disorders across the lifespan. Nature reviews. Neuroscience 20(1):49–65. https://doi.org/10.1038/s41583-018-0088-y

Madlinger-Lewis L, Reynolds L, Zarem C, Crapnell T, Inder T, Pineda R (2013) The effects of alternative positioning on preterm infants in the neonatal intensive care unit: a randomized clinical trial. Res Dev Disabil 35(2):490–497. https://doi.org/10.1016/j.ridd.2013.11.019

O'Brien K, Bracht M, Robson K, Ye XY, Mirea L, Cruz M, Ng E, Monterrosa L, Soraisham A, Alvaro R, Narvey M, Da Silva O, Lui K, Tarnow-Mordi W, Lee SK (2015) Evaluation of the Family Integrated Care model of neonatal intensive care: a cluster randomized controlled trial in Canada and Australia. BMC Pediatr 15:210. https://doi.org/10.1186/s12887-015-0527-0

Petty J (2017) Kangaroo mother care' helps preterm babies survive … but offers benefits for all. The Conversation. https://theconversation.com/kangaroo-mother-care-helps-preterm-babies-survive-but-offers-benefits-for-all-71644

Pickler RH, McGrath JM, Reyna BA, Tubbs-Cooley HL, Best AM, Lewis M, Cone S, Wetzel PA (2013) Effects of the neonatal intensive care unit environment on preterm infant oral feeding. Res Rep Neonatol 2013(3):15–20. https://doi.org/10.2147/RRN.S41280

Pineda R, Guth R, Herring A, Reynolds L, Oberle S, Smith J (2016) Enhancing sensory experiences for very preterm infants in the NICU: an integrative review. J Perinatol 37(4):323–332. https://doi.org/10.1038/jp.2016.179

Pineda R, Guth R, Herring A, Reynolds L, Oberle S, Smith J (2017) Enhancing sensory experiences for very preterm infants in the NICU: an integrative review. J Perinatol 37(4):323–332. https://doi.org/10.1038/jp.2016.179

Sanders MR, Hall SL (2018) Trauma-informed care in the newborn intensive care unit: promoting safety, security and connectedness. J Perinatol 38(1):3–10. https://doi.org/10.1038/jp.2017.124

Santhakumaran S, Statnikov Y, Gray D et al (2018) Survival of very preterm infants admitted to neonatal care in England 2008–2014: time trends and regional variation. Arch Dis Child 103:208–215

Schwichtenberg AJ, Christ S, Abel E, Poehlmann-Tynan JA (2016) Circadian sleep patterns in toddlers born preterm: longitudinal associations with developmental and health concerns. J Dev Behav Pediatr 37(5):358–369. https://doi.org/10.1097/DBP.0000000000000287

Shaw RJ, Deblois T, Ikuta L, Ginzburg K, Fleisher B, Koopman C (2006) Acute stress disorder among parents of infants in the neonatal intensive care nursery. Psychosomatics 47(3):206–212

Soleimani F, Azari N, Ghiasvand H et al (2020) Do NICU developmental care improve cognitive and motor outcomes for preterm infants? A systematic review and meta-analysis. BMC Pediatr 20:67. https://doi.org/10.1186/s12887-020-1953-1

Spittle A, Orton J, Anderson PJ, Boyd R, Doyle LW (2015) Early developmental intervention programmes provided post hospital discharge to prevent motor and cognitive impairment in preterm infants. Cochrane Database Syst Rev 11:CD005495. https://doi.org/10.1002/14651858.CD005495.pub4

Thaise A, Roque F, Lasiuk GC, Radünz V, Hegadoren K (2017) Scoping review of the mental health of parents of infants in the NICU. J Obstet Gynecol Neonatal Nurs 46(4):576–587

van den Hoogen A, Teunis CJ, Shellhaas RA, Pillen S, Benders M, Dudink J (2017) How to improve sleep in a neonatal intensive care unit: a systematic review. Early Hum Dev 113:78–86

Vanderbilt D, Bushley T, Young R, Frank D (2009) Acute posttraumatic stress symptoms among urban mothers with newborns in the neonatal intensive care unit. J Dev Behav Pediatr 30(1):50–56

van Tilborg E, de Theije CGM, van Hal M, Wagenaar N, de Vries LS, Benders MJ, Rowitch DH, Nijboer CH (2018) Origin and dynamics of oligodendrocytes in the developing brain: Implications for perinatal white matter injury. Glia 66(2):221–238. https://doi.org/10.1002/glia.23256. Epub 2017 Nov 14. PMID: 29134703; PMCID: PMC5765410

Weber A, Harrison TM (2019) Reducing toxic stress in the neonatal intensive care unit to improve infant outcomes. Nursing Outlook 67(2):169–189. https://doi.org/10.1016/j.outlook.2018.11.002

Werth J, Atallah L, Andriessen P, Long X, Zwartkruis-Pelgrim E, Aarts RM (2017) Unobtrusive sleep state measurements in preterm infants–a review. Sleep Med Rev 32:109–122

Williams KG, Patel KT, Stausmire JM, Bridges C, Mathis MW, Barkin JL (2018) The neonatal intensive care unit: environmental stressors and supports. Int J Environ Res Public Health 15(1):60. https://doi.org/10.3390/ijerph15010060

Wraight CL, McCoy J, Meadow W (2015) Beyond stress: describing the experiences of families during neonatal intensive care. Acta Paediatr 104:1012–1017

16

Hypoxia, Hypoglycemia, Hypothermia; The Three Hs - A Global Perspective on Early Care of the Newborn

"A Global Perspective on Hypoxia, Hypoglycemia and Hypothermia"

Judy Hitchcock

16.1 Introduction

When I mentioned to a colleague that I was writing this chapter "A global perspective on hypoxia, hypoglycemia and hypothermia" and wondering where to start, she said,

> Well, that's easy, just keep them *Pink, Sweet and Warm*!!

And there you have it, this chapter in a nutshell!

No matter where you are in the world, the principle is the same. However, where you are born in the world makes a huge difference to surviving the transition from in utero; where these primary needs are perfectly met, to independent life where, paradoxically, the infant is totally dependent on others for survival. How much experience and education the supporting care giver has, makes all the difference to mother and infant outcomes.

We are fortunate to be educated in neonatal resuscitation skills; such knowledge inspires confidence when assisting the neonatal nurse practi-

tioners and consultants with managing a compromised infant. We have an emergency trolley with everything in logical order to hand, to deal with the unexpected in a timely fashion. We rely upon the very latest technology to provide us with accurate monitoring of vital signs, we rely upon blood gas analysis machines to provide instant information about the effectiveness of circulation and the breathing on gas exchange. We rely on the x-ray technician for confirmation of invasive lines and tubes and diagnostics of conditions; but most importantly, we rely on each other; we all work together, supporting each other as much as the infant being stabilised, to provide an optimal outcome to a compromised start.

Now imagine not being in a hospital with the level of clinical governance that we expect; not surrounded by state-of-the-art intensive care equipment (Fig. 16.1) and certainly not supported by an educated team of clinicians and technicians.

It may even be that those supporting infant delivery and providing care may not be recognised as neonatal nurses or midwives but may have a generic title of "nurse" and be expected to provide whatever care they can with minimal formal training in the needs of the infant. It is a sad

J. Hitchcock (✉)
Capital and Coast District Health Board, Wellington, New Zealand

Council of International Neonatal Nurses, Inc. (COINN), Yardley, PA, USA

J. Petty et al. (eds.), *Neonatal Nursing: A Global Perspective*, https://doi.org/10.1007/978-3-030-91339-7_16

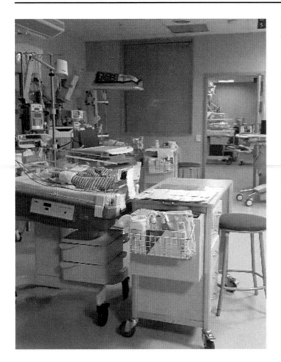

Fig. 16.1 Modern intensive care equipment

hypoxia, hypoglycaemia and Hypothermia. These resources can be found WHO I Survive and thrive: transforming care for every small and sick new-born

> **Key "Think Points" for Learning**
>
> - Keep them **Pink.** Ensure infant breathing is adequate to maintain oxygenation and understand consequences of ineffective respiratory effort causing **Hypoxia.**
> - Keep them **Sweet.** Ensure infant glucose levels are maintained for energy, understand the consequences of low blood sugar and prevent **Hypoglycaemia.**
> - Keep them **warm.** Ensure that the infant is kept warm, not affected by heat loss and cold stress, ensuring **Hypothermia** is prevented.

fact that global statistics for and infant death remain stubbornly high and are the focus for targeted improvement of the Sustainable Development Goals, (SDGs) recognising birth is high risk to term babies and their mothers, let alone premature babies. Infant mortality is still extremely high and reflects the need for the third goal from the SDGs, which aims by *2030* to *end preventable deaths of newborns and children under 5 years of age, with all countries aiming to reduce neonatal mortality to at least as low as 12 per 1000 live birth* and under-5 mortality to at least as low as 25 per 1000 births.

It's a big ask, not least with the impact of the SARS-Covid 2 pandemic compromising this target, amplifying the challenges faced, particularly in low-income countries, to provide access to neonatal care. However, progress is continuing in earnest and underpins the recently updated World Health Organisation (WHO) guidelines for Care of Sick and Small Newborn infants. Within these guidelines, written in conjunction by COINN board members, are comprehensive modules for managing thermoregulation, blood sugar levels and respiratory effort and the consequences of

Impressed with the simplicity of Pink, Sweet and Warm; a golden nugget, easy to remember and use in management of the newborn; I googled the phrase to give due credit to reference and found several articles mentioning it and wondered why I hadn't heard it before; as it is obviously a succinct learning prompt that has been around for years, even mentioned in article from 2003! http://mncyn. ca/wp-content/uploads/2013/08/volume23.pdf

The article provides a simple synopsis of the principles but, more importantly, it also recommended the "New" S.T.A.B.L.E. course being introduced, a mnemonic (Fig. 16.2) for Sugars and Safe Care, Temperature, Airway, Blood pressure, Lab work and Emotional support.

S.T.A.B.L.E. is now a recognised course, fundamental in delivering the principles for managing the newborn, compromised infant and over 25 years since it was first shared! I can remember bringing back a S.T.A.B.L.E. prompt card to my Special Care Nursery in Whanganui, New Zealand, to display behind the open-resuscitaire hot box, to prompt us when involved with stabilising an infant for transfer to the Wellington NICU, our tertiary centre. I think that was in 2004, after the Sydney COINN conference!

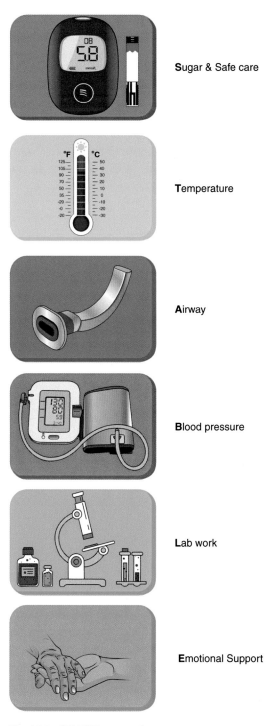

Sugar & Safe care

Temperature

Airway

Blood pressure

Lab work

Emotional Support

Fig. 16.2 STABLE mnemonic

Today, the S.T.A.B.L.E. course is a recognised global teaching resource and one that COINN endorses and offers at conferences as an addi-

tional skills workshop. It is a short course and one I took in Perth, Australia and thoroughly recommend for really nailing the management of the compromised infant, especially ameliorating the effects of the three partners in crime: Hypoxia, Hypoglycaemia and Hypothermia manifestations that without being held in check, will rapidly have dire consequences for the infant. A thorough understanding of these consequences can be found in a vast abundance of research, references and scholarly reviews; but for the purposes of this chapter, references will be underpinned by the WHO modules and the STABLE course.

There can be any number of physiological and environmental reasons that impact on infant stability, such as a shocking birth, prematurity or an infection to name but a few. Even with an effective heartbeat and circulating blood volume, stability can be compromised by the interplay of hypoxia, hypoglycaemia and hypothermia. The presenting infant is a far cry from being vigorous, pink, sweet and warm; but is pale, cyanosed, has poor tone and requires assistance with respiratory support. Skilled clinicians follow the neonatal resuscitation algorithm and provide respiratory support, as indicated to effectively improve breathing effort. This stabilisation management runs like a well-oiled machine; bloods are taken to establish gases and blood sugar level, and a glucose infusion commences to maintain energy levels and prevent the consequences of potential hypoglycaemia. The resuscitation follows the algorithm, and the team confidently ameliorates the consequences of a poor start which, in less favourable circumstances, lead to hypoxia, hypoglycaemia and hypothermia, and the negative cascade of consequences.

16.2   The Pink, Sweet and Warm Infant

Let's consider the pink, sweet and warm infant, and appreciate birth as transformative, enabling an independent new life and simultaneously creating new parents when the baby is born. Their lives will never be the same again, and nothing else will seem to matter as much as this little scrap of humanity, already filling up their hearts with so much love that they feel they could burst with happiness. The anticipation, pure joy and relief, when that all important first breath effectively opens up those lungs for the first time and the baby cries, is enough to bring us all to tears, because it is nothing short of a miracle, a pink and vigorous miracle at that.

A well-worn cliché it maybe, but there's nothing more joyful than the sound of a newborn baby, vigorously crying before being placed skin to skin with mum to keep warm, rooting to latch at the breast, already independent and hungry. It's all so natural, amazing and rather a given that everything will simply "go to plan for a normal birth"; and so it does for many of those fortunate enough to give birth in a first world country, ably assisted by a midwife or obstetrician; but for many women around the world, childbirth remains seriously high risk, whilst for the infant the risks lie in a phenomenal sequence of changes that must occur to ensure a successful transition to extrauterine life.

However, *Hypothermia, Hypoglycaemia and Hypoxia* are partners in crime when it comes to putting a spanner in the works and disrupting this finely tuned sequence of events. They are the three greatest challenges to the newborn infant successfully transitioning to extrauterine life. All are held in check by an effective beating heart and circulating, oxygenated blood volume; providing that all important first breath to inflate the lungs and initiate spontaneous breathing is effective. When followed by a hearty cry. The transition to pink and vigorous is simply "mission accomplished".

Let's pause from waxing lyrical for a moment and appreciate just how safe standards of obstetric care globally, have dramatically improved infant mortality; and yet there is still a need for the SDGs to highlight the ongoing priority for access to skilled health care providers at delivery, with the necessary education to support a compromised infant, especially understanding the ongoing neonatal care likely to be needed to restore blood gas values, blood sugar levels and baby's temperature, to within acceptable parameters for the gestation of the baby.

In a first world tertiary setting, we are used to clinical governance underpinning our practice and that those involved in the provision of care for mother and baby, are educated to a high level of proficiency in neonatal nursing. The environment is clean, and equipment is sterile to minimise the risk of cross infection. We have fabulous, open resuscitation cots (Fig. 16.3) that provide ease of access and a warm environment, whilst stabilising the infant during interventions and assessment, including being weighed and having x-rays taken with minimal handling. These given norms are simply not the case in under-resourced, geopolitically challenged hospitals and birthing environments.

16.3 The Blue, Hungry and Cold Infant

Let's leave the picture perfect stable infant, pink, vigorous, breast feeding and keeping warm against mum and consider a concerning alternative scenario, not in a first world birthing environment, where stabilising the compromised infant is managed as a matter of skilled routine, following the neonatal resuscitation protocol guidelines, (in the appendices for reference) but in a setting without access to technology and limited experience or knowledge in management of the sick, shocked or small newborn infant; how the three detrimental factors, hypoxia, hypoglycaemia and hypothermia manifest and how to mitigate them in an under-resourced setting.

Hypothermia is a preventable condition that has a well-documented impact on morbidity and mortality, especially in preterm infants. A normal core temperature is between 36.5C and 37.5C (97.7 F and 99.5 F) The WHO defines levels of mild moderate and severe hypothermia in infants as follows.

- Mild: Core temperature between 36 and 36.4 C (96.8- 97.6F).
- Moderate: Core temperature between 32-35.9C (89.6-96.6F).
- Severe: Core temperature less than 32C (less than 89.6F).

Fig. 16.3 Intensive care open cot

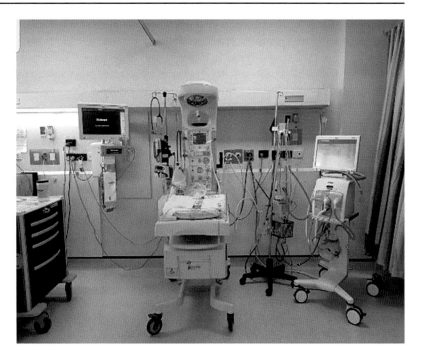

Fortunately, hypothermia is the one factor that can be limited by ensuring that the birthing environment is warm to minimise the potential for cold stress. Simple and yet effective measures must be taken to prevent conduction heat loss, such as being placed on cold surfaces when being weighed, when the infant can simultaneously lose heat through radiation, and ensuring there is no convection loss of heat from a potential draft such as the air conditioning. It is essential to dry the infant, to prevent heat loss through evaporation of moisture, and wrap in a warm towel before placing skin to skin with mum, which not only keeps the infant warm but also helps to regulate breathing and facilitate breastfeeding the infant.

Kangaroo mother care (KMC) is widely researched and when equipment, such as an open resuscitaire or incubator are not available, nursing the infant skin-to- skin in KMC, underpinned by extensive research, has proven positive stabilising benefits, aside from obviously providing vital warmth. Furthermore, when Mum is not well enough for KMC, Dad is just as important for providing warmth and comfort. Isn't it interesting how placing baby skin-to-skin is of benefit to stabilise the transition from birth, wherever baby is born in the world, and is ideal for main-taining warmth, once the infant is effectively breathing independently?

Maintaining infant temperature within expected parameters, limits the cascade of physiological events that cold stress can have on the infant; where receptors in the skin and deep tissue play an integral role in maintaining normal temperature, as the cold infant responds to stress to conserve heat. Cold stress initiates a number of reactions to minimise heat loss but in order to mount these responses, the infant metabolic rate must increase; brown fat must be metabolised, and all stress responses increase the utilisation of oxygen and glucose. With unprotected heat loss, the infant temperature is capable of dropping 0.5-1C degrees every minute; it does not take long for signs of hypoxia and hypoglycaemia to become evident.

16.4   What Are the Signs of Hypothermia?

In contrast to the pink, warm and vigorous infant, the cold infant conserves energy and is quiet, has cool extremities, is pale and peripheral cyanosis may be evident, as central warmth is conserved.

This could also indicate that the baby is significantly hypoxic, with altered respiratory rate and effort apparent. Jittery movements could also indicate low blood sugars.

Be aware of the dusky, pale, quiet, lethargic infant with altered respirations because those three "H" conspirators' are present, causing the infants' metabolism to work harder to maintain acid-base balance by compensating and correcting effectively. This can only be for a short time before there's a need for supportive intervention. Keeping the baby warm will minimise the negative cascade that invariably follows with hypothermia and the cause of metabolic acidosis.

16.5 What Is this Negative Cascade?

When the infant becomes hypothermic, metabolic rate, oxygen consumption and glucose utilisation increase. Severe hypoxaemia may lead to hypoxia which means there is insufficient oxygen required for normal cell function. If the infant must rely on anaerobic metabolism, lactic acid production and glucose consumption will increase, dropping the pH of the blood. Hypoglycaemia may eventuate from increased glucose utilisation and depletion of glycogen stores. Since glucose is the primary energy source for the brain, level of consciousness will diminish, respiration will slow, and oxygenation will suffer. If not reversed there is significant risk of cell damage but at worst, it could mean death, but not if we keep the infant PINK, SWEET and WARM.

16.6 How to Keep the Infant Warm

If possible, nurse the infant in an incubator according to age and gestation for temperature regulation, in a neutral thermal environment and for ease of observation, providing developmental care measures, such as containing the infant with nesting boundaries, and minimising stress factors like loud noises.

Imagine the challenges in a low resourced setting where this is not possible. The most effective measure is to minimise heat loss and reduce the energy being expended, which brings us back nicely to the benefits of skin to skin, because without any such equipment, the ideal warm, comforting and stabilising environment is KMC, especially if there is no alternative for respiratory supportive measures, skin to skin KMC will help reduce respiratory distress.

Imagine, just for a minute, knowing what the infant needs to effectively be supported through a compromised start to life, but not having the necessary equipment or supply of oxygen to help. Preventing hypothermia is one thing but preventing hypoxia is far more challenging for compromised infants born in low-income and under-resourced countries. In extreme respiratory distress and in direct contrast to our well, pink, vigorous baby, the infant will have poor tone, be dusky, cyanosed, in fact have a **pale blue** tinge. Without the availability of blood gas analyser, health providers are dependent on observational skills and recognising when an infant is compensating to maintain normal biochemistry values.

16.7 Hypoxia

Prior to formally establishing hypoxia through blood gas analysis, there is room for observational skills to assess the infants' respiratory effort. If there has been significant compromise during birth, then the baby will obviously be in a poor state, exhibiting compromised respiratory effort, colour and tone; and require significant resuscitation to establish spontaneous respirations and restore stability.

Understanding the basic interventions needed to rescue the infant from a shocking birth, can make all the difference to survival and is the underlying commitment from the WHO, to reach those health care providers in low-resourced countries (LIC) and provide access to learning modules that provide confidence in managing the compromised infant in a stressful situation. The Sick and small newborn infant modules referenced here when completed).

This has been the goal behind the Helping Babies Breathe (HBB) programme, developed in collaboration with WHO and is part of the Helping Babies Survive (HBS) initiative that endeavours to teach LIC health providers an understanding of the immediate interventions needed for infant resuscitation skills. Described as "The Golden Minute", interventions provide the fundamental difference between life and death. Resources are available on-line, but are dependent on access to a computer, not to mention a reliable national grid to power it. Accessibility to these resources has been increased with the launch in Nairobi in February 2021, of the Helping Babies Survive newborn care training and data collection app that supports evidence-based programmes such as HBB. Widespread adoption and use of smartphones now enable instant access to fundamental information at point of care.

Learning that rubbing the infant dry is a primary intervention and serves the dual purpose of preventing heat loss through evaporation, whilst simultaneously stimulating the infant to breath, closely followed by ensuring the airway is effectively supported and open, is a fundamental skill, an obvious intervention once the anatomy of the infant airway is understood, but without such knowledge, there may be significant delay before the lungs are inflated and effective breathing has started. Being able to access education to teach the use of a bag and mask to resuscitate an infant, will have a significant impact on positive outcomes and improve those SDGs statistics and without such access to education, the potential for hypoxia and a poor outlook is high.

16.8 What Is Hypoxia?

A low level of oxygen in the circulating blood, impacting negatively at a cellular level is a state of Hypoxaemia, the precursor to Hypoxia where oxygen level to the tissues falls below the minimum physiological levels required for cell function. This ultimately leads to a metabolic acidosis, as a result of anaerobic metabolism and the increase in the production of lactic acid.

Hypoxia is a clear indicator that the infant has experienced anaerobic metabolism secondary to shock, such as a compromised birthing event, the consequences of severe hypothermia or severe hypoglycaemia; impeding cardiac output and resulting in impaired oxygen and glucose delivery to the tissues. There can be other causes such as congenital heart, sepsis or inborn errors of metabolism, but the primary culprits are the troublesome trio and close observation of the infant is paramount to thwart the negative consequences. There are multiple reasons for impaired oxygen assimilation, generally described as respiratory distress; and why observation of respiratory rate and effort are so important. Similarly, noting the infant's colour is an obvious indicator of poor oxygenation. Deoxygenated blood is darker and gives a pale, bluish tinge to the skin.

Infants experiencing respiratory distress exhibit increasing work of breathing and become tachypnoeic, exceeding the normal rate, which is between 30- 60 breaths per minute (S.T.A.B.L.E Respiratory rate chapter), This is associated with the infant exhaling more carbon dioxide to alleviate increasing metabolic acidosis. If work of breathing is compromised, use of accessory muscles increases to assist with ventilation of the lungs. There is nasal flaring and audible grunting, whereby the infant tries to increase functional residual capacity of the lung, when the alveoli are collapsed and require more respiratory effort to open.

In a well-resourced setting, management is undertaken by skilled clinicians, who understand blood gas interpretation from the results supplied by the lab technician and are competent to manage the respiratory support to improve oxygenation, such as using ventilators, Hi-Flo and continuous positive airways pressure (CPAP); but when there is no lab and all that is available are observational skills, options to support effective breathing are limited.

With the luxury of pulse oximetry monitoring, the percentage of oxygenation can be monitored accurately. The red bi-polar sensor saturation probe measures the redness of the circulating blood. In a state of hypoxia, being less saturated with oxygen, the blood is less red and records at a lower percentage value; but the true indicator of impaired respiratory gas exchange is established with blood samples, from which can be deduced the impact of poor oxygenation on glucose metabolism and the biochemistry values that are inextricably linked and accurately indicate a metabolic acidosis. It is worth bearing in mind here, how reliant we are on confirmed values to manage the compromised infant. Understanding and interpreting reported values are invaluable skills and I find the S.T.A.B.L.E. tool helpful to distinguish the difference between respiratory and metabolic acidosis or alkalosis.

In a low-income, poorly resourced country, the ideal would be to monitor a compromised infant with a pulse oximeter to establishing the oxygen saturation, as would providing supplemental oxygen if indicated and available, with clinical governance underpinning oxygen therapy and delivery mode, but without a blood gas analyser to confirm the gas values, knowing how to protect and position the infant to maintain the airway, whilst also endeavouring to keep the infant sweet and warm, will help with resolving transient tachypnoea of the newborn and limit the negative consequences of hypoxia.

Keeping the infant warm is manageable with KMC; however, the biggest challenge for the infant is to maintain sufficient energy levels, because whilst increased work of breathing is evident, feeding is not recommended until the infant is stable. It is a huge conundrum, because without an alternative means to maintain the energy requirements, the infant will tire and have no energy to feed and the negative cascade will spiral down, hypoglycaemia will eventuate and exacerbate the deteriorating situation.

16.9 What Is Hypoglycaemia?

Hypoglycaemia refers to low blood sugar levels (BSL), which impact on availability of glucose for energy at a cellular level. It is vital that blood sugar levels are maintained to meet all the energy requirements after birth, especially for the infants' brain, which unlike the liver, skeletal and cardiac muscle, cannot store adequate amounts of glucose in the form of glycogen and needs a consistent steady supply of glucose to function. Before birth, the infant is prepared for extra uterine life by conserving energy stores of glucose in the form of glycogen and relies primarily on placental transfer of glucose and amino acids to meet energy demands. However, once born and the umbilical cord is cut, this ready supply of energy is interrupted, and the infant must rely on enzymes to convert the stored supply of glycogen back into glucose molecules to meet an independent need for energy. The ability to achieve this successfully depends on an adequate supply of glycogen stores. Inadequate glycogen stores are easily depleted increasing the risk of hypoglycaemia.

16.10 Managing Hypoglycaemia

The PINK vigorous, term infant will let everyone know when hunger sets in! That urgent cry cannot be ignored, everything stops to breastfeed the infant and effectively restore energy levels sufficient to allow three to four hours rest before feeding again. However, the seriously compromised, term infant with respiratory distress, cannot and should not feed until stable because they have poor suck, swallow, breath coordination, which in turn can delay gastric emptying. The distress increases energy consumption and the potential for aspiration of the stomach contents into the lungs.

The "sick or small infant" is challenged to meet the necessary intake required to maintain sufficient energy levels and is at serious risk of hypoglycaemia. Even more challenging is the premature infant who will have a multiplicity of complex needs, further compromising and impacting on their energy reserves depending on gestation. Understanding the underlying reason for hypoglycaemia, will determine the management protocol undertaken to maintain blood sugar levels within the acceptable parameters required for a sustained growth trajectory; and necessary until the infant can fully breast feed independently. This can range from simple measures of buccal dextrose gel, to complex nutritional support of total parenteral nutrition (TPN) and lipids for extremely premature infants.

The otherwise well infant, who is just sleepy and not interested in feeding, can be managed with expressed colostrum as available, given via syringe, and regular BGL samples, according to the guidelines in place. Conservative and effective management with buccal administration of dextrose gel, provides enough energy to keep the BSL values positive until the infant becomes more alert and starts to breastfeed with great purpose. The onset of hypoglycaemia is averted without invasive management of an intravenous dextrose infusion.

The seriously compromised symptomatic infant, who requires stabilisation, will have an Intravenous infusion of glucose commenced to maintain blood sugar levels and fluid requirements; with blood sugar analysis at regular intervals to ensure values remains above 2.8 mmol, a value recommended in the S.T.A.B.L.E programme. This value varies slightly depending on evidence adopted, where I currently work the value is 2.6 mmol. The BSL can be managed by analysing a drop of blood from a simple heel prick or, for definitive value accuracy, through point of care analysis or plasma glucose lab confirmation. Now, consider how infants at risk of hypoglycaemia can be managed without access to these resources. How technology dependent we are in first world settings for managing BSL values at point of care, how fortunate to have lab technicians providing accurate blood values and skilled clinicians providing intravenous access for dextrose infusions.

What can be done to minimise the risk of hypoglycaemia in under-resourced countries? Symptomatic Hypoglycaemia is hard to isolate from manifesting symptoms of Hypothermia and Hypoxia, although neurological signs of jitteriness, tremors, hypotonia, irritability and lethargy may be more significant. Basic interventions can do much to minimise the consequences of hypoglycaemia by keeping the infant skin to skin with

mum, minimising the energy expenditure and limiting the potential negative cascade of hypothermia and hypoxia.

How we effectively disseminate the knowledge and skills to all those involved in the care of the infant, will help achieve the SDG goal for a reduction in global infant mortality statistics. Harnessing the advances in digital technology, especially the access to education, such as the HBS app, will promote confidence in providing infant resuscitation skills, remembering the vital importance of "The Golden Minute" and to keep the infant

"PINK, SWEET and WARM".

Glossary

Adenosine triphosphate (ATP) For every molecule of glucose completely metabolised, 38 molecules of ATP are produced: 2 from Glycolysis to pyruvic acid and 36 molecules from metabolism of pyruvic acid to ATP via Krebs citric acid cycle, a complex biochemical chain of events that provides the infant with energy and removal of the bi-product carbon dioxide, which is exchanged in the lungs and breathed out.If there is poor respiratory effort, with consequential low oxygen content in the cells, metabolism of glucose is incomplete. Only 2 molecules of ATP are produced for every molecule of glucose that is metabolised to pyruvic acid, which is then metabolised into lactic acid. This is why an elevated lactate level, low pH, Low bicarb value on a blood gas result is important, as it provides an indication of anaerobic glycolysis; a response to poor oxygenation of the blood and why hypoxia and hypoglycaemia are inextricably linked.

Brown fat Brown fat helps to maintain infant temperature. The term infant has a store of brown fat to help maintain temperature, whereas the preterm infant does not. Brown fat requires oxygen and glucose to metabolise, so naturally an infant who is hypoglycaemic, has poor or depleted glycogen stores and/or is hypoxic will not be able to metabolise brown fat to maintain temperature and keep warm.

Glycolysis Gylcolyisis is the primary step in the breakdown of glucose for cellular respiration.Ideally, with an uncompromised respiratory effort there is an excellent supply of oxygen at the cellular level, allowing for the complete metabolism of glucose into ATP.

Glycogen Glycogen is a store of energy. In a term infant, glycogen accounts for approximately 5 to 8% of the liver and muscle weight and 4% of cardiac muscle weight (STABLE 2013 edition) Inadequate glycogen stores are easily depleted in a compromised infant, increasing the risk of hypoglycaemia. High risk groups are premature infants who miss out on the third trimester when glycogen stores are laid down.

Hypoglycaemia Hypoglycaemia refers to Low Blood Sugar levels, which impact on availability of glucose for energy at a cellular level.

Hypothermia Hypothermia is defined as a cold infant with a temperature reading below expected values for age and gestation; and is the one condition that is preventable and yet can have a serious detrimental effect on infant stability if it goes unchecked. It can be caused by environmental factors such as getting cold at delivery or physiological factors such as prematurity, or metabolic disorder.

Hypoxia Hypoxia is the term used to describe an inadequate oxygen level to the tissues below the physiological levels required for cell function.

Hypoxaemia Hypoxaemia describes a low level of oxygen in the circulating blood, impacting negatively at a cellular level.

Krebs citric acid cycle Krebs citric cycle is a complex biochemical chain of events that provides the infant with energy and removal of the bi-product carbon dioxide, which is exchanged in the lungs and breathed out.

Further Reading

Helping Babies Breath (HBB) programme. https://www.aap.org/en-us/advocacy-and-policy/aap-health-initiatives/helping-babies-survive/Pages/Helping-Babies-Breathe.aspx#:~:text=Helping%20Babies%20Breathe%20teaches%20the%20initial%20steps%20of,to%2047%25%20and%20fresh%20stillbirths%20by%2024%25%20

Helping Babies Survive HBS app. https://pubmed.ncbi.nlm.nih.gov/33004639/

Kangaroo care. WHO I Care of the preterm and low-birth-weight new-born

PINK, SWEET AND WARM. http://mncyn.ca/wp-content/uploads/2013/08/volume23.pdf

S.T.A.B.L.E. About – The S.T.A.B.L.E. Program (stableprogram.org)

WWW. WHO Newborn health (who.int)

Nursing Mana: Intuitive Effects on Nurse and Patient Care

17

Leilani Kupahu-Marino Kahoano,
Myrahann K. Kanahele-Gerardo, Susan Kau,
and Alakai Georgiana N. Kahale

L. K.-M. Kahoano (✉)
Hawaii Healthcare | Cradles and Crayons Pediatric
Nursing Agency, Ewa, HI, USA

Mālama o Nā Keiki | Caring for Hawai'i Neonates
(C4HN), Honolulu, HI, USA

Alliance of Global Neonatal Nursing (ALIGNN),
Honolulu, HI, USA

Queen Julia Kapiolani Hawaiian Civic Club
(QJKHCC), Honolulu, HI, USA

Council of International Neonatal Nurses, Inc.
(COINN), Yardley, PA, USA

M. K. Kanahele-Gerardo
Mālama o Nā Keiki | Caring for Hawai'i Neonates
Kekaha, Kauai, HI, USA

Queen Julia Kapiolani Hawaiian Civic Club
(QJKHCC), Honolulu, HI, USA

S. Kau
Kapiolani Medical Center for Women & Children
Caring for Hawaii Neonates, Honolulu, HI, USA

Queen Julia Kapiolani Hawaiian Civic Club
(QJKHCC), Honolulu, HI, USA

A. G. N. Kahale
Lei Poina ole - Poe Niihau (people of Niihau), A
Program of Mālama o Nā Keiki | Caring for Hawai'i
Neonates Kekaha, Kauai, HI, USA

Queen Julia Kapiolani Hawaiian Civic Club,
Honolulu, HI, USA

17.1 Introduction

Mana is innate to indigenous cultures, especially the Hawaiian people. This partially explains why these islands have drawn upon many to seek her spiritual essence. The word Hawai'i also holds the answers as to why ancient Hawaiian ancestors were intuitively skilled scientists, spiritually guided and their "inherited" mana passed through the cells and blood of the Hawaiian descendants today. Many have found they can feel the connection to our ancestors by choosing to "acquire" mana through education and hone into their "inherited" knowledge.

> **Key "Think Points" for Learning**
> - It is important to consider intuition as a way we can learn about people and the best way to care for them.
> - Intuitive knowing is important in nursing, to work alongside knowledge generated from research-based evidence.
> - Understanding this intuitive perspective from a specific cultural setting enhances our global awareness and understanding relating to caring for the "person."

J. Petty et al. (eds.), *Neonatal Nursing: A Global Perspective*,
https://doi.org/10.1007/978-3-030-91339-7_17

17.2 Intuition

Intuition is defined in Merriam-Webster's Dictionary (2019) as: (1) quick and ready insight (2) a: immediate apprehension or cognition b: knowledge or conviction gained by intuition c: the power or faculty of attaining to direct knowledge or cognition without evident rational thought and inference. "Intuition Prosociality" explains prosociality in two categories: (1) Prosocial behaviors, (2) Prosocial outcomes (Zaki and Mitchell 2013). Both categories include intuition and evolved controlled behaviors that benefit the well-being of others and uphold prosocial norms. One of the behaviors is "automaticity"—the speed and immunity to the presence of distractions (Bargh and Chartrand 1999). These behaviors were natural to native Hawaiians and have become a necessary traditional practice in modern times for the professional nurse, especially relating to care of high-risk babies. The next sections are formed from reflections on my growth as a registered nurse (RN) and neonatal nurse (Leilani Kupahu-Marino Kahoano).

17.3 Mana

Mana in Hawaiian refers to energy from the spirit or a healing power (Pukui and Elbert 1986). As a "Novice" nurse advances to "Expert" level nursing, a part of the competency needs to include the intuitive assessment in patient care. This type of internal data collection complements the clinical, evidence-based, information and technology. As an "Advanced Beginner" nurse in the Neonatal Intensive Care Unit (NICU) caring for micro-premature babies (gestational ages 23–28 weeks), in the 1990s, this registered nurse (RN) learned the importance of intuitively sensing subtle patient changes showing before technology and laboratory results confirmed a patient was sick. This discovery set in motion "Why is mana important to our babies' assessments?" "Can this innate sense be taught to others?" "Does the spirit of a culture influence nursing actions?" The neonatal intensive care unit (NICU) of the past was constantly filled with sensory overload in patient areas and cluster care was not yet a NICU standard. By intentionally studying a 23-week patient

in the 1990s, the process of a deeper awareness of common behaviors and/or individual responses to many of our primary patients began. Years of 12-hour shifts and one-to-one assignments allowed for observing, documenting, and becoming "one" with these patients who spent months in the NICU. To "feel" their needs and "listen" to their voices no matter the presence of many distractions became more natural as my nursing experiences evolved over the 20 years. The speed at which I began to trust my intuition went from second guessing my observations and gut feelings to confidence in seconds when advocating for our littlest patients in emergency situations.

17.4 Inherited Mana

Hawaiians are classified into different categories: Kanaka Maoli, Native Hawaiians, Keiki o ka 'Aina, Hawaiian with blood quantum, and other categories continue to be established. For the purpose of this chapter, we shall refer to the Kanaka Maoli—the Native Hawaiians born into a lineage of families prior to the arrival of Western civilization. As my own family genealogy became clearer, the word "mana" resonated in all areas of personal and professional life. We may not have realized how much of our past is important to the present—at the cellular and blood levels, we are our past and that inherent quality is key to supporting babies thriving. This exploration revealed unexpected facts of a family member possessing the highest authority of spiritual power in leadership for ancient Hawai'i. His name was misunderstood after Christianity arrived; however, today, it has been revealed his prophetic nature and indigenous knowledge healed, guided, and altruistically unified Hawai'i. This confirmed the Western concept of "Intuitive Prosociality" that existed as "mana", an ancient Hawaiian tradition and can be an inherited gift.

A profound mo'olelo (story) is King Kamehameha III—born as a still birth in 1814; however, versions of his birth explained he was almost 30 minutes with obvious breaths. Na Kahuna (priests) and high-ranking royalty were present to pray over this baby until his breath returned. He becomes the longest reigning royal leader of Hawai'i—nearly 30 years and the greatest changes occurred during this time. Another mo'olelo includes the people of Ni'ihau who were raised, and continue today, without the modern conveniences of the Western World. They believe that their prayers made together to God is the la'au kahea—the medicine healing from God only. Their innate sense of medical treatments, birthing practices, caring for premature births, and mother for the first month are great examples of this inherited mana—Kahua Mana.

As a neonatal intensive care unit (NICU) and Hospice nurse, arterial blood gases (ABGs) were able to prove the impact a nurse has on the physiology of a high-risk baby. The skills and competence of nurses and their abilities to connect with patients can impact the length of hospital stay, medication needs, ventilation changes, and overall responsiveness to multi-disciplinary changes—how we prepare the baby for all activities can result in positive or negative outcomes. In the early 2000s, a 23 weeker who was now 25 weeks gestation, Baby G, had arterial blood gases (ABGs) on the same day and this registered nurse (RN) was the primary nurse who had been off shift for several days:

1700: Ph 7.1, PCO2 69, PO2 37, BE -6. Patient had ventilation changes and Sodium Bicarbonate was given. The Day nurse was assigned this patient and was noted to not be one of the primary nursing team members. The nurse's attitude at the end of the shift was reported to be overwhelmed and stated that it "was a bad baby today."

2000: 12-hour shift change; 1:1 assignment. There was a request for a new ABG drawn before touching the patient for his first assessment as this RN was the primary nurse for this assignment. The isolette was opened. The arterial line was calibrated and the nurse introduced self to the baby with aloha, sharing encouraging words of a good shift together. The endotracheal tube (ETT) was preoxygenated in anticipation of suctioning via a Ballard system. Then the isolette was closed. Some minutes were allowed for the baby to remain stable before the new ABG drawn as pre-approved by the senior nurse and neonatologist as this team understood how to affect the baby's return to stability.

2015: Ph 7.1, PCO2 69, PO2 37, BE -6. No changes in patient physiology from the 1700 ABG. Next, this RN requested if senior nurse and neonatologist would approve no ventilation or medication changes until a post-assessment ABG was done—approved. Physical assessment was undertaken with compassionate care—a kind of connecting that focuses on the neonate, handling every aspect of assessment with intentionality that requires gentle, slow movements to create the spiritual connection with the baby. The entire assessment was 20–30 minutes in length with a strong focus on spiritually, mentally and emotionally "connecting" so the remainder of the shift could be used to improve this baby's acidotic condition and move toward stability for the next shift. When the assessment was done, time was allowed to pass before drawing a new ABG.

Between 2130 and 2200: Ph 7.4, PCO2 39, PO2 37, BE -0.9. Dramatic changes excited the team as it was the first time in days this baby exhibited a major change. The patient was allowed to settle into the next hours with minimal ventilation and medication changes. The medical team agreed to work with the nurse's plan to allow the baby to naturally stabilize, then add ventilation and medication changes, if necessary. It became obvious the baby could partner in this medical plan. If he was allowed to be carefully assessed and cluster care was included, we witnessed he could correct his acidotic state toward a healthier stability. Over the coming days, with the return of this same RN for the 12-hour night shifts, the baby had strengthened, and overall physiology improved with less mechanical and pharmacology changes. How can we translate this innate understanding to nursing schools and new graduate programs?

17.5 Acquired Mana

There is a need to design an intentional clinical program including all team members: Physicians, nurses, respiratory therapists, X-ray technicians, parents, community nurses who will care for this baby after discharge—i.e. any team member that will have their caring hands on a high-risk baby to develop an understanding to provide care that affects and maintains physiological, spiritual, social/emotional stability. This could have a major impact on the service provision of hospitals, decreased hospital admission days, increase in the nursing workforce, the inclusion of indigenous cultural knowledge, and so much more. Intuitive knowledge can be developed through education, daily interactions, and mentoring as examples of acquired mana.

17.5.1 Ho'omakaukau: To Get Ready!

Ho'omakaukau means "To get ready" and to prepare for the next steps. When we awaken, the gift of gratitude is given for opening our eyes, having our breath and the privilege to give kahu (sacred care) our babies, families, and colleagues. Moving through each moment becomes very intentional so when arriving at work, we are ready to step into our babies' space, ready to be present for their needs. They become our leader throughout the day so that we answer and respond to what they really need versus what we want them to have for their care. Sometimes, our desire to comfort in ways that makes us comfortable or how we have taken care of our own babies may not be what truly comforts or meets the needs of babies on a NICU. Before rushing into the tasks of the day, a gentle introductory touch upon the baby's bottom or head and/or a gentle voice to say "We're together and I believe we can do our best together" can make all the difference to having a smoother day. Even the sickest baby can feel that this simple, yet, compassionate gesture changes their own attitude—this is Ho'omakaukau!

17.5.2 Makaukau: Ready!: Being Present

Makaukau—we are now ready to begin— we have taken care of all needs to set our day ahead, we are ready by the shift report received, have checked our medications, reviewed last night's charting notes, anticipated the upcoming examinations, wiped down room equipment, checked patient room boards and more—so much in the first 10–15 minutes can set the tone of the day and reduce the nursing stress one feels when unprepared. The baby feels our stress of rushing through the tasks that must be done. Often two or three babies within the first hour of our shifts in our care can feel our own stress. How we prepare ourselves by taking that extra step of preparation can make the unexpected changes during the shift easier to handle. This seems so intuitive to do, yet, it is a habit that must be built over time so that it becomes second nature to do. Makaukau!

17.5.3 Ho'oponopono: To Make Right

It is important to start each day with gratitude for what we can do, not what happened yesterday and cannot be changed. However, we do have the ability with minamina—an action of valuing relationships, projects, privileges to care for the tiniest patients—to choose respect over harboring negativity and pono, to do the right thing, avoiding any moments left unfinished. Like Hospice care, when a patient is able to come to peace with unfinished business or make right the relationships that hindered growth, their spirit can move forward to a better place. This same gift is applicable to patient care; humbly making right those areas that allow us to give our babies every detail of attention they deserve in the hours we are committed to them. Ho'oponopono is a Hawaiian lifestyle of conflict resolution that allows for peace in the most chaotic moments. The NICU is constantly in ebb and flow of uncertainty when a new, critical, admission arrives. Ho'oponopono allows the purest of patients to enter into a space of all being in the right mindset to instill positive external energies into patient care.

17.5.4 Lokahi: Harmony

Lokahi is the result of minamina and ho'oponopono. A natural balance flows through the nurse and the team members when we take the time to value relationships by asking for forgiveness or giving forgiveness, so we both can be released from any future negativity. Lokahi is especially important as some babies enter into the world already challenged by the pregnancy or birthing process. They count on us to be completely ready to tend to every need for their day together. Lokahi is a balance that requires dedication to the process of keeping calm when suddenly a patient takes an unexpected turn toward life or death.

17.5.5 Ho'olewa: Releasing the Mana and Intentional Recognition

Ho'olewa—we celebrate the life of those who have passed. This is especially important to recognize the value of a baby who occupied a patient room, especially for weeks or months. The standard practice after a baby passes is to quickly turn over the room so a new admission or a transfer patient can settle in. Housekeeping personnel enter the room, clean, and prepare for the next patient. Other team members may enter to prepare supplies and restock cabinets. Respiratory team members check the oxygen equipment. Imagine how many people enter this room after a discharge, especially after the death of a patient. Do we ever take time to have a blessing of the room? Do we utilize our pastoral care to consider the energies left by a family, medical team, or the baby? Ho'olewa is important to recognize a little spirit once was in this room, the sorrow of their family members, and the need to ho'oku'u, i.e. to set free and noa, anything left from the previous person entering this space. The intentions of the next team preparing the space can enter knowing they are helping to release the past and preparing for the next little one, to count on us to be fully present for their needs. This is especially important if the same nurse needs to take on another patient. The patient deserves to enter the room with new energies so patient care can truly start anew. Ho'olewa gives a moment of sacredness and reverence for this little life who has departed or has been discharged to home. Either way, we let the next patient and team start fresh. In Hawai'i, we place a kukui lei outside the door as a way of making the room right; kukui represents life, medicine, light, and much more. This quiet way of immediately letting all know this room is being blessed for the patient, family and team can be simple to ho'olewa our tiniest patients.

17.5.6 Ola: Life

Ola is life and the span of our babies' lives can be brief or they can live to an older age. We may never see this baby ever again; however, for the time we have shared in their life, you have made a lifetime difference because your presence, skills, knowledge, and mana have impacted their care during the most fragile developmental stage of their lives. Being a practitioner valuing the natural, intuitive, knowledge of elders, it has been important to maintain a balance of "inherited" and "acquired" knowledge to provide the best bedside care.

17.5.7 Ho'ihi: Respect Leading to Filial Piety

Ho'ihi means respect and Filial piety is the respect of parents, elders, and those loved ones very dear to us. This is a natural cultural mannerism and traditional lifestyle that expects the younger generation to treat our elders with reverence. This character trait enhances our patience to care for the natural changes of life—Dementia and Alzheimer's are not seen as a disease, it is more a part of life's changes. This same care is transferred to our high-risk babies in that we observe what they are able to do and be naturally in their world to help them thrive.

17.5.8 Inoa: Name

It is believed that one's name leads us to the path of our life's purpose. In naming a baby, it is important a "kupuna" or "tutu" or one that had a ho'ailona (vision) privileges a baby with a carefully intentioned name for life. Additional names could be added over the lifetime depending on significant events. In Hawaiian culture, it was believed names could cause life or death to a person; thus, even more important who gives the name and the mana they live will affect the future of this baby. This gift of naming is not taken lightly and is a serious responsibility for the person gifting the baby's name. An example is a baby who was given a name that was defined as "sin, offense" in the literal sense; however, in the "kaona"—the veiled meaning, the elders knew this name could cause the demise of this baby in later years. An elder, "tutu lady," encouraged the mother to add "Lei o" to the beginning of this name so the baby could be protected against any harm or become what the negatives of this name represents, without the leading words of protection. The parents listened and added "Lei o" to which the young man is now in his 60s and has maintained a very humble life. Native Hawaiians have been known for insightful wisdom.

17.5.9 Mea 'Ai: Food

A study in the 1950s by the University of Hawai'i, "Poi in Hawai'i," proved how important poi was to the digestive system of not only babies, but also adults with cancer or digestive issues (Derstein and Rada 1952). The natural scientist, innate to ancient Native Hawaiian people, figured out, through the gift of Mana (spirit) and Aloha (God), what plants healed or harmed. Recognizing that kalo could be turned into poi and could become the staple for Native Hawaiians was similar to potatoes for the American and Irish people. Food is an important cultural tradition that brings families together. This applied to the babies being connected intimately by the same poi bowl mixed with water and often offered as the first food for babies, especially high-risk ones. Babies were fed in the haumana style; an elder or parent chewing the food first, then placing a small amount in the baby's mouth to prevent choking and passing on the "mana" of this person to the baby.

17.6   Native Mind, Heart and Spiritual Scientists

In ancient Hawai'i, the society had a natural lifestyle of understanding of how the body needed to develop in the physical brain and heart; simultaneously, the kino (body), na'au (gut), and mana (spirit). How they raised their babies from pregnancy to adulthood was a kuleana (responsibility) of the entire 'ohana (family) and extended 'ohana (extended family and friends). Many babies were naturally brought up with the simplicity of life, encouraged to discover the world around them, and given the next tasks according to their natural abilities, not their chronological stage of development. The Native Hawaiians referred to the na'au as the heart and brain, whereas the Western medi-

cine viewed the brain as the primary center for processing all information. The anterior fontanel was treated with natural herbs to protect and grow the brain. However, the na'au was considered the first brain—it required being fed first in order for the rest of the body to develop and function properly. It was also understood that the gut had a spiritual connection with the heart, physical brain, and entire body. How it was nurtured spiritually and physically included aloha (love) and ho'oponopono (forgiveness). In the Western society, we understand the development of the brain is affected by experiences and needing a strong foundation. In Hawaiian child development, spirituality is what creates the strong foundation and in Western early child development, the brain is the primary focus including social-emotional-mental. By combining the two understandings of early child development, the future baby has a greater chance of being raised with a new kind of resilience, coping skills, physical development, academic achievements, environmental responsibilities, and much more. Lessening "toxic stress" can begin in the NICU by setting up family programs that take advantage of the time a baby is admitted and introduce learning to provoke a self-assessment of parents and/or primary caregivers. There is always something new that can be learned relating to current knowledge; this is important as part of the innate lifestyle of the ancient Hawaiians. Our monarchs are good examples of knowledge discovery and spiritual enrichment. The basic social-emotional skills of "Executive decision making and self-regulation" can be a beautiful beginning of collaboration between nurse, parents, and baby. Infant mental health needs to include infant spiritual health so we can contribute to the future of healthier communities.

The *"Serve and Return"* metaphor in early childhood development is like tennis. In my opinion, if the volley of positive or negative information is long enough and frequent, a longer lasting impression is made in the brain and heart. The bursts of shorter volleys and less intense returns would seem easier to heal with early and strong interventions. However, if the spirit of a keiki is very strong and becomes in conflict with its physical self, eventually the spirit and the ego are imbalanced. On the outside, the keiki may have learned to cope, yet, internally a quiet struggle is growing, often unbeknownst to the parents and in adult years, even to oneself. The COVID-19 pandemic revealed how many people were affected as adults and this trickled down to the children and youth. The spiritual aspect of who we are and how it made us feel as a community was revealed, the longer this period of time lasted. We better understand how a spiritual foundation is important to the physical and physiological development of a baby.

17.6.1 Kahu/Kahuna: Spiritual Healer/Prophetic guidance

The responsibility of the Kahuna in the past was prophetic, healing and known as the "physician" as Western culture recognizes. They were also responsible for the spiritual wellness of an 'ohana' or community. Kahuna pale keiki or Kahuna ma'i keiki were terms this RN heard in younger years as her grandmother Kahana was a Registered Nurse for over 33 years; however, she also recognized the ways of old in her quiet ways. To this day, there are some who worked with Kahana and remembered her to be the nurse sent into the patient rooms when other team members were unable to calm a patient or encourage medication compliance.

17.7 Mo'oku'auhau: Genealogy

17.7.1 Filial Piety

Hawai'i is known for its care of elders and their children. This nurturing of many first babies was automatically the responsibility of a pre-designated grandparent or "kupuna"—elder. In ancient times, it was custom to "hanai"; to adopt a baby legally and raise this baby as one's own. The baby took on all the kuleana (responsibilities), were taught and at times were returned to the birth family in the teen or young adult years. This type of upbringing was especially known in the hula world. A young one could live with his or her kumu (teacher) or grandparent and the 24 hour living together would instill all behaviors needed through this spiritual upbringing. In return, this deep respect for the elder protected the adult in their aging years, as well as carried on traditions exactly as given at birth. Living with the bible was the first book of instruction and guidance used as the foundation of learning, and daily praying together for all things granted to live in this life. This solidified the deep respect for the elders and this mana was passed on to the younger ones and would be held with high regard for their lifetime. The relationship was even more deeply cared for after the passing of this elder.

17.8 Nursing School Curriculum

Standard nursing school curriculum has to focus on teaching the art and science of nursing. Teaching theoretical models of care and emphasizing safe, high-quality care are important. But also important are the cultural and spiritual aspects of care. It is uncommon in some countries to have courses that are dedicated to transcultural nursing and spirituality; however, in Hawai'i, courses are in place and more prevalent. Respect and sensitivity especially linked to our Hawaiian heritage is important to providing quality care. Many native Hawaiians believe in lokahi or the balance of physical, mental, and spiritual aspects of a person in order to understand health and illness. This balance is important to restore if health is to prevail. Another important concept stressed in our nursing education is Ohana or family. For neonatal nurses, the concept of family is essential as we care for the family-baby unit. During nursing education, this concept of Hawaiian core values can enhance the developmental care we strive to provide for every baby.

17.9 Infant Mental Health

The concept of infant mental health is not new but for Hawaiian neonatal care it is an extension of Lokahi and Ohana. It encompasses social and emotional development of the baby which is dependent on the family interaction. The Association for Infant Mental Health in Hawai'i (https://aimhhi.org/) is dedicated to supporting infants from birth to 5 years of age through building trust and security. This organization stresses that the baby's first relationships either nurture or hinder the way the surrounding environment is explored. The values of the association are to "foster positive relationships" and to "listen" to parent voices. By observing and listening to the family and by teaching them how to recognize their baby's cues, positive and negative, nurses can help them and confidently provide care, promote trust and security. Infant mental health also means that mental health specialists need to be available to families, as a NICU stay is extremely stressful. If they do not have help with coping and decreasing their stress, the baby will feel this stress and become insecure. Infant and family mental health is an important and integral part of neonatal care.

17.10 Pu'ukohola Heiau

Pu'ukohola Heiau translates to the temple on the hill of the whale. It is found on the Big Island of Hawaii. This is a sacred site where ceremonies are held. Temples and rituals associated with Hawaiian culture such as the hula are taught to native Hawaiian children as part of the educational process. A collaborative program between Chaminade University School of Nursing, University of Hawai'i Pharmacology and Native Hawaiian School of Medicine physicians and other native Hawaiian groups re-enacts a period of Hawaiian traditions at Pu'ukohola and set up a two-day community health screening for the local people of Kohala. For many who come for their annual physical assessment will only seek treatment here, as they still follow their traditions of only Native Hawaiians caring for them. Before Covid, the plan was to begin seeing perinatal, neonatal and pediatric patients. The hope is to resume this program in 2022 and have a full 'ohana (family) screening program to be set up for earlier identification of the common medical concerns in the Native Hawaiian communities: examples are cardiac problems, obesity, diabetes and ongoing neonatal concerns.

17.11 Uniki Training

Uniki training to teach a person how to become Kumu Hula or hula teachers takes years, often takes decades to truly pass on the spiritual essence of traditions. Hula is a form of passing knowledge from one to another. It is not just a dance. It incorporates dance, dress, use of plants, music, and the following of strict protocols or the preserving of ancient rituals. This training teaches ancient traditions and culture. Children begin this training before birth depending on one's family lineage. The hula is a spiritual experience that promotes healing, deepens the relationship between one's passion, work, personal and community contributions. To be selected as a student of this formal training transfers traditional knowledge into my nursing practice over the decades; the result has been powerful. There is an equal balance of being responsible to the Native Hawaiian traditions and nursing practice to bring forth the best patient care and outcomes. In relation to evidence-based medicine, just as these rituals are important to honor my Hawaiian roots, so are the traditions of nursing important for my professional life. One example of this is the White Coat Ceremony.

17.12 White Coat Ceremony

The Arnold P. Gold Foundation established funding for nursing schools to hold White Coat ceremonies. Dr. Gold, a pediatrician, dedicated his career to providing humanistic care. In 1993 he established the first White Coat ceremony for medical students just beginning their professional journey (https://www.gold-foundation. org/). It established a rite of passage from being a college student to becoming a medical professional student, when the white lab coat is earned to signify a commitment to humanistic and not just technological or physical care.

Nurses many years ago also had rites of passage through their education; receiving a cape, a student nursing cap, a nursing pin, and finally a black stripe on the cap. But as times changed, these rituals were lost. Dr. Gold along with the American Association of Colleges of Nursing (AACN) expanded the White Coat ceremony to include nursing students in 2014. Schools of nursing could apply for funding for the first year. After that time, the school was to maintain the ceremony. Here in Hawaii, now schools of nursing hold this ceremony to commemorate the movement into the student's first clinical experience. This rite of passage upholds the tradition of moving forward to become a professional nurse. It also incorporates the Hawaiian values of respect, trust, and spirituality as well as a commitment to the Hawaiian people to provide respectful, integrative care. It demonstrates that Hawaiian traditions and values can be, and are aligned with, good high-quality care.

17.13 Conclusion

This chapter reflects some of the traditions of Hawaii and how these values and traditions can, and should, be incorporated into neonatal nursing care. For the new family unit Ohana is at the heart of all we do. Physical neonatal care is not enough. It must include sensitivity to the spiritual and mental health needs of the family unit.

Mana Statement
Mana is the spiritual life force energy that is all present in our universe. It is initiated at the time of conception and continues to flow throughout the developing fetus—"its lifeline" through the placenta.

The spirituality and its cultural components of energy continue when the infant is born. The mana is nurtured and embraced by invisible bonds. The acquired/learned behaviors along with religious beliefs and practices of healing help shape/strengthen one's spiritual energy.

We as caregivers need to be culturally sensitive and aware of the intrinsic values of the mana. By being healing "mediums" to the mana, we will guide the infants and their families to begin their journey to becoming a new family unit.

Susan Kau RNC-NIC[1]
June 21, 2021

References

Bargh JA, Chartrand TL (1999) The unbearable automaticity of being. Am Psychol 54(7):462–479

Derstein V, Rada EL (1952) Some dietetic factors influencing the market for poi in Hawai'i. In: Agricultural economics, pp 31–43

Merriam-Webster (2019) Merriam-Webster dictionary, 12th edn. Merriam-Webster, Springfield, MA

Pukui MK, Elbert SH (1986) Hawaiian dictionary revised and enlarged edition. University of Hawaii Press, Honolulu

Zaki J, Mitchell JP (2013) Intuitive prosociality. Curr Dir Psychol Sci 22(6):466–470. https://journals.sagepub.com/doi/10.1177/0963721413492764

[1]Celebrating 40 years as an NICU RN at Kapiolani Medical Center for Women and Children and on the Caring for Hawai'i Neonates Board.

Global Research to Advance Neonatal Nursing and Neonatal Outcomes

18

Wakako Eklund

18.1 Introduction

The World Health Organization (WHO) designated the year 2020 to be the "Year of the Nurse and the Midwife," and further extended this designation in European regions to carry the momentum and emphasize the significant role nursing played in the year of the COVID-19 pandemic (Nursing Times 2020; WHO 2021d). WHO then prioritized the themes of "Protect, Invest, Together" by designating the year 2021 as the "International Year of the Health and Care Workers" (WHO 2021c). At the time of this writing in March 2021 and into 2022, the COVID-19 pandemic has infected over 120 million people and taken 2.67 million lives worldwide making it one of the most rare global phenomena (Johns Hopkins University and Medicine 2021).

The impact of the pandemic on perspectives toward global nursing research may be greater in significance than ever anticipated, prior to the pandemic. Nursing research may now have an increased opportunity to describe what we do,

who we are, and what impact we have to our patients to the global audience if strategic efforts are to be made. Research results can advocate for further investment in nursing by global, regional, or national leaders. This chapter will not only discuss the impact of the pandemic on neonatal nursing research, it will also cover the topics that are important in today's society and global research culture. Considering modifiable factors impacting health disparity in the specific area of practice or involving patients' families as key collaborative members in the future research are some of the important topics to be discussed.

W. Eklund (✉)
Pediatrix Medical Group of Tennessee, Nashville, TN, USA

School of Nursing, Bouvé College of Health Sciences, Northeastern University, Boston, MA, USA

Council of International Neonatal Nurses, Inc. (COINN), Yardley, PA, USA
e-mail: wakako.eklund@pediatrix.com

Key "Think Points" for Learning
- Global research collaboration is not new; however, the current environment may have increased the need for, and value of, global research, offering numerous opportunities.
- Neonatal nurses' spirit of inquiry often comes from the day-to-day interactions with the newborns and families under their care.
- The reader should consider the content discussed as "hot topics", to reflect on your own practice environment and search for opportunities to improve care, policy, working environment, and the family's experience in clinical settings.

© The Editor(s) (if applicable) and The Author(s), under exclusive license to Springer Nature
Switzerland AG 2022
J. Petty et al. (eds.), *Neonatal Nursing: A Global Perspective*,
https://doi.org/10.1007/978-3-030-91339-7_18

18.2 Strength of Global Collaboration

18.2.1 Challenged by the Unexpected: Global Spirit of Inquiry

The pandemic has gravely impacted how the entire world functions. How families and infants are cared for suddenly changed. Nurses on the frontlines had neither evidence-based guidelines nor opportunities to conduct research to build the evidence during the pandemic. They had to provide care and protect the infants and families in their care. Nurses, however, were requested to modify their practice by the authority of each health facility as a part of the organizational strategy to minimize the COVID-19 impact. Often these changes occurred without any specific regard to the individual infant or the family needs. Practice modifications included limiting parents' presence in the newborn settings/neonatal intensive care units (NICUs) in visiting frequencies or duration, thus denying or limiting breastfeeding or Kangaroo Care opportunities. These modifications also led to decreasing opportunities for necessary education to empower parents due to limited time parents are given at the bedside. Nurses often anecdotally questioned why? What impact would their presence have on our operations or the infants and their families both now and long term? The Journal of Neonatal Nursing COINN News Pages featured COVID-19 reflections submitted by global neonatal nurses, nurse researchers as well as educators from August 2020 to February 2021. Every publication indicated struggles and challenges (COINN 2020a, b; Petty 2020, 2021). Parents/families, clinicians, nurse researchers, educators, and students, none were immune to the pandemic-related changes and many asked, how would this practice change impact the outcomes for the NICU babies and families, or students in educational settings?

Parents were suddenly infrequently seen in many NICUs. In some NICUs, parents were completely banned for periods of time. One US-based study reported a significant decrease in NICUs with 24-hour parental presence and reported a decrease in parental presence during the rounds, highlighting the increased barriers against family members as they attempt to directly engage with the care team or to have shared decision making (Darcy Mahoney et al. 2020). Another US-based study reported an increase in maternal involvement, even when the mother was COVID-19 positive as more evidence became available toward the later period of the pandemic in the summer of 2020. The long duration of restricted parental presence, however, (which is still restricted in many part of the globe due to delta and omicron that continued into 2022) or even the decrease in specialized services critical for developmental needs continue and are highly concerning in terms of infant and family outcomes (Ahmad et al. 2021). Both the short- and long-term impact of pandemic-related newborn/NICU care practice modifications must be monitored by global collaborative research teams to determine the impact over time. Parents, nurses, as well as the physician colleagues all wondered what benefits do babies receive through these modifications in proportion to the potential harm caused by not having parents nearby frequently? What negative impact would we see including the impact of potentially and temporarily reduced breast milk production, and how it may lead to reduction in successful breastfeeding at 6 months or 12 months of age? Each and every question that emerges in a nurse, mother, father, or any other professionals who surround the infants and families is a valid research question. Now is the time that nurses, even those who did not feel they had any interest in research, felt the spirit of inquiry that has led to research questions, raising awareness of how "relevant" research is to every neonatal professional. Anyone can initiate research.

18.2.2 Nursing Efforts to Gain Evidence to Guide Practice

The COVID-19 pandemic may have created an opportunity for nurses in all settings to realize the power of research inquiry to propel what we question "today" into what we do best "tomorrow." It may be an opportunity to open a dialogue with students or novice nurses to embed in them the value of questioning about what they do daily in a constructive way. In recently conducted work, nurses were observed to be seeking for evidence to guide practice.

According to Semaan and colleagues, who conducted a global survey to assess maternal and newborn health professionals' experiences early in the pandemic, nurses demonstrated active efforts to find evidence, although limited evidence was available (Semaan et al. 2020). A total of 714 responded from 81 countries, both from high-income and low-income countries (63% high income). Nearly half of the respondents were nurses or midwives. The great majority (92%) indicated that they made a personal effort to update themselves by researching even in absence of regional or national guidelines. The findings of this study also underscored the important research questions that rise from the nurses and other professionals on the frontlines in absence of evidence, especially in response to the 'knee-jerk' reactions seen globally to universally limit the family presence in NICUs, or separate COVID-19 positive mothers from their infants all together. These research questions shall now be outlined.

18.2.3 Suggested Research Areas

Many neonatal nursing professionals, including the author, questioned and often debated with colleagues that we had no evidence that current modifications would not cause more harm than good, with long-term implications to the infants and families. Promotion of breastfeeding, Kangaroo Care or family-centered care practices and the global adoption of these effective practices had been primarily the results of neonatal nurses' efforts in the past decades in various global regions. Nursing professionals are positioned to address such topics by discussions, collaborative initiatives, and conducting joint research/quality improvement projects. Readers are invited to refer to Chaps. 15 and 16 of this book, where further discussions on relevant topics are found.

Numerous manufacturers have endeavored to make COVID-19 vaccines to be available and numerous countries have released emergency authorizations to start vaccinations starting in late 2020. Disparity in vaccination is a serious concern, thus, targeted efforts are being made to deliver large shipments of vaccines to Africa and other global regions (Lancet Commission and on Covid-Vaccines and Therapeutics Task Force Members. 2021) (WHO 2021a). It would take, however, a significant duration of time before the vaccine eligibility as well as the availability extends globally to achieve the level of herd immunity. Therefore, continued research endeavors are necessary to refine the care we give while we remain under the "new normal."

A simple sweeping review of the general impact of the pandemic alone has led to several areas of research/quality improvement opportunities for consideration where nurses can lead:

- Education: development of and evaluation of improved web-based interactive learning formats or simulation modules to fortify maternal/child health education that allows uninterrupted delivery, no matter where the students are. Considerations for high-income and low-income regions cannot be possible without a global collaboration.
- Workforce development: enhanced global sharing of expertise to accelerate the workforce development and to increase professional training opportunities are needed to prevent further shortages of neonatally trained professionals both at the staff levels or advanced level.
- Researcher training in higher learning: increased global exploration on how best to equip graduate, post-graduate and PhD programs to expand the distance learning platform, thereby preventing the disruption of students' enrolment is highly desired (some global regions, such as Asia has minimal offerings for doctoral level nursing education and most required relocation at the time of this writing).
- Indirect impact of pandemic-related practice modifications to (1) neonatal neurodevelopmental factors such as delayed feeding

achievement, delayed discharge, delayed development of mature sleep-awake cycles, (2) short- and long-term psychosocial impact on parents/siblings (bonding, attachment, mental health post-NICU or post-grieving experience of losses).

- Promotion of advanced practice neonatal professionals globally: (1) how advanced practice policy expansions (e.g., tele-medicine recognition for NPs in North America) impact the healthcare access and what the feasibility of similar policy expansion may be in other global regions, (2) exploration to identify the gap in neonatal/family care in global regions where advanced practice can bring improvement in care quality, access as well as in outcomes.
- Vaccine roll out equity to neonatal nurses globally: disparity should not exist in nurses' vaccination status and, although this would take time, global efforts to examine the vaccination level among neonatal nurses requires vigilant follow up (some areas have prioritized only in adult healthcare areas and may not elect the nurses in neonatal/maternal care to be prioritized for vaccination).

18.2.4 Recent Examples of Global Research Data as a Collected Voice

The year of pandemic also highlighted the shared similarities and strengths among global nursing and related communities, rather than the differences known in nursing educational/training systems or the organization of healthcare delivery systems. Semaan and colleagues' work explored the COVID-19 impact on healthcare professionals who care for newborn and families. This work is one example of the power of global data. Multiple rounds of survey analysis were organized by global collaboration coordinated by the Institute of Tropical Medicine in Antwerpen, Belgium. This survey, which was offered in 12 languages, brought data from both high-income and low-income countries, describing how the lock-down and other changes such as visiting restrictions for families brought on by the national or regional policies affected the work environment, patient access to care or care quality. Reported results highlighted the global nature of the 2020–2022 pandemic which made the global approach logical in order to gain the full picture of the experiences of healthcare professionals (Semaan et al. 2020). Similarities of challenging experience appear to speak louder than the regional differences, highlighting the value of collaboration.

18.2.5 Global Multi-Stakeholder Collaboration: International Neonatal Consortium

Nurses are increasingly invited and involved with global multi-stakeholder efforts to improve neonatal care in recent years. One example is of the International Neonatal Consortium (INC) which was launched in 2015 (Turner et al. 2016). INC's mission is to unite the effort of multi-stakeholders who are relevant in the research to develop new therapies for neonates. The development effort for neonatal-specific therapies has lagged behind that of adults and older children for decades. A work titled, "Tiny and Forgotten: a Call for a Focused Neonatal Policy Reform" describes how various policy efforts were made in the past in both North America and Europe; however, it has not sufficiently impacted to benefit the neonates (Bucci-Rechtweg and Ward 2019). Neonatal clinical trials are expensive, viewed as highly risky by funding organizations, and numerous other barriers exist to bring truly neonatal-specific new therapies to the NICU. INC consists of not only drug/device manufacturers, research organizations, medical professionals, global regulatory organizations, but also families who had premature infants in NICU (whose children are the research target population) and nursing professionals. Nurses are often at the bedside to care for the infants who are enrolled in clinical studies; they are tasked to make necessary documentation, support parents or recognize and report adverse events. INC has conducted numerous global projects since its inception in 2015 which contributed to developing various tools and guidelines to propel the neonatal research. Nursing members were involved to provide input with nurse perspectives. Further, nurse members played a significant role in several projects, including one to develop the neonatal-specific adverse event grading system (Salaets et al. 2019). The nursing professionals from multiple countries contributed to the Delphi process to clarify and refine the definitions of various neonatal-specific conditions as they relate to the adverse event scale.

Nurses were also actively involved in the design, development, and implementation of a global multi-stakeholder parallel survey to explore the communication/education practices surrounding neonatal clinical trials in NICUs. This work began in 2017. A parallel survey developed with each stakeholder group in mind was provided to address family, nurse and physician respondent groups separately. Nursing was the largest group who contributed to the data for this global survey. A collaborative manuscript was published recently (Degl et al. 2021). At the time of this writing, numerous nurse members are actively serving on various committees alongside other stakeholder members with new global projects to address important topics, such as health disparity.

18.3 Hot Research Topics in 2021/2022

18.3.1 Health Disparity

Global health leaders have long focused on prioritizing efforts to mitigate disparity/inequality in healthcare resources, access, and health outcomes that are linked to socioeconomic status, location of residence/birth, age, gender, or nationality/ethnicity/race. Global action plans by the World Health Organization, such as "Born too soon; Global Action on Preterm Birth" (WHO 2012), or the currently active efforts, "Every Newborn Action Plan" (WHO 2021b), or recently launched, "Global Alliance for Newborn Care" (GLANCE 2019) initiated by the European Federation of Care of Newborn Infant (EFCNI) specifically focus their efforts to address the dis-

parity in maternal health, preterm births, stillbirths, and infant/neonatal mortality with the goal of making high-quality care given by neonatally trained professionals available to support every newborn and his or her family. COINN has long endorsed numerous global initiatives by serving on various committees and on the boards to represent neonates and neonatal nurses while supporting research, or actively engaging in critical discussions. Robust global research in this area is highly important in the twenty-first century, and neonatal nurses must acknowledge the existing disparity in their own areas to explore opportunities where improvements are needed. It is also important to recognize the indirect impact that COVID-19 may have had, further impacting the existing disparity.

Disparity does not only concern the low-income verses high-income regions. Even within one region, significant disparity exists. Efforts have been made to increase awareness for health disparity in neonatal/perinatal settings by discussing this issue at national and international conferences or by publications (Eklund 2020; Sigurdson et al. 2018). Both quantitative and qualitative research studies have been published. The Vermont Oxford Network (VON), which consists of health professionals and families at more than 1000 health centers around the world, support quality improvement efforts in neonatal care. Recent publication titled, "Vermont Oxford Network for Health Equity: potentially better practices for follow through," recommends the following actions that are needed for a change: 1. Promote a culture of equity, 2. Identify social risks of families and provide interventions to prevent and mitigate those risks, 3. Take action to assist families after discharge (transition to home), 4. Maintain support for families through infancy, 5. Develop robust quality improvement efforts to ensure equitable, high-quality NICU and follow-through care to all newborns by eliminating modifiable disparities, and 6. Advocate for social justice at the local, state, and national levels. Some families would require a specific level of support or unique set of resources than others to achieve a safe transition to home (Vermont Oxford Network 2020; Horbar et al. 2020).

Many countries are challenged to know how best to care for various patient groups, especially with increased immigration, or influx of refugee population. This offers opportunities for research to identify the needs and how best to meet the needs of any population that may be at risk of disparity. Language/cultural barriers alone create communication challenges leading to possible disparity in care quality. Insufficient provision of bedside education or emotional support due to language barriers leads to parents taking infants home unprepared, even worse, with inadequate or even inaccurately understood information (Eklund et al. 2018). The stress imposed on the families with sick newborn (s) can have immediate and long-term impact. Parental experience of acute stress or post-traumatic stress disorder has been recognized as a reality in the NICU environment even when parents speak their own language; thus, significant efforts have been made to design educational tools for neonatal professionals (Hall et al. 2020). The impact of the unfamiliar environment some families are placed in, and the extent of the psychological or mental health disparity must not be overlooked. (There is a short case study presented in Chap. 11 regarding a foreign-born mother who delivers a premature infant in Okinawa, Japan.)

To demonstrate the need for further research or quality improvement efforts, a few recent statistics from the USA and UK are presented in the following section. Various factors are linked to disparity, emphasizing the need to identify modifiable risks broadly in line with nurses' perceptiveness.

Pregnancy-related death rate (n/100,000 live births) in the USA from 2007–2016 was higher for Black (41) and American Indian/Alaskan Native women (30) than for white women (13) (CDC 2019). Age also mattered in this study, reporting a four-fold death among black women for 30–34-year-old category compared to white women. High school educated women in this study had twice as high pregnancy-related mortality than college educated women (21.6 vs 10.9), thus, education matters. The black infant mortality in the USA in the 2017 was twice that of white infants (10.9 vs 4.7 per 1000 live birth) (Kaiser

Family Foundation 2020). Preterm birth rate in the USA in 2017 was 9.9%; however, the black preterm birth rate was higher (14%) than the preterm birth rates for white (9.1%) or Hispanic (9.6%) population (Manuck 2017). In the United Kingdom, socioeconomic differences and ethnicity also lead to disparity. Stillbirths rate between January 2014 to December 2015 was found to increase as socioeconomic/deprivation quintile increased from the least to the most (28.9–49 per 10,000 births). The deprivation scores are based on "the Children in Low-Income Families Local Measure" to describe the least deprived/quintile 1 to the most deprived/quintile 5 (Best et al. 2019). When ethnicity was reviewed, statistically significant stillbirth risks were found among Asian (RR = 1.72, 95% CI 1.60–1.85), Black (RR = 2.18, 95%CI 1.98–2.4), and for those mixed ethnicity (RR = 1.15, 95% CI 1.02–1.29). The national overall neonatal mortality rate was 15.9 per 10,000 live births during the same period. Again, the neonatal mortality rate increased as the deprivation quintile increased from the least to the most (12.8–20.7 per 10,000 live births), and again, it was more common among Asian (RR = 1.47, 95% CI 1.31–1.66), Black (RR = 1.49, 95% CI 1.26–1.77) than white ethnicity (RR = 1.37, 95% CI 1.21–1.55). The researchers state that both stillbirth and neonatal mortality rates were lower in this report than what had been reported between 2000 and 2007; however, it emphasizes the need for identification of strategies to further address the current disparity.

Some countries do not have many ethnic groups residing in the country; however, the recent pandemic may have accentuated the existing socioeconomic disparity among young families of child-bearing age, elucidating the fragility of the society. Also, even in those regions, such as Japan, where immigrant population was once not a prominent part of the society, a gradual but steady increase in immigrant population has become more noticeable in the last decade in various regions, meaning the neonatal healthcare professionals must consider how best to care for non-Japanese patients. Nurses' commitment in addressing this potential or actual disparity by collaborating with policy makers, family members, and other committed stakeholders globally will hopefully bring about positive results.

18.3.2 Health Policy and Advocacy to Impact Neonatal Care/ Neonatal Nursing

As the previous section demonstrated, global, national, and regional health policy drives the priority for newborn/maternal health when a certain global campaign is launched, and goals are set. In order to achieve the health-related outcomes, such as what the "Every Newborn Action Plan" is designed to accomplish, national level or regional level efforts are prioritized in terms of resources (WHO 2021b). In every region, health policy influences the quality of care that infants and their families receive, and it is the policy that impacts nursing practice at every level. Policy also impacts the priority as national leaders and lawmakers make decisions to allocate the investment. There are numerous policy and advocacy opportunities for neonatal nurses, and this is a highly important research area. It is beyond the scope of this chapter to detail potential research opportunities or introduce where to get started. There are, however, critical actions that one can take to gain familiarity to the policy and advocacy realm, even today:

- Join a local, national, or international neonatal professional organization and get involved.
- Explore within the organization if there is a policy and advocacy committee.
- Learn which regional or national regulation governs your nursing practice and understand how policy impacts one neonatal nurse today.
- Explore if there is a policy column in any nursing journal available in your area.
- Join the parent support organization to support the advocacy efforts.

Many neonatal nurses have advocated for various elements of neonatal nursing, or neonatal care by contributing to developing standards at the local health facility, regional health department, national health ministry, or at the international organizations. COINN has been busy advocating for neonatal nurses and neonates. Much work is needed to propel neonatal nursing forward to ensure quality care can be provided for newborns and families.

18.3.3 European Research Priorities

A three-round Delphi study to identify neonatal nursing research priorities was conducted by a European research team. A total of 75 nurses from 17 European countries responded to this study. Out of the eight priority domains (Wielenga et al. 2015), the top four included the following: neonatal pain/stress management, family-centered care, nursing practice, and quality and safety. Global efforts such as this highlight the key areas and that global/collaborative research efforts can strategically and effectively deploy resources with the vision to improve outcomes. Without these types of concerted efforts, it would not be possible to continue to build the evidence that guides practice aiming for even better outcomes.

18.3.4 Enhanced Collaboration with Family/Patient Organizations in Global Research

Patient-centered research requires a strong perspective of, and involvement by, patient or family members. Patient-Centered Outcome Research Institute (PCORI) is a US-based non-profit organization that promotes research efforts which improve outcomes important to patients in neonatal settings; this refers to families of neonates (PCORI 2021). A family-led organization, the NEC Society based in the USA has successfully received funding awards from PCORI more than once and organized professional conferences involving family members, researchers, industry partners, and clinicians to propel research aimed at NEC prevention (NEC Society 2019, 2020). The family as the central figure within a research team is highly encouraged and should be considered more frequently to ensure that patients' values are sufficiently recognized and incorporated into the future of neonatal research design and quality improvement projects. The European Federation of Care of the Newborn Infants (EFCNI) has also led patient-centered neonatal initiatives of global scale, such as Global Alliance for Newborn Care (GLANCE 2019), which initiated the *Zero Separation* Campaign in response to the increased parents/infant's separation caused by the pandemic (GLANCE 2020). Various parent organizations, specific to families of small and sick newborns, such as European-based EFCNI or US-based NICU Parent Network (NICU Parent Network 2019), are valuable partners to neonatal nursing and nurse researchers, since more family sensitive outcomes must be considered in any research. Increased studies must be targeted to improve the family outcomes for our small and sick newborns regardless of where they are born in our global regions. The task may sound daunting, but it must begin with small collaboration, one connection at a time, to ensure that the future of neonatal nursing and neonatal health remain bright.

18.4   Conclusion

Global research needs have received increased attention and awareness due to the COVID-19 pandemic. Research needs encompass clinical/practice-related topics as well as policy and education. Use of social media, or web-based meeting platforms all contribute as tools to connect neonatal nurses globally. By recognizing the needs for the global collaboration, expertise can be effectively and strategically gathered to maximize the team's strength in designing research, conducting research, translating the research results, implementing new strategies, and disseminating the evidence-based information into various global regions. The pandemic, while it was not a welcome visitor to the world, must be regarded as an opportunity for neonatal nurses and the enhancement of future research endeavours. Neonatal nurses must continue the momentum to describe what we do, who we are, and what impact we have in improving neonatal and family outcomes effectively, so that our work can be a powerful advocate to initiate continued and greater investment in nursing on a global scale. We need all of us to be involved in some way, no matter which region of the world we come from.

References

Ahmad KA, Darcy-Mahoney A, Kelleher AS, Ellsbury DL, Tolia VN, Clark RH (2021) Longitudinal survey of COVID-19 burden and related policies in U.S. neonatal intensive care units. Am J Perinatol 38(1):93–98. https://doi.org/10.1055/s-0040-1718944

Best KE, Seaton SE, Draper ES, Field DJ, Kurinczuk JJ, Manktelow BN, Smith LK (2019) Assessing the deprivation gap in stillbirths and neonatal deaths by cause of death: a national population-based study. Arch Dis Child Fetal Neonatal Ed 104(6):F624–F630. https://doi.org/10.1136/archdischild-2018-316124

Bucci-Rechtweg CM, Ward RM (2019) Tiny and forgotten: a call for focused neonatal policy reform. Ther Innov Regul Sci 53(5):615–617. https://doi.org/10.1177/2168479018821922

Center for Disease Control and Prevention (CDC) (2019) Racial/ethnic disparities in pregnancy-related death- United States, 2007–2016. https://www.cdc.gov/mmwr/volumes/68/wr/mm6835a3.htm

Lancet Commission on Covid-Vaccines and Therapeutics Task Force Members (2021) Urgent needs of low-income and middle-income countries for COVID-19 vaccines and therapeutics. Lancet 397(10274):562–564. https://doi.org/10.1016/S0140-6736(21)00242-7

Council of International Neonatal Nurses (2020a) Council of International Neonatal Nurses (COINN) news page. J Neonatal Nurs 26(4):232–236. https://doi.org/10.1016/j.jnn.2020.05.007

Council of International Neonatal Nurses (2020b) Council of International Neonatal Nurses (COINN) news page. J Neonatal Nurs 26(5):299–303. https://doi.org/10.1016/j.jnn.2020.07.008

Darcy Mahoney A, White RD, Velasquez A, Barrett TS, Clark RH, Ahmad KA (2020) Impact of restrictions on parental presence in neonatal intensive care units related to coronavirus disease 2019. J Perinatol 40(Suppl 1):36–46. https://doi.org/10.1038/s41372-020-0753-7

Degl J, Ariagno R, Aschner J, Beauman S, Eklund W, Faro E, Iwami H, Jackson Y, Kenner C, Kim I, Klein A, Short M, Sorrells K, Turner MA, Ward R, Winiecki S, Bucci-Rechtweg C, International Neonatal Consortium (2021) The culture of research communication in neonatal intensive care units: key stakeholder perspectives. Journal of Perinatology: Official Journal of the California Perinatal Association 41(12):2826–2833. https://doi.org/10.1038/s41372-021-01220-5

Eklund WM (2020) Health disparity in perinatal/neonatal settings: what can neonatal nurses do? Adv Neonatal Care 20(6):426–427. https://doi.org/10.1097/anc.0000000000000815

Eklund WM, Westcott M, Grogan C (2018) Culturally sensitive, family-centered care: unique needs of the military families serving abroad. Adv Neonatal Care 18(6):425–428. https://doi.org/10.1097/anc.0000000000000572

GLANCE (2019) Every baby born receives the best start in life Worldwide. https://www.glance-network.org/

GLANCE (2020) Zero separation. Together for better care! Keep preterm and sick babies close to their parents. https://www.glance-network.org/covid-19/campaign/

Hall SL, Sorrells K, Eklund WM (2020) Caring for babies and their families: providing psychosocial support in the NICU: an innovative online education tool to empower neonatal nurses to support NICU families. Adv Neonatal Care 20(4). https://journals.lww.com/advancesinneonatalcare/Fulltext/2020/08000/Noteworthy_Professional_News.2.aspx

Horbar JD, Edwards EM, Ogbolu Y (2020) Our responsibility to follow through for NICU infants and their families. Pediatrics 146(6):e20200360. https://doi.org/10.1542/peds.2020-0360

Johns Hopkins University & Medicine (2021) Coronavirus resource center. In: COVID-19 Dashboard by the center for systems science and engineering. https://coronavirus.jhu.edu/map.html

Kaiser Family Foundation (2020) Infant Mortality Rate by Race/Ethnicity. https://www.kff.org/other/state-indicator/infant-mortality-rate-by-race-ethnicity/?currentTimeframe=0&sortModel=%7B%22colId%22:%22Location%22,%22sort%22:%22asc%22%7D

Manuck TA (2017) Racial and ethnic differences in preterm birth: a complex, multifactorial problem. Semin Perinatol 41(8):511–518. https://doi.org/10.1053/j.semperi.2017.08.010

NEC Society (2019) NEC Symposium 2019. https://necsociety.org/2019/06/06/2019-nec-symposium/

NEC Society (2020) NEC Society Receives $250,000 Research Capacity Award. https://necsociety.org/2019/08/16/nec-society-receives-250000-research-capacity-award/

NICU Parent Network (2019) NICU Parent Network. https://nicuparentnetwork.org

Nursing Times (2020) Europe will extend year of the nurse and midwife into 2021. https://www.nursingtimes.net/news/2020-international-year-of-the-nurse-and-midwife/europe-will-extend-year-of-the-nurse-and-midwife-into-2021-17-09-2020/

Patient-Centered Outcomes Research Institute (PCORI). (2021) Improving Outcomes Important to Patients. https://www.pcori.org

Petty J (2020) Council of International Neonatal Nurses (COINN) news page. J Neonatal Nurs 26(6):358–363. https://doi.org/10.1016/j.jnn.2020.09.007

Petty J (2021) Council of International Neonatal Nurses (COINN) news page. J Neonatal Nurs 27(1):63–65. https://doi.org/10.1016/j.jnn.2020.11.010

Salaets T, Turner MA, Short M, Ward RM, Hokuto I, Ariagno RL et al (2019) Development of a neonatal adverse event severity scale through a Delphi consensus approach. Arch Dis Child 104(12):1167–1173. https://doi.org/10.1136/archdischild-2019-317399

Semaan A, Audet C, Huysmans E, Afolabi B, Assarag B, Banke-Thomas A et al (2020) Voices from the frontline: findings from a thematic analysis of a rapid online global survey of maternal and newborn health professionals facing the COVID-19 pandemic. BMJ Glob Health 5(6). https://doi.org/10.1136/bmjgh-2020-002967

Sigurdson K, Morton C, Mitchell B, Profit J (2018) Disparities in NICU quality of care: a qualitative study of family and clinician accounts. J Perinatol 38(5):600–607. https://doi.org/10.1038/s41372-018-0057-3

Turner MA, Davis JM, McCune S, Bax R, Portman RJ, Hudson LD (2016) The international neonatal consortium: collaborating to advance regulatory science for neonates. Pediatr Res 80(4):462–464. https://doi.org/10.1038/pr.2016.119

Vermont Oxford Network (VON) (2020) VON for Health Equity: Potentially Better Practices for Follow Through. https://public.vtoxford.org/health-equity/potentially-better-practices-for-follow-through/

Wielenga JM, Tume LN, Latour JM, van den Hoogen A (2015) European neonatal intensive care nursing research priorities: an e-Delphi study. Archives of disease in childhood. Fetal and Neonatal Edition 100(1):F66–F71. https://doi.org/10.1136/archdischild-2014-306858

World Health Organization (WHO) (2012) Born too soon. Global Action on Preterm Birth 2013. http://www.who.int/pmnch/media/news/2012/201204_borntoosoon-report.pdf

World Health Organization (WHO) (2021a) COVID-19 vaccine doses shipped by the COVAX Facility head to Ghana, marking the beginning of global rollout. News

World Health Organization (WHO) (2021b) Every Newborn Action Plan. https://www.who.int/maternal_child_adolescent/newborns/every-newborn/en/

World Health Organization (WHO) (2021c) Year of the Health and Care Workers 2021. https://www.who.int/campaigns/annual-theme/year-of-health-and-care-workers-2021

World Health Organization (WHO) (2021d) Year of the Nurse and the Midwife 2020. https://www.who.int/campaigns/year-of-the-nurse-and-the-midwife-2020

Part III

Final Words

Key Messages and the Way Forward

19

Julia Petty

This book has discussed the role and work of neonatal nurses across the globe, for the World Health Organizations (WHO) regions, taking a representative from each region to illustrate evidence-based practices relating to care and optimizing outcomes for babies and families. It is hoped that we have bought together both differences and commonalities in nursing care applied to our own patient groups in order to share practices and learn from each other. This is a key and vital message from our book. We believe that a book written by COINN members will enable our collective voice to be heard, aligning with our core values and goals in relation to promoting neonatal nursing as a global speciality through evidence, research, and education of neonatal nurses. Our core values and goals are outlined below.

Core Values

- excellence in newborn care: through evidence, research, and education of neonatal nurses.
- advocacy for high quality newborn care: by promoting global health of newborns and their families.

- respect for diversity: by integrating cultural norms and values among the care of newborns and their families.

COINN Goals

C: Connect neonatal nurses globally and share knowledge, skills, and resources.
O: Optimize newborn survival and health.
I: Impact global policy for newborns, families, and neonatal nurses.
N: Network: with other healthcare professionals and organizations.
N: Necessitate neonatal nursing education and its pivotal role to health outcomes of newborns and families.

Importantly, as this book was partly written amid the COVID-19 pandemic that swept the world in 2020, this hugely significant event must be included in any current literature aimed at informing healthcare professionals about optimum care delivery. During the coronavirus pandemic, a full lockdown was imposed, including closure of workplaces, schools, and universities to protect population health. We were mandated to leave home only to shop for necessities or to exercise once a day, and to seek medical help only when required. Neonatal healthcare staff as part of a wider healthcare team were required to wear personal protective equipment, affecting

J. Petty (✉)
Department of Nursing, Health and Wellbeing, School of Health and Social Work, University of Hertfordshire, Hatfield, Hertfordshire, UK

Council of International Neonatal Nurses, Inc. (COINN), Yardley, PA, USA
e-mail: j.petty@herts.ac.uk

J. Petty et al. (eds.), *Neonatal Nursing: A Global Perspective*,
https://doi.org/10.1007/978-3-030-91339-7_19

communication and preventing close contact with the parents of the babies in our care. Parents were faced with restrictions to visitation and contact with their babies leading to vital initiatives such as "Zero Separation" (Global Alliance for Newborn Care (GLANCE), 2020). The future impact of mitigation measures within specific, vulnerable groups such as neonates and families are yet to be seen (Green et al., 2020; 2021a; 2021b). Therefore, it is fitting in a book that discusses global neonatal care delivery, to address the potential impact of the pandemic, and indeed what is now a vital part of future planning in relation to the neonatal nursing workforce.

The global nursing workforce has made, and continues to make, a substantial contribution during the COVID-19 public health emergency. The key role of the neonatal nurse must be seen within this context. We must continue to be a voice and an advocate for our vulnerable patients and their families in line with inclusive practice. Advocacy acts to *"ensure that people, particularly those who are most vulnerable in society, are able to have their voice heard on issues that are important to them, defend and safeguard their rights, and have their views and wishes genuinely considered when decisions are being made about their lives"* (Royal College of Nursing, 2017). In normal circumstances, poor populations lacking access to health services are left most vulnerable during times of crisis. Misinformation and miscommunication disproportionly affect individuals with less access to information channels, who are thus more likely to ignore government health warnings. Failure to consider vulnerable populations may not only exacerbate the barriers to healthcare these populations already face but may act to deepen health inequalities (Ahmed et al., 2020). During this unprecedented time, policy makers must ensure that strategies to address the pandemic do not further marginalize vulnerable populations. We, as a vital specialty within healthcare as a whole, must address inequalities by tackling the social determinants of health, defined as circumstances in which people are born and live in, along with the systems put in place to deal with illness shaped by a wider set of influences: economics, social policies, and politics.

We are ideally placed to play a vital role in information dissemination across the globe, in any setting, in the following ways:

- Neonatal nurses must continue to advocate to ensure governments prioritize the information and communication requirements of our vulnerable patient group.
- Develop and disseminate educational materials on basic hygiene practices and infection prevention.
- Use digital technology to overcome issues related to social distancing.
- Provide culturally sensitive language translations for the purpose of communicating health information.
- Build on relationships with community institutions and religious groups to ensure the provision and dissemination of evidence-based information.
- Nurses should be provided with the time and autonomy to build on relationships with community institutions and religious groups to ensure the provision and dissemination of evidence-based information.

As well as supporting and advocating for those at the highest risk of the effects of COVID-19 in society (World Health Organization, 2020a), we also need to be prepared for any potential further disaster outbreaks (WHO, 2020b). Education is a key part of this preparation. Historically, the role of public health nurses focused on the management of sanitation and infectious disease. The World Health Organization has recognized the need to bridge this gap, highlighting the requirement for infection prevention and control knowledge, and its application in healthcare settings to secure outbreak preparedness and response (WHO, 2020a). When outbreaks occur, it is crucial that nurses can liaise with health protection teams to commence next steps including pathogen identification, appropriate treatment, and prevention of further infections (Corless et al., 2018). In order to do this, nurses need to have knowledge about notifiable infectious diseases, their symptoms, modes of transmission, and ways to break the chain of infection. This education should commence in pre-registration nursing programs (Burnett, 2018). An enhanced understanding of the skills and competencies which underpin health protection would advance the nursing contribution during pandemics, and allow nurses to protect themselves, as well as the communities they serve; in our case the neonatal community.

The neonatal nurse also has a vital role within preventative health as part of multidisciplinary health protection teams—formed of nurses, practitioners, doctors, surveillance and administrative staff, to provide international and local support to prevent and reduce the impact of infectious diseases, hazards and major emergencies. Following the Ebola outbreak in 2014, the measles outbreak in 2018, and more recently COVID-19, health protection has been given an increasingly high profile and recognized for its specialist knowledge and skills. Despite this, health protection training continues to be reserved for those nurses who choose to pursue this specialty as a career in health protection, post-registration.

The rapid integration of health protection training within pre-registration nursing programs would support the nursing workforce in managing the potential increase in infectious diseases. In addition, with several coronavirus vaccines now in development, urgent health protection training for the nursing workforce will ensure they are prepared to lead on the delivery of vital vaccination campaigns.

Providing nurses with the skills to identify vulnerable populations and their diverse healthcare needs, alongside increased knowledge on the fundamentals of health protection, will mean they are well placed to act as advocates, uphold the rights of these vulnerable groups to maintain their dignity, safeguard against discrimination, and protect against inequities in healthcare provision. The means to achieve this include ensuring the delivery of accessible, accurate, and evidence-based health information during periods of crisis (Inter-Agency Standing Committee (IASC), 2020). Throughout the COVID-19 response, an array of health-related information about COVID-19 has been presented in various media channels, including social media, television broadcasts, radio, postal and text message alerts (Ofcom, 2020). The failure to deliver this information in readily accessible and understandable formats to vulnerable groups, including people living with disabilities, refugees and migrants, older people, and people from black and minority ethnic (BME) backgrounds has been deemed a human rights concern (Human Rights Watch, 2020).

People living with disabilities may have inequities in access to public health messaging due to specific communication needs (IASC, 2020). Refugees and migrants may have problems with access to publicly available preventative information and health and social care services due to their legal status, discrimination, or language barriers (IASC, 2020). Similarly, people from BME backgrounds may not speak English as a first language and information provided may not be culturally sensitive, which may impede the person using any health-related advice provided (Paakkari and Okan, 2020). The health literacy of these groups also warrants consideration. This underpins the rationale to ensure the delivery of accessible, plain language health-related communications, presented in easy-read formats.

In ensuring the inclusion of vulnerable groups during the ongoing COVID-19 response and reducing the health inequalities they may continue to be subject to, several approaches can be employed by the nursing profession. Nurses can first advocate to ensure governments prioritize the information and communication requirements of those in vulnerable groups. They can highlight the need for multiple forms of communications in accessible formats such as Braille, large print and text captioning for the hearing impaired (IASC, 2020). Further actions include the development and delivery of educational materials on basic hygiene practices and infection prevention. With advances in digital technology, such as social media, nurses can use these communication channels to overcome issues related to social distancing.

In addition, nurses must be provided with the time and autonomy to take advantage of, and build on the links they hold with community institutions and religious groups during periods of crisis. Community and religious leaders are primary sources of support, guidance, comfort, and healthcare for the communities they serve (WHO, 2020c). They can provide spiritual and pastoral support during public health emergencies and advocate for the needs of vulnerable groups. By communicating transparent, evidence-based steps to prevent COVID-19 to religious and community leaders, nurses can promote the dissemination of helpful information, reduce fear and stigma, and promote health-saving practices in formats that individuals can understand and are more inclined to act on and share (WHO, 2020c).

COVID-19 mitigation strategies must be inclusive of vulnerable groups to ensure the maintenance of their human rights and reduce inequities, rather than exacerbate them. Nurses, as advocates, play a crucial role in this process. Investments to enhance the knowledge and skill sets of nurses will not only present positive outcomes now but will secure preparedness for future outbreaks. If any lesson has been learnt from this public health emergency, it is that the costs of inaction are immense. The world will most likely see another pandemic in the future.

In summary, COVID-19 mitigation strategies must be inclusive of vulnerable groups and ensure existing inequities are reduced rather than exacerbated. Neonatal nurses play a crucial role in this process. In relation to the future, we now need to evaluate the current skills and knowledge held by the global neonatal workforce and what it needs to cope with future potential outbreaks (Purba, 2020). Such issues warrant urgent consideration from government, nurse leaders, and policy makers across the world to ensure long-term investment is made to support the profession and to ensure nurses are well equipped to effectively respond to future outbreaks. This must include a focus on meeting the needs of vulnerable groups and advocating on their behalf to reduce inequity in access to healthcare, health protection, and cultural inclusion.

Finally, it is vital that neonatal nurses, midwives, and other healthcare professionals are adequately informed and educated about the potential impact of COVID-19 mitigation measures on neonatal practice (Green et al., 2020; 2021a; 2021b). We need to be a continued voice for our profession, an advocate via publications within the neonatal nursing field, which to date are limited. It is hoped we can encourage nurses to write about their experiences and the impact of this pandemic on our field of nursing. With this point in mind, the book will finish with some thoughts and reflections from staff, all valued COINN colleagues, who wrote about their experiences of the impact of COVID-19 on themselves, their fellow staff and the families they care for. These selected quotes from a writing project "COVID-19: Neonatal Nursing in a Global Pandemic" (Neonatal Nurses Association (NNA), UK, 2020) highlight what is required in relation to the way forward for neonatal nursing to have hope for the future, to continue to embrace positive change (Shaw et al., 2021) and to optimize the outcomes of the babies and families that we care for so passionately.

Hope:

The stress of the NICU is made even more traumatic in this time of uncertainty. I continue to be concerned for what seeing only half a face in a baby's earliest experience might mean for their development. I see looks of confusion on my patients' faces, but I know that the care I provide and the tone of my voice and compassion through touch is felt by my patients. I still see smiles from the babies and that gives me hope (USA, clinical nurse).

I feel hopeful that by retaining our humanity through a collective effort and empathy with one another and our colleagues across the globe we can protect our tiny precious patients, their families and each other (New Zealand, clinical nurse)

Embrace positive change with education:

It is important now to analyze how we as educators can support clinical teams to achieve this. The future requires all those working in education institutions to seek new ways of offering distance learning that keeps the students engaged, motivated and ensures that CPD education equips healthcare teams with the knowledge they require to offer both safe care and drive change (UK Educator).

As we understand the changes ahead and how to map out the neonatal pathway through COVID-19, we need to ensure that as a community of neonatal nurses and midwives that we do not let the impact impair our ability to care or portray that emotion to parents when they may feel alone and scared at a vulnerable stage of their parenthood. We need to ensure that COVID-19 has the smallest impact on neonatal care (Northern Ireland, Advanced Neonatal Nurse Practitioner (ANNP).

This "community" applies to the global community of neonatal nurses and the valued allied health professionals that we work with across the world. To adapt the words of WHO (2020d) who speak of "strengthening" nursing and midwifery, and ensuring neonatal nurses and midwives are enabled to work to their full potential;—this is one of the most important things we can do to achieve universal health coverage and improve health globally of the babies and families in our care. We will continue to strive to be the voice of neonatal nurses across the globe and to educate for the good of our babies and families anywhere in the world (COINN, 2019a; 2019b).

References

Ahmed F, Ahmed NE, Pissarides C, Stiglitz J (2020) Why inequality could spread COVID-19. Lancet Public Health 5(5):e240

Burnett E (2018) Effective infection prevention and control: the nurse's role. Nurs Stand 33(4):68–72

COINN (2019a) News Pages. https://www.coinnurses.org/newsletter

COINN (2019b) Competencies for global neonatal nursing https://coinnurses.org/wp-content/uploads/2019/05/COINN-Core-Competencies-2019.pdf

Corless IB et al (2018) Expanding nursing's role in responding to global pandemics. Nurs Outlook 66(4):412–415

Global Alliance for Neonatal Care (GLANCE) (2020) Zero separation: together for better care. https://www.glance-network.org/news/details/zero-separation-global-campaign/

Green J, Petty J, Bromley P, Walker K, Jones L (2020) COVID 19 in babies: knowledge for neonatal care. J Neonatal Nurs 26(5):239–246

Green J, Petty J, Whiting L, Fowler C (2021a) Exploring modifiable risk-factors for premature birth in the con-

text of COVID-19 mitigation measures: a discussion paper. J Neonatal Nurs 27(3):172–179

Green J, Staff L, Bromley P, Petty J, Jones L (2021b) The implications of face masks for babies and families during the COVID-19 pandemic: a discussion paper. J Neonatal Nurs 27(1):21–25.

Human Rights Watch. (2020) World Report. https://www.hrw.org/world-report/2020

Inter-Agency Standing Committee (IASC) (2020) COVID-19 Resources Relating to Accountability and Inclusion. https://interagencystandingcommittee.org/covid-19-resources-relating-accountability-and-inclusion

Neonatal Nurses Association (NNA), UK (2020) COVID-19: Neonatal Nursing in a Global Pandemic. https://nna.org.uk/covid-19

Ofcom (2020) UK's internet use surges to record levels. https://www.ofcom.org.uk/about-ofcom/latest/media/media-releases/2020/uk-internet-use-surges

Paakkari L, Okan O (2020) COVID-19: health literacy is an underestimated problem. Lancet Public Health 5(5):e249–e250

Purba AK (2020) How should the role of the nurse change in response to Covid-19? Nursing Times [online] 116(6):25–28

Royal College of Nursing, UK (2017) Three Steps to Positive Practice A rights based approach when considering and reviewing the use of restrictive interventions. https://www.rcn.org.uk/professional-development/publications/pub-006075

Shaw C, Gallagher K, Petty J, Mancini A, Boyle B (2021) Neonatal Nursing during the COVID-19 Global Pandemic: A thematic analysis of personal reflections. J Neonatal Nurs. 27(3):165–171. https://doi.org/10.1016/j.jnn.2021.03.011

World Health Organization (2020a) Social determinants of health. Key concepts. WHO. https://www.who.int/health-topics/social-determinants-of-health#tab=tab_1

World Health Organization (2020b) Infection Prevention and Control in Health Care for Preparedness and Response to Outbreaks. https://www.who.int/csr/bioriskreduction/infection_control/background/en/

World Health Organization (2020c) Practical considerations and recommendations for religious leaders and faith-based communities in the context of COVID-19. WHO, Geneva. https://www.who.int/publications/i/item/practical-considerations-and-recommendations-for-religious-leaders-and-faith-based-communities-in-the-context-of-covid-19

World Health Organization (2020d) Strengthening Nursing and Midwifery to achieve health for all. https://www.who.int/campaigns/year-of-the-nurse-and-the-midwife-2020/get-involved/key-messages

Index

A

Accreditation Commission for Education in Nursing (ACEN), 5
Advanced neonatal nurse practitioners (ANNP), 56, 58
Africa, 87, 91
American Academy of Pediatrics (AAP), 3
Arterial blood gases (ABGs), 162
Australia
    Covid-19, 35
    education, 33, 34
    neonatal nursing, 33, 35
    neonatology, 33
    parent support organizations, 35
    professional organizations, 34
    training, 34
Australian and New Zealand Neonatal Network (ANZNN), 34
Australian healthcare system, 31, 32
Australian population data, 31, 32

B

Biculturalism, 39
Black and minority ethnic (BME), 185
Brain development, 137
Brazelton neonatal behavioral assessment scale (BNBAS), 139
Brazil, neonatal care, 23
    education, 27, 28
    evidence-based practice, 28, 29
    hospital organization, 25–27
    professional associations, 27
    public health policies, 24, 25
Brown fat, 155

C

Canada, neonatal care
    assessment, 17
    education, 13
    family-integrated care, 15
    five decades, 14, 15
    management, 18
    organization, 12, 13
    social justice, 20
    training, 13, 14
Canadian Association of Neonatal Nurses (CANN), 12
Canadian Neonatal Network, 19
Canadian Nurses Association (CNA), 11
Cardiopulmonary resuscitation (CPR), 131
Cerebral function monitoring (CFM), 54
Clinical nurse specialists (CNSs), 14
CN education in neonatal intensive care (CN-NIC), 99
Community-based neonatal approach, 122
Community health workers (CHWs), 122–124
Competency assessment programme (CAP), 44
Congenital hypothyroidism, 25
Continuous positive airway pressure (CPAP), 50, 89, 90, 157
Council of International Neonatal Nurses, Inc. (COINN), 75, 88, 96
COVID-19, 35, 91, 171–174, 183–186
Critical care, 13
Cultural awareness, 40

D

Data collection, 60
Devolved nations, 53–55
Direct antibody test (DAT), 54
Disaster preparedness, 103
Disparities, 67
District Health Information System (DHIS), 81
Doctor of Nursing Practice (DNP), 5, 14

E

Education, 4, 173, 183–186
Electroencephalography (EEG), 138
Endotracheal tubes (ETT), 77
Enhanced neonatal nurse practitioners (ENNP), 56
European federation of care of the newborn infants (EFCNI), 175, 178
European Foundation for the Care of Newborn Infants, 67, 178
European qualification framework (EQF)., 69

Evidence-based practice (EBP), 101
Extreme low birthweight (ELBW), 9

F
Families in recovery (FIR), 20
Family and Infant Neurodevelopmental Education
        (FINE), 59
Family-integrated care (FICare), 57, 61, 68
Filial piety, 167

G
Gestational age (GA), 135
Global regulatory organizations, 174

H
Hawaiian, 166
Health disparity, 171, 175, 176
Health policy, 177
Helping babies breathe (HBB), 157
Helping babies survive (HBS), 157
High dependency unit (HDU), 32
Ho'ihi, 165
Ho'olewa, 164, 165
Ho'omakaukau, 163
Ho'oponopono, 164
Hospital Episode Statistics (HES), 60
Hypoglycaemia, 151–154, 156, 158, 159
Hypoplastic left heart syndrome (HPLH), 9
Hypothermia, 151–157
Hypoxaemia, 157
Hypoxia, 151–154, 156, 157

I
Idiopathic respiratory distress syndrome (IRDS), 71
Indirect impact, 173
Infant, 24, 25, 30
Infant mental health, 167
Inoa, 165
International Council of Nurses (ICN), 75
International neonatal consortium (INC), 174
Intravenous push (IVP), 97
Intuition, 161

J
Japan, neonatal care, 93, 94, 103, 104
    bereavement care, 105
    cultural challenges, okinawa, 104, 105
    education, 97, 98
    evidence-based practice, 101, 102
    NICU, 95, 96
    organization, 95
    practice regulation, 97
    professional associations, 96
    reflection, 107
    training, 98–100

Japanese academy of neonatal nursing (JANN), 96, 99
Japanese association of nursing programs in universities
        (JAMPU), 100

K
Kahuna, 166
Kangaroo method (KM), 24
Kangaroo mother care (KMC), 18, 91, 114, 122, 124, 155

L
Lebanon, 111–113, 116
    care and design, 112, 113
    developmental care, 115
    discharge planning, 116
    feeding, 115
    intravenous lines, 115
    neonatal staff, 113, 114
    pain management, 116
    physical parameters, 114
    sepsis, 114
    thermoregulation, 115
    transport, 113
Lokahi, 164
Low birth weight (LBW), 112, 122
Low-resourced countries (LIC), 156

M
Magnetic resonance imaging (MRI), 71
Makaukau, 164
Mana, 161, 162
    acquired, 163
    inherited, 162, 163
Migrants, 185
Minimally invasive surfactant therapy (MIST), 49
Minimizing stress, 136
Miscommunication, 184
Misinformation, 184

N
National Association of Neonatal Nurse Practitioners
        (NANNPs), 3, 5
National health service (NHS), 53, 54
National neonatal research database (NNRD), 60
National Transport Group (NTG), 60
Neonatal abstinence syndrome (NAS), 6, 9
Neonatal care, 3, 6, 9, 10, 15, 16, 88, 90, 92
    Brazil, 23–29
    Canada, 11, 13–15, 17, 18, 20
    education, 4
    evidence-based practice, 5
    Japan, 93–95, 98–101, 103, 105, 106
    New Zealand, 39–43, 45, 46, 48–50
    1980s and 1990s, 7, 8
    1960s and 1970s, 7
    organization, 4
    reflective practice, 6

Russia, 73–78
South Africa, 81–85
training, 4, 5
2000s, 8, 9
United Kingdom, 53–58, 62, 63
Western Europe, 67–69, 71
Neonatal data analysis unit (NDAU), 60
Neonatal healthcare staff, 183
Neonatal intensive care unit (NICU), 7, 8, 25, 32, 50, 76, 87, 112–114, 127, 136, 141, 143, 144, 162
    adequate nutrition, 143, 144
    brain development, 136, 137
    comfortable positioning, 141
    environment, 140, 141
    family integrated care, 144
    newborn hospitalization, 128
    patient and family centered care, 129
    preventing stress, 141, 142
    protecting skin integrity, 143
    protecting sleep, 137–140
    reflective practice, 132
    skin-to-skin contact, 145
    sleep disruption, 137
Neonatal life support (NLS)., 59
Neonatal networks, 55, 56
Neonatal nurse, 184, 185, 187
Neonatal nurses association (NNA), 186
Neonatal Nurses' Association of Southern Africa (NNASA), 82
Neonatal nursing, 3, 5, 23, 87, 88
    career progression, 58, 59
    education, 3, 24, 88
Neonatal resuscitation, 101, 102
Neonatal stress, 137
Neonatal survival, 122, 124
Neonatal transportation, 44–47
New Zealand, neonatal care, 39
    cultural awareness, 40
    cultural safety, 40
    nursing education, 42, 44
    organization, 44–48
    three-point model of care, 42
Nongovernmental organizations (NGOs), 90
Non-invasive prenatal genetic testing (NIPT), 102
Nurse Entry to Practice programme (NetP), 43
Nurse practitioner (NP), 8, 14
Nursing school curriculum, 167

O
Ola, 165
Operational delivery networks (ODN), 55
Optimum environmental care, 146
Orogastric tube (OG), 143

P
Pandemic, 171–173
Participation, 40
Partnership, 40, 127, 129

Patent ductus arteriosus (PDA), 17
Patient and family centered care (PFCC), 127, 130
    collaboration, 129
    dignity and respect, 129
    implementation, 129–131
    information sharing, 129
    participation, 129
Patient-centered outcome research institute (PCORI), 177
Pediatric nursing societies Europe (PNAE)., 67
Perinatal Problem Identification Programme (PPIP), 81
Peripherally inserted central catheter (PICC), 28
Phenylketonuria, 25
Phototherapy, 54, 55
Policy and advocacy, 177
Poly cystic ovarian syndrome (PCOS), 37
Positive end expiratory pressure (PEEP), 54
Prematurity across, 62
Preterm, 13, 18, 19
Prevention of mother-to-child transmission (PMTCT), 84
Professional Development and Recognition Programme (PDRP), 43
Protecting skin integrity, 143
Protection, 40
Pu'ukohola Heiau, 167, 168

R
Rapid Mortality Surveillance (RMS), 81
Refugees, 185
Reproductive collaboration, 102
Research organizations, 174
Researcher training in higher learning, 173
Russia, neonatal care, 73
    challenges, 75
    competencies, 74, 75
    evidence-based practice, 75
    nursing education, 74
    organization, 73, 74
    professional associations, 75
    reflective practice, 76–79
Russian Nurses Association (RNA), 74

S
SARS-CoV-2, 63, 64
Skin-to-skin contact (SSC), 18, 122, 124
Social injustice, 20
South Africa, neonatal care, 81
    education, 82
    evidence-based practice, 84, 85
    organization, 83, 84
    training, 82, 83
South African Demographic Health Survey (SADHS), 81
South African Nursing Council (SANC), 81, 82
Special care baby units (SCBU), 32, 50
Special care unit (SCU), 32
Stabilization, 47
Sustainable development goals, (SDGs), 152

T
Thermoregulation, 115
Total parenteral nutrition (TPN), 143, 159
Training, 5
Transitional care (TC), 55

U
Umbilical venous catheters (UVCs), 70, 71
Uniki training, 168
United Kingdom (UK), neonatal care, 53
    continuing professional development, 59
    data collection, 60
    education, 57
    evidence-based practice, 59
    family-integrated care, 61
    multidisciplinary team, 56, 57
    organization, 55
    parental mental health, 61

professional registration, 58
training, 58

V
Vermont oxford network (VON), 175
Vulnerable populations, 184

W
Well-baby nursery (WBN), 32
Western Europe, neonatal care, 67
    education, 68, 69
    evidence-based practice, 70
    training, 69, 70
Whakamarietia, 41
White coat ceremony, 168
Workforce development, 173

Printed in the United States
by Baker & Taylor Publisher Services